Everyday Pediatrics for Parents

A Thoughtful Guide for Today's Families

For Prospect - Sierra School with best wishes,

Elmer R Grossman, MD

Elmer R. Grossman, M.D.

CELESTIALARTS
Berkeley, California

AUTHOR'S NOTE: When you read this or any other book on a medical topic it is important to keep in mind that the information and advice being given is of the most general nature. I am sitting at home in Berkeley, California, writing about the problems of children as I have experienced them during my years in practice. I have not met you or your children, and there is no way that either of us can know how accurately my ideas will fit your circumstances. Books like this cannot be substitutes for your own doctor's observation and judgment. This book does not attempt to tell mothers and fathers how to be parents. I have attempted to make it a source of ideas and suggestions for ways to think about and understand your children's growth, behavior, and problems of illness.

CELESTIAL ARTS PUBLISHING
P.O. Box 7123, Berkeley, CA 94707

Cover and Text Design: Greene Design
Cover Photo: Andree Abecassis

Printed in the United States

Library of Congress Cataloging–in–Publication Data

Grossman, Elmer R.
    Everyday pediatrics for parents / Elmer R. Grossman
      p. cm.
    Includes index.
    ISBN 0-89087-813-7
    1. Children--Diseases. 2. Children--Health and hygiene.
    3. Pediatrics--Popular works. I. Title.
    RJ61.G918 1996
    618.92--dc20

                                  96-26803
                                    CIP

First Printing, 1996

1 2 3 4 / 99 98 97 96

Acknowledgments and Dedication

It seems to me that a book like this is the fruit of an old tree. I'm responsible for what I write, but my ideas reflect who I am, and that is a matter of time and history. My parents taught me that humanity is a family affair, and they showed me trust by letting me make my own decisions about life. My teachers, from elementary school to the University of California at Berkeley, introduced me to the world of critical thought. In medical school, my professors oversaw my rites of passage into our profession, about which I initially had considerable reservations, but which I came to love. They showed me in practice and by precept what it meant to be a doctor. I learned what it meant to be a pediatrition under the tutelage of Moses Grossman, Mary Olney, Sidney Adler, Marshall Klaus, and Helen Gofman. My partners in the Berkeley Pediatric Medical Group, our warm and wonderful office staff, and our extraordinary family of patients helped me to continue to learn about pediatrics and about life. And during all those years I have drawn sustenance and love from friends and family. Without that support I would have little to give and nothing to say.

Writing this book has given me an exciting and absolutely delightful three years. The last several months has been further enlivened by working with my terrific editor Veronica Randall, whose expert enthusiasm is matched by her wit and appreciation of my prose! Every chapter benefited from the critical scrutiny of two practicing mothers (of the two sets of twins on the front cover), my daughters Marianna Grossman Keller and Cam Sutter. I am grateful for their many suggestions which have made this a more practical and useful book, and for their willingness to devote so many hours of their busy lives to the task. The chapters on young and middle-aged children benefited from the questions and comments of my daughter Deena Tyrrell Grossman and her husband Larry Tyrrell (the parents of my eldest granddaughter, also on the front cover). The contibutions of my wife Pam, a practicing grandmother, have been innumerable. Her readings and re-readings have resulted in clearer expositions, fewer repetitions, and, in general, less fog and confusion. In hundreds of hours of discussion, she has helped me to stay focused on the needs of the parents who will read the book. Somehow she has endured what she calls author's widowhood and managed to stay sane, loving, and supportive. With love and gratitude, I dedicate *Everyday Pediatrics for Parents* to her.

Table of Contents

Preface

Does anybody really need another book on child care? Without any doubt, there are really plenty of good, basic books on raising children, so why have I written another one, and why should you or any other parent read it? I thought long and hard about these questions before deciding to embark on this project. The short answer is that I wanted to make parents think about the issues of their children's development, their health care, the families in which their children would be raised, and the society into which they are born.

My particular point of view reflects my four decades of pediatric practice in a variety of medical settings including county and community hospitals, the United States Air Force, Kaiser Permanente Medical Group, Children's Hospital in Oakland, and the great medical center of the University of California in San Francisco. But the heart and soul of my medical experience has been a third of a century I spent with the Berkeley Pediatric Medical Group, a small private practice partnership in the exciting, challenging, wonderful little city of Berkeley, California. Our patients, the staff, and my partners at Berkeley Peds have taught me a great deal of what I know about everyday pediatrics. I have also had the privilege of teaching medical students and young doctors at our local medical school and other teaching hospitals. Continued contact with the medical young and their academic elders does have the effect of keeping one at least a little bit humble. Having had one foot in academic life and the other in the world of private practice has enabled me to see the foibles and appreciate the strengths of both.

In 1959, when I entered practice the definition of pediatrition was the expert to whom parents looked to provide the *answers*. Since then, I have come to believe that often the most valuable service I can offer parents is asking them the right *questions*. Frequently, these questions have shown them alternatives and options of which they have not been aware, helped them to look freshly at the problem. That is the point of *Everyday Pediatrics for Parents*. This is not a one-volume encyclopedia covering every aspect of child health and development. Such a book would be beyond my abilities and would be too heavy to hold! This modest book raises the questions about child care in health and disease that have seemed important to my patients and to me over the last forty years. I won't tell you how to raise your children or live your lives; instead I'll ask you to *think* about your possibilities and your choices.

Despite my attempts to be objective, you will probably notice that I am guilty of a certain amount of preaching. My sermons tend to have two recurrent themes. The first is the necessity for skepticism about everything you will ever read or be told concerning the health and growth of children; there is a lot of nonsense floating around. The second theme is the virtue of simplicity. Fancy theories, complex explanations, and overly zealous medical interventions are often equally ill-founded and unnecessary. "Small and simple is beautiful" is not a bad slogan for a pediatrician's book.

Introduction

Handbooks for parents on how to care for their children are certainly nothing new. Ten separate books on child care were published in England alone in the year 1600, and doctors and other "experts" have been writing on this endlessly complex and fascinating topic ever since. Dr. Elmer Grossman stands out in this rather large field not only because of what he is, but also because of who he is.

For many years I sent both medical students and resident physicians-in-training to observe, absorb, and reflect on how Elmer Grossman practiced medicine. Not only did I want them to see a master clinician in action, I wanted them to see firsthand his unusually sensitive and caring manner with children and their parents. Elmer truly listened to his patients, paid close attention to parental observations, insisted on giving adequate time to each visit, and communicated with great patience, clarity, and above all, respect. Visiting the Berkeley Medical Group was a special and inspiring experience for these young doctors, many of whom expressed the hope that they could use Dr. Grossman as a model for their future practice.

The Department of Pediatrics at the University of California also recognized his unique talents. He took time from his busy schedule to serve on its faculty ever since completing his pediatric residency training there in 1958, and he has been a Clinical Professor of Pediatrics since 1980.

Now that Dr. Grossman has retired, we are indeed fortunate that his wisdom, humor, and humanity come through every page of his new book. Although we can no longer make a personal appointment with the Doc, *Everyday Pediatrics for Parents* is the next best thing. His commitment to you, the reader, is as strong and clear as ever. It gives me great pleasure, both professionally and personally, to recommend this invaluable resource to every family in America.

—*Marshall Klaus, M.D.*

Chapter 1

The Possibilities of Parenthood

One of the few good reasons for watching television is nature programming. Some intrepid soul with a camera takes you undersea to watch colonial sponges, or inside a termite colony to watch the interaction of the insects, or onto the African plains to witness the cooperative pup-rearing of wild dogs. One watches transfixed, and marvels at the wisdom of the natural order which gives rise to these amazing cooperative endeavors. And, every so often, there comes the shock of recognition, when one sees the parallel to the human experience of raising our children. Particularly in America, we have become so used to thinking about ourselves as separate individuals, and about our families as unique entities, that we need to be reminded that the human condition is as colonial as a sponge, and as organized as a hill of termites. At least, that is how it looks to me as I undertake the medical care of children, watch family life, and observe the community in which I live.

It is only within this large, natural framework that our apparently deliberate choices to have children make any sense at all. From the viewpoint of a solitary individual or a mated, married couple, becoming parents is obviously a nonrational activity. If we were really driven by the need to maximize personal pleasure in our lives, would we undertake parenthood? It entails spending considerable sums of money which we could otherwise lavish on ourselves. It means devoting unlimited hours, day and night, for two decades or more, to the care and feeding of the young. And parenthood means, as one of my mordant pediatric partners used to say, giving hostages to fortune.

But we do undertake parenthood, irrationally and with gusto. We are driven by our biology just as the sponges and termites and wild dogs are driven by theirs. I will never forget the abrupt intensity of longing for a baby that overcame my wife and myself during my internship year. The Korean War was still going on, and we knew that I would be in the service and sent overseas within a few months; in short, it was no time to start a child. But if we saw a baby at the supermarket or passed a mother and infant on the street, we stopped and stared and yearned for one of our own. We had become mechanisms for blending our genetic inheritance into individuals of a new generation.

The Goals and Roles of Parenthood

Since you are a parent or plan to become one, what do you plan to do with the possibilities? This question carries some implicit assumptions: first, that the constraints of circumstance are loose enough that you actually have some choices, and second, that you will decide to let deliberate thought and discussion take the place of custom, habit, and hormones in arranging this part of your lives. Neither of these assumptions is particularly likely to be true. Most of us fall into the familiar patterns of life in which we were raised and with which we are surrounded. But change is in the air regarding family functioning, and some of us are not so enamored of our own upbringing as to feel bound to inflict it on a new generation of parents and kids. If the family backgrounds of the two people forming a new union is relatively similar, the new structure which emerges will probably feel fairly familiar and comfortable to both. It is likely to be built along a pattern close enough to those in which each was raised to allow a considerable degree of automatic decision making. The resultant growth will not necessarily require much tinkering or pruning to assume a familiar form. Of course, this peaceful scenario will be far from reality if either partner has had a family which was a hateful and destructive mess. When one has survived and escaped from such an environment, one is unlikely to consciously want to recreate it anew. But in these circumstances, many couples flounder. They may swing wildly to another extreme of intrafamily relationship style, rejecting the despised accustomed ways. Or they may attempt to figure out, with head and heart, a method of living that begins to meet their present needs.

The graduates of even the best and most nurturing families are likely to enter their new relationships with a variety of impractical expectations, prominent among which is the idea that a new family grows automatically and without effort. Until you try it yourself, you cannot understand the difficulty of making a new family structure take root. And of course the advent of the first child throws everything into a cocked hat. Suddenly there are new roles to fill, and the old roles become obsolete. The partners must again redefine themselves and their places in the enlarged family.

As if this were not enough, one or both of every nesting pair of humans has the additional task of flying off to make a living. When one of you remains at home, your life experiences begin to diverge drastically from the mate who is out foraging in the world. Remaining at home carries the real risk of a sense of dependency, of loss of identity, and a weakening of the sense of yourself as a person of any worth outside the four walls of your home. If you are the one entering the larger arena of a job or career, your sense of self grows and changes as you take on new and challenging tasks. Forging a new professional identity can take over your life to the exclusion of everything else. Some of the pressures are external; the medical intern, the newly hired lawyer, the assistant professor without tenure, the youngest salesman on the floor—all of them are expected to work too many hours and too many nights. The internal pressures are just as demanding: The drive to master the field, to prove your skills, to become established and secure—these push and pull as effectively as the knowledge that the eyes of the supervisor or the department head or the chief resident are watching. After a while, the seventy-hour weeks begin to erode the marriage; there is only so much time and energy to go around, and the family's share gets smaller and smaller. If both of you work outside the home and become similarly engulfed by work, the hazard is that neither of you will have time or energy for the other or for your children. Raising kids *and* maintaining a marriage *and* working outside the home are tasks that require continuing effort, energy, and attention; it is both foolish and dangerous to act as if no harm could come from ignoring their requirements.

Who Does What in a Family? The context of this question is clear: Since mothers now work away from home more often than not, what does it mean to be a mother? Who will do the tasks that stay-at-home moms have done in the past? And how about fathers? Why haven't they always done an equal share of the child care in the past? Why shouldn't they take it on now? One currently fashionable answer is that men are really not much different from women, but since they are bigger and stronger, they have forced women to stay home and do the hard work of producing, nursing, and raising the children. This argument is convincing only to those who have failed to notice that the structure of women's bodies makes pregnancy and breast feeding a lot easier for them than it would be for men. It is also necessary to ignore the differences in the behavior and interests of the sexes at every age beyond early infancy. Politically incorrect? No doubt—but as a father and pediatrician who tried to raise four children in a gender-neutral fashion, let me give the following report: Little girls are not much interested in dump trucks, by and large, and the doll play of little boys tends to violence rather than tender, loving care.

Just recently, friends of ours gave a doll to their 5-year old grandson and a toy truck to their 7-year old granddaughter. The children looked at their gifts briefly and then Sam threw the doll over to Sarah, saying "That's hers", and retrieved the truck from his sister. Sam and Sarah's parents, who had diligently tried gender-neutral toys for years, were not the least surprised. The reality of the human condition includes both biological and social factors that weigh against the unisex theory of parenting. Men do not have either the biological or social experience of being pregnant and giving birth. Watch mothers and fathers during the period surrounding the birth of a baby, and note their differing responses to the new-born. The baby has been, quite literally, a part of the mother, and her reactions to her infant have an intensity which is unique to her sex. Men generally don't seem to care all that much about infants. Sound sexist? It's based on the observation of the responses of adults to babies. When they were infants, I often took my twin granddaughters out in their stroller. Nearly every women who had the good fortune to pass these charming children would stop and smile and comment to me about them. Very rarely, in fact almost never, would a man glance at them and smile. I know an argument can be made that this is learned behavior, that men and boys have been taught to be disinterested. But I just do not see the evidence that my sex has it's collective brain hard-wired for nurturing parent-hood in the way that is, fortunately, the case for women.

The good news is that most of us males do eventually learn to be passable parents, but it may take a while and patience is required. The man who expects to love his brand-new baby with the unconditional joy he sees on the face of his wife may be disappointed. These observations lead to **Grossman's Law of Family Life: *The sexes really are different.*** Failure to heed this law leads to following predictable scenarios: Some young women will decide that they really prefer being mothers to struggling in the high-testosterone crucible of business; and some young men will find that staying at home and being househusbands is not their notion of a fulfilling mission in life. Working couples who decide to share equally in the tasks of child rearing and housekeeping tend to report that, despite everyone's best intentions, mothers continue to bear a disproportionate load at home. No doubt there are multiple causes for this regrettable reality, including culturally supported masculine sexist pig-ism, and perhaps some residue of archaic feminine subservience, equally supported by certain aspects of the culture. However, it would be unwise to ignore the possibility that biological differences exist that help shape our perceptions of what is important and useful activity. It is true that in some species of birds, the males stay home and incubate the eggs, but human males are not commonly built to that design.

How Do Parents and Families Change Over Time? When I was a very young child, the world of adults seemed stable and the adults themselves unchanging. It seemed to me that once I reached adult status, I too would become a finished product. It was a considerable shock to discover that change was a constant. Every few years I noticed that I had become significantly different in a variety of ways. It was scary, confusing, and exciting. If you have had similar childhood illusions about the grownup world you may be surprised to discover that families change, too. The young mother who delighted in staying at home with her babies may find herself growing restless when the kids go to preschool; she begins to think seriously about re-entering the job market. The young man who was consumed by his newly minted career may begin to look at his rapidly growing children and decide that it is time to invest more time and energy in them. There are inevitable changes in the marriage relationship as well. During the early years of parenthood, the demands of young children added to the pressures of work can push a couple apart. The unexamined marriage may become tattered around the edges if it is ignored for too long. There are also the predictable cycles of personal change that interact with family life. The mid-thirties can be a time of turmoil as men and women, no longer quite so young, reassess the trajectory of their lives. The midlife crises of the forties are justly infamous as well. All this means that family patterns are never set in concrete. We may not welcome the winds of change, but we should expect them.

Time—Why Is There Never Enough of It? Why do we run so fast in this country? Did you know that Americans actually sleep about an hour less each night than we did thirty years ago? We also appear to have less peaceful, "down" time in which to decompress be simply human. Our "free" time comes at a high price, filling up with commuting, carpooling, shopping, running errands, and overtime hours at work for extra income. It is a costly pattern in terms of family life. As we think about how to live together, how and where to work, and who will do what at home, we need also to look at the time constraints with which we surround ourselves. Raising children means being present for them, and being present means having time and energy and patience. Chronic sleep deprivation and overtiredness is not a good prescription for maintaining a happy family. It's time to take stock of where we are and where we are going, and make some conscious decisions about how we spend our brief and precious hours on earth.

Chapter 2

Dealing with Doctors

Do you really have to deal with us, or can doctors be avoided altogether? For any number of excellent reasons, a substantial number of people certainly try to keep their distance from the medical profession. After all, we are widely perceived to be an expensive, inconvenient, uncomfortable, and even dangerous group, wielding excessive power, and prone to frequent and fatal error. Which of these unpleasant attributes is emphasized depends on a variety of factors. Control is the issue for some parents who are accustomed to being in charge of their lives and resist asking for assistance. Any number of times I've gotten a phone call from a parent telling me that Junior has had a fever of 103 degrees for several days; perhaps it might be time for a visit? Most parents would have called days before. Sometimes the issue is socioeconomic distance; poor people soon learn that middle class doctors often seem not to understand them and even more often fail to make themselves understood. It does not take many unsatisfactory interchanges between uncomprehending doctors and patients to sour everyone on the encounter.

What Medicine Can Do, and What It Can't

Despite all of this, I continue to believe that physicians and other medical people have quite a bit to offer. The treatment of acute injury and serious medical emergencies needs no defense. Except for a few religious groups of assorted persuasions, there is general agreement on the utility of medical intervention in these instances. Even practitioners of alternative systems of healing send us patients with broken legs, convulsions, coma, and the like.

For less obviously life and limb threatening events, the case is less clear. A very large number of injuries will heal by themselves, and an equally large proportion of acute illnesses get better on their own. The contributions of the doctor can be to alleviate pain and other symptoms, sometimes to speed healing, and often to relieve anxiety by explaining what has happened and how nature will right the matter. In these murky cases, the use of medicines is common and usually justified, but the costs and hazards of the investigations and the treatments needs consideration as well. In chronic illnesses, and with other disabling conditions where cures are distant or even unreachable, the physician's role is both more modest and more problematic. In these situations, we doctors may be able to do less good, and we are at increasing risk of doing harm.

In the practice of pediatrics, half of our time is spent in the care of well children. Here our roles are even less well defined. We have taken over, or been thrust into, functions of advice-giving and skill-teaching that once were the purview of the elders of the tribe. A few decades ago when most pediatricians were male, someone in our profession described us as grandmothers with bow ties. Since most of us have not been particularly well trained in grandmothering, this has not been a wholly happy situation. Consider also the effect of giving advice in general. The presumably knowledgeable professional person tells the patient (or client or customer) what the facts are and what should be done about them. This is an interchange with a real potential for injuring the seeker of advice. If I go to you for help, I define myself as weaker, more needy, a suppliant; in giving (or selling) me advice, you increase your status, your power, and your authority over my life. This is a transaction which many people prefer to avoid.

Doctor Substitutes. Of the various available methods of avoidance, using a doctor substitute is most popular. Commonly, this will be a nurse or nurse practitioner. Nurses are accurately seen to be more accessible than many physicians. They tend to speak in a more easily understandable fashion, using less unintelligible medical jargon, and their services are less expensive. They are likely to present themselves as equals rather than as social superiors. Without question, nurses can handle a substantial portion of routine health care needs, especially when the nurse's role is relatively tightly defined. The Plunkett nurses of New Zealand who handle all the well child care in that country are excellent examples. In our country there are nurses who carry major responsibilities in specialty clinics dealing with diabetes or high blood pressure, or other medical problems. The problem with a nurse doing a doctor's work seems to me to be this: The doctor's work is sometimes unexpectedly and unpredictably very difficult indeed. At any rate, after four years of medical school and four more years of pediatric specialty training and four decades of pediatric practice I continued to find it so.

Another increasingly popular choice is to leave Western medicine altogether, and seek a practitioner of an alternative system of medicine. As a more or less orthodox physician, this has always posed a problem for me. I have the sneaking suspicion that many of them know truly useful things. Some have been able to help patients whom I have been unable to help with the tools of Western medicine. But they have in common one, to my mind, fatal flaw, which is the nearly total disinclination to submit themselves and their methods to the rigors of Western scientific observation. Consequently, these practitioners are literally flying blind—and their patients are flying right along with them. There are some exceptions; a few careful studies have been carried out in homeopathy, chiropractic, and traditional Asian medicine, but not nearly enough to allow objective judgment. Patients who submit themselves or their children to the manipulations, exotic herbs, massages, diets, miscellaneous potions, and laying on of hands by the alternative healers need to be aware that, as consumers, they are truly on their own. No Food and Drug Administration, no hospital ethics committees, and no tradition of scientific study stands between them and some quite unusual notions of disease and treatment.

Finding the Right Doctor. This is not such an easy or straightforward matter. For one thing, you may have little or no choice. Your health insurance may limit the group of available physicians; there may be few, if any, doctors in your area; financial considerations will severely limit physician availability for the poor until we reform the American health care system. Next is the question of type of doctor: generalist (family practitioner), pediatrician, or internist? The family doctor has had training in a broad range of medical areas; adult medical care, uncomplicated obstetrics, some surgery, and some pediatric training are all part of the family doc's background. For the majority of medical problems, the family doctor is an appropriate source of care. The advantages of one-stop shopping for the whole family are obvious: It's all under one roof, and the doctor's knowledge about a particular family is all in one brain. The internist has been trained in the medical problems of adults; no obstetrics or gynecology, no surgery at all, no pediatrics. The internist's depth of information about adult disease is likely to be greater than that of the family doctor, but adult medicine is all the internist is well trained to do. Despite this handicap, some internists will include children and adolescents within their practices, perhaps assuming that these young people can be thought of as miniature adults. Those of us in pediatrics consider this an error. We pediatricians have much less training and competence in adult disease; we generally learn to do simple skin surgery and our obstetrical training is minimal. What we do know is the special nature of illness in childhood, and we have some familiarity with the general field of child growth and development. Our three or more years of specialty study after we earn our M.D.s are exclusively devoted to kids and adolescents. Sometimes this extra knowledge makes a considerable difference.

It may seem self-evident that where the doctor has been educated should be of considerable importance; surely a degree from a prestigious school followed by residency training at a fancy hospital must mean a higher quality of physician? Well, no. The fancy schools and famous hospitals have made their reputations honestly, but nearly always it is in medical research, and in high-tech, "tertiary care," super-specialized medical treatment. This has exceedingly little to do with the quality of instruction provided for medical students and resident physicians. In short, it may be interesting to read the diplomas on your doctor's office wall, but they are not the medical equivalents of a Consumers' Report rating.

There are no official ratings for primary care doctors which could assist you in your choice. When my patients are about to move to another area, and ask me for a referral, I can look up the names of pediatricians in their new town, but not much more. My advice is always the same: Ask *everyone* for information about their own doctors. Ask your child's new teacher, your new boss, the lady standing behind you in the supermarket checkout line. Get all the opinions you can and see if some patterns emerge. If there is a medical school in your new area, call the secretary of the department of pediatrics and ask for the names of the part-time or volunteer clinical faculty who practice in your community. These are doctors whose reputations are sufficiently high that they are entrusted with part of the responsibility for the training of young physicians. When you find a doctor you like, use her as your entrée into the rest of the medical community. As a practitioner, she has the best chance of knowing the real scoop on her colleagues.

Get–Acquainted Visits and Shopping Around. If you must choose a new doctor too quickly because of a sudden illness, your initial choices may be limited, and you may find yourself more or less committed to someone you really don't like or don't trust. To avoid this kind of forced choice, it is better to find the doctor you want *before* you need a doctor at all. It is well worth the investment of one or more get-acquainted visits with doctors about whom you have heard good reports. I have to say that this is by no means easy or cheap. Some physicians hate comparison shoppers; they don't like being thought of as commodities to be chosen or rejected. A brief conversation with the doctor's receptionist will generally make this apparent. Furthermore, you may have to pay for these visits out of your own pocket. Health insurance carriers may look askance at bills for this kind of visit, and it may take several such visits to find the physician who suits you. What you are looking for may be difficult to define; I think it is a matter of the music more than the words. Look for a comfortable style. This will depend on your own past experience with doctors, and your views of professional relationships. And your first choice may turn out to be a mistake; if you see a doctor often enough to form a negative opinion of him, find a new physician and leave. All of us in medical practice have patients who leave; we may hate being rejected but, as the old medical aphorism goes, there are worse ways to lose a patient.

Chapter 3

Wellness Care

How did we get into this business, anyway? When you stop to think about it, there is nothing inevitable about the connection of well child care with pediatric practice. In many parts of the world, asking a doctor about feeding, growth, development, and general well child supervision will be rewarded with puzzled silence or offhand dismissal. Dealing with the healthy isn't considered the doctor's field. In this part of the world, however, these issues are within the doctor's purview. After all, if the doctor is consulted about diet during disease, why not about diet in health? If asked about urinary tract infections, why not about bed wetting? But added to this connection are two other very American factors: our faith in science as the fount of wisdom, and the loss of grandparents and other stable family sources of information about raising children.

The problem here is the discrepancy between the doctor's old role as dispenser of medical advice and the new role of expert on the care and feeding of children. As the source of information on disease, the doctor presumably knows a great deal more than the patient and has some objectivity as an observer of the process of disease from which the patient is suffering. Both patient and physician agree that the doctor is an authority, although the fact that doctors

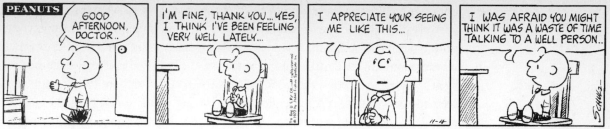

disagree is widely understood. As a source of information on the ordinary concerns of parents raising their children, the doctor is on much shakier ground. For one thing, not all that much is known about child development; it is a relatively new science. For another, some doctors are largely unfamiliar with the available information. Our training programs do not all give adequate attention to well child care. Until we have experience with the children in our own families, our understanding may be thinly academic at best, based neither on sound science nor on practical wisdom. One of my partners commented that she still blushes when she remembers the advice she gave in the years before she became a mother herself. To make matters even worse, the doctor's views are often no more than the ordinary prejudices of his or her age, sex, and social class. When I am consulted about the treatment of menstrual disorders, I draw on clinical science; when the same adolescent asks me about contraception, my answers are likely to vary depending on my religion, my age, whether I have teenaged children myself and whether any of them has ever gotten pregnant. Even if we were all masters of an established academic field of well child care, even if we all had the firsthand experience that comes from parenthood, our authority in well child matters would *still* be limited. That is because the choices we make as parents depend on our own personalities and on the goals we have for our children.

Doctors need to understand when we are using the usual "medical model" of diagnosis and treatment, and when we are using the "wellness care model" of analysis of the problem and exploration of alternative solutions. Let's take the example of the child who cuts himself, loses some blood and develops an iron deficiency anemia; the diagnosis is straightforward and so is the treatment. The medical model will fit very nicely. In contrast, the child who has iron deficiency caused by a diet limited to cows' milk and apple juice presents a different problem. In either situation, the anemia can be cured with iron drops or tablets, but the bottle addict will relapse unless changes are made in the diet. Success often depends on the doctor figuring out why the old diet was allowed. Sometimes all that is needed is information about nutrition; sometimes the underlying problem is one of family relationships. I've seen bottle addiction in families where parents were unable to set limits, where exhausted mothers used bottles to get the baby through the night so that she could sleep, and where a parent seemed to want to keep the child from growing up. The doctor can't change these behaviors with a prescription for iron. But he can try to help the family understand where the problem lies. When the source of the difficulty is understood, the solution may be obvious; otherwise, the doctor's task is to help the family examine their options. While both responsibility and authority remain clearly with the family, the doctor becomes a facilitator and the medical model is no longer sufficient.

This changes the doctor-patient relationship in a fundamental way. When I first began to practice well child care, I had the uncomfortable feeling that I was shifting gears back and forth between two different and conflicting modes. If the child was sick in some clearly somatic way, I was the old fashioned doc, making a diagnosis and prescribing treatment. "Here is the problem: solve it my way." When the problem was behavioral or developmental, I became the neutral explorer and mediator. "Here is the problem; do we all see it in the same fashion? How might you folks deal with it, so that you can solve it your way?" One interesting side effect of this dichotomy was to make it easier for me to share authority in "medical" matters as well. In the long run, doctors need to admit that most health and disease rest in the hands of the patients rather than the medical profession. This is sometimes obvious; do I choose to smoke cigarettes or not? Sometimes it's a little more complicated. My friend Walter needed his damaged heart valves replaced last year. His surgeon gave him the choice of mechanical valves, with an increased risk of strokes, or pig valves, with the likelihood of wearing out sooner. It was a nice example of acknowledging that the patient had a stake in the choice.

Parents (and children when they are old enough) have the right to choose. Do we treat this ear infection, with the attendant risks of adverse drug reactions, or observe without treatment, with the chance of chronic ear disease and other complications? Do we immunize the child? There are lots of choices along the way, and we doctors are not going to approve of all the decisions our patients will make. The wellness care mode of practice makes it clear to me that this patient is not my child, and his parents' choices are not my choices, but most of the time, that's all right. Under certain circumstances, I think that the doctor should retain the old role and former authority of the physician. This may entail being stern and directive with a family paralyzed by conflict or indecision. On rare occasions, I've had to report a family to a child abuse agency. When non-compliance becomes neglect, the counselor's role must give way and the doctor must become the child's advocate.

What seems to work best for me is a melding of the old "Doctor Authority" and new "Doctor Facilitator." I don't find it necessary to outline the pros and cons of treating every case of impetigo or acute appendicitis, but I have gotten used to remaining open to discussing the options for handling many "organic" problems. It is no longer a stretch to move into the facilitator mode when the issue is how to deal with a sleep problem or obesity. So in this unexpected way, my experience with wellness care has changed the way I function as a physician in general. Sometimes I miss the old *Father Knows Best* medicine, but in truth a more democratic style seems to fit me and my families more comfortably.

On the other hand, some parents may find the facilitator style too indecisive and may actually prefer a physician with a more authoritative approach. That's fine, too. What you are looking for is a good fit between the doctor's style and your needs as a patient or a parent. Evaluate your family's requirements, and don't settle for a poor fit.

The Elements of Wellness Care

When I undertake the wellness care of a new baby in my practice, I set myself several tasks. First is the overseeing of the physical health and development of the baby. I need to know as much as possible about the family's history of health and disease to be alert to problems which may arise with this child. I examine the baby with care to evaluate her physical condition. During the years that follow, repeated physical examinations will allow me to observe and study her growth and development so that any abnormalities can be dealt with at an early stage.

Second is the overseeing of the child's emotional or psychosocial growth. Here I am involved in a rather different undertaking. There is a very large range of perfectly normal human behavior, and as a medical observer watching some behaviors unfold over time, I need to remain clear about what is within that range and what isn't. This may sound simple, but, believe me, it isn't. Our ability to predict the outcome of a child's personality development is fairly primitive, and our power, as parents or as pediatricians, to alter it is even more questionable. This is the basis for my skepticism concerning the whole enterprise of "anticipatory guidance." This fancy term refers to the practice of telling parents what to expect at various stages of their children's growth, with some words of wisdom about handling the anticipated problems. Maybe it is useful, maybe not. I have certainly dispensed my share and more of advice on child rearing and its vicissitudes; sometimes the advice has been accurate and even heeded. But kids are individuals and families are unique; "one size fits all" does not work any better in pediatric practice than it does in buying shoes.

The third task in well child care is to be ready and willing to listen to parents' concerns about their children. I may have planned to talk about home safety at the visit of the 8-month old and his mother, but if she wants to talk about a collapsing marriage or a senile relative or a financial crisis in her family, I can be useful only if I set my plans aside and attend to her needs.

Prevention of disease is the fourth task of well child care. I am immensely grateful that my career in pediatrics has coincided with the increased availability of immunizing agents against some of the infectious illnesses most dangerous to children. When I became a doctor in 1953, we could protect our patients against only four common childhood infections: diphtheria, pertussis (whooping cough), tetanus, and smallpox. I'll never forget working as an intern on the hospital's contagious diseases service. One whole room was filled with polio patients, paralyzed by their disease and kept alive only by the iron lungs in which they lived. I can visualize with painful clarity that circle of respirators. The adults and older children were encased from the neck down in massive steel cylinders eight feet long, their motors softly pumping air in and out. The smaller children and babies were in half-sized versions of the same devices. Often there was a mother or a father sitting next to the child, reading to him or feeding him dinner. The advent of every summer's polio season brought completely justified anxiety to every parent in the country. I will never forget the immense excitement and joy we all felt when Jonas Salk's polio vaccine was announced.

As of 1996, we now have effective vaccines against measles, rubella, mumps, chicken pox, hepatitis A and B, and meningitis (and other deadly infections) caused by the bacterium Haemophilus influenzae type b. A milder whooping cough vaccine is coming into use, and a new, safe rabies vaccine is now available. There is also a moderately effective vaccine against influenza for older adults and highly susceptible people of any age. Smallpox has been eradicated from the earth, making the somewhat hazardous smallpox vaccine a thing of the past. These are the triumphs of public health and medical science.

I've gone on at some length about disease prevention by vaccines because human memory seems to be short, and there is resistance to the use of vaccines on the part of some laypeople and even a few physicians. Most Americans have never seen a patient suffocating from the membranes of diphtheria in the throat, or a baby in convulsions because of brain damage from whooping cough, or a child dying from polio, or a person blind, deaf, and brain damaged because of the mother's case of rubella during pregnancy. We have traded these wholesale horrors for a small number of bad reactions to immunization shots. Without doubt, there is risk attached to every immunizing vaccine ever made. Equally without doubt, the odds for ourselves and our children are in favor of vaccination, rather than running the risks of disease. (For more detail concerning the various immunizing agents, see Chapter 37.)

Information Excess. As soon as your pregnancy is visible, you become the target for advice from every corner. Your friends, your neighbors, your family, and total strangers will give you unsolicited and often contradictory advice. Your mailbox will overflow with advertisements, magazines, and newsletters even before you come home from the hospital with your newborn. Everyone is an expert in how you should raise your baby, what shots she should get and why, what to feed her and when. Much of this advice is obviously commercially motivated; there is a lot of money to be made on parents and babies. Perhaps this is the easiest to protect yourself against, since the motivation of the seller is so clear. It is more difficult to fend off the well-meaning experts each of whom wants you to do things their way. Physicians are among the worst offenders in the advice sweepstakes. Some doctors have publicly opined that pregnant women should gain only 15 or 20 pounds during pregnancy, while others have advised much greater weight gains. Caffeine during pregnancy has been damned by some and ignored by others. Some insist that only heavy alcohol consumption is risky, others advise not to drink at all. The list of conflicting opinions is endless.

In the marketplace of ideas, as elsewhere, it is a case of "let the buyer beware." I may as well admit that the ideas I espouse in this book are not an exception to this rule. I try my best to be accurate and sensible, but infallibility has not be granted to my profession, so read with care.

Chapter 4

Being Pregnant

Up until the last century, the passage from childhood into adult life was rapid. Sexual maturity in the teen years was followed by marriage and mating, not necessarily in that order. Early childbearing was inevitable; the only safe, partially effective method of contraception was prolonged breast feeding. The other major factor limiting the number of children in a family was infant and childhood mortality from disease, injury, and famine. For most young women, life was a series of pregnancies and hard work from an early age. The notion of a long period of adolescent development with deferred adult duties and rights was unheard of.

Today's young American woman often begins menstruating just before her teens, and she is likely to be fertile quite soon thereafter. Since the social pressures against early sexual intercourse have weakened, the girls most likely to become pregnant in their teens are those who have had little or no sex education, who have less access to a variety of contraceptive methods, and who live in cultural settings where early pregnancy is increasingly accepted.

For the young women who can and do protect themselves from pregnancy, or who can arrange an abortion if need be, the options are wholly different: a long adolescent period of formal education; delayed adult status, usually with prolonged dependence on parents for financial support; late marriage; later and limited childbearing. And a substantial number of women are faced with THE CHOICE: Career or Children or Both. All of these variations effect the ancient theme of motherhood. One is the discontinuity in the life of that new phenomenon, the woman in her thirties who is about to have her first baby. She knows a great deal more about the world than her great-great-grandmother knew, but she has often been out of touch with the other, older world of childbearing and child rearing. Her life as a young adult may have been wholly divorced from the patterns of family, pregnancy, breast feeding, and everyday mothering that typified her forebears. The typical experience of the human female is now a rather mysterious area, full of unknown threat and worrisome possibility. It should be no surprise if her pregnancy is marked by a considerable degree of anxiety.

There is plenty to be anxious about. Can she afford to stay home and be a full time mother? Does she want to? If she stays home for a month or a year or several years, what will be her chances of returning to a career? How long will her job wait for her? Will she find the tasks and limitations of the maternal role bearable? Who will she be if she is "only" a mother? The women's movement has brought these questions into public consciousness, but, needless to say, not to a public consensus.

As if this were not sufficient cause for worry, what about day care for her child if and when she does return to work? "Who will raise my baby?" is hardly a comfortable question to be mulling over during a night of restless sleep just before the baby is due. We will return to the topic of day care in Chapter 8.

Most women will have some anxious moments about the health of the baby they are carrying. Dr. Helen Gofman, one of my wisest teachers, told me that I should examine every newborn infant at the mother's bedside so that she can see for herself that her baby is perfect and healthy. If the baby does have a problem, the mother will get an immediate understanding of it. Nowadays, the Medical Anxiety of the Week usually concerns pregnancy and the health of fetuses. The rapidity with which one published study is contradicted by the next has led to some appropriate cynicism, but, in my opinion, not enough. I hate to say this about my own profession, but some of us doctors have an unfortunate tendency to shoot off our mouths. Perhaps we get excited by an apparent finding in a piece of our own research, or we may be unduly fond of a particular theory, or we are given to a bit of unjustified self-promotion. In any event, sometimes physicians rush into print with new information which turns out later to be wrong or unfounded. Often the information is brand new, just reported at some medical conference, and not yet subjected to the scrutiny of the rest of the profession. When new research has been published in a reputable medical journal, there has at least been the probability of careful perusal by independent referees who are experts in the field.

The situation deteriorates further when the sources are self-appointed experts with little or no scientific training. The public has little protection from this onslaught and the reality is that pregnancy may make us unusually vulnerable. We want so powerfully to protect the babies we are growing. The admonition to do or purchase this or avoid that is hard to ignore. The appropriate rule to apply is **Grossman's Law of Medical Advice: *Ask if it is really true.***

Medical Care During Pregnancy

You may have more choices than you think. First of all, who will be your medical adviser during your pregnancy: a midwife, a family doctor, or an obstetrician? In much of the industrialized world, this is the realm of mid-wives, who are typically nurses with extra training and experience. In recent years, midwives have become an increasingly popular choice in America. They approach pregnancy as a normal process, rather than some sort of illness to be worried over and treated. Midwives are likely to be less rushed than doctors, and they are often perceived to be more psychologically available. As women, and often as mothers themselves, they may be easier for a pregnant woman to talk to than the typical, commonly male, physician. Finally, they usually charge less. Obstetrician/gynecologists have dominated big-city obstetrical care for many years. Their training tends to stress the problem aspects of pregnancy, and their general approach can sometimes give a pregnant women the feeling that her doctor considers her a medical disaster waiting to happen. This may not contribute to a calm pregnancy. To make matters worse, the explosion of malpractice suits in the United States today has forced many physicians to practice defensive medicine. This means doctors are doing tests and procedures, not because they are medically indicated, but as protection against potential legal attack. In the management of pregnancy, this has helped popularize monitoring during labor, frequent use of operative delivery by Caesarean section, and other intrusive procedures of little or no proven utility. Happily, a number of OBs are attempting to moderate this excessively pathological point of view. The third alternative is the family doctor or general practitioner. Their training and experience in obstetrics will be less extensive than that of an OB, but a GP's more inclusive view of the pregnant woman and her family makes this type of care particularly valuable. In the unusual instance where an obstetrical specialist's help is required, the family doctor will have a back-up consultant available.

No matter what sort of medical professional you choose to assist your pregnancy and delivery, you will benefit from childbirth education classes. The same basic approach is shared by the several varieties of preparation for childbirth instruction: They demystify pregnancy and delivery. Women who know what is happening and how to cooperate with the process will generally have easier and shorter labors, with less need for pain relieving medications. This is better for both mothers and infants. (It's better for the fathers, too.)

Where Will Your Baby Be Born? Home births have become the exception in this country, but they still have their place and their enthusiastic supporters. When all goes well with a pregnancy and delivery, a home birth can be a lovely event. The happiest house calls I have ever made have been to visit the new baby and family shortly after the birth at home. I recall one family whom I found all in or on the parents' bed; the mother dozing, the father with the newborn wrapped in a blanket, asleep on his chest, the two older kids next to him. It was like coming into a den of friendly bears. The only problem with home deliveries is the lack of instant medical help if an obstetrical emergency occurs. Although it is rare that a few minutes delay makes a difference, there is no denying the fact that it can. Birthing centers have been developed in an attempt to meet this problem. They are typically free-standing units, often converted dwellings, with as homey an atmosphere as possible, and a close relationship with a nearby hospital and its emergency service. Another alternative is the family-centered birthing services within hospitals. This is a relatively new concept that attempts to counter the institutionalization of patient care by addressing the expressed needs of patients and their families. It is surprisingly hard to achieve, but it can be done.

Mothering the Mother. Not so many years ago, it was common custom to admit a woman in labor to a hospital, send her husband home, and pretty much abandon her to labor. A nurse or doctor would check her progress from time to time, but often she was left isolated, frightened, and in pain. It was a stupid and cruel procedure, and we now know better. Loving and knowledgeable company before and during childbirth makes an enormous difference. The presence of family members is basic; the baby's father, the mother's own mother, maybe both. In addition, many mothers receive support from birth coaches who stay with her throughout her labor, helping her to carry out natural childbirth techniques, and generally acting as her advocate in dealing with her medical attendants or with hospital procedures. Sometimes the birth coach is the baby's father, sometimes a woman friend, sometimes a paraprofessional with experience in childbirth. Doulas are women who accompany the mother during her labor. They may take an active role like the birth coach, or they may simply be a supportive presence. The effect of birth coaches and doulas is similar; labors are often shorter and C-sections are strikingly less common when a birth coach or a doula is present. They are a welcome antidote to the high-tech obstetrics that used to be the rule. (Doulas and how they can help are described in *Mothering the Mother*, by Marshall H. Klaus, John H. Kennell, and Phyllis H. Klaus. Reading, MA: Addison Wesley, 1993.)

Involving the Family. The concept of **family-centered childbirth** is decidedly more than a question of where the birth takes place. It encompasses the whole decision-making process surrounding pregnancy and childbirth, and implies that the entire nuclear family can be involved in planning for and caring for the new baby. The old American pattern of fathers having little to do with their babies and young children has begun to wane in response to a host of new social factors. Among these is the sense that emotional distance from his children is costly to the father himself, as well as to his children. Although he may not have felt drawn to parenthood in the same way that many women crave becoming mothers, young men often find the pregnancies of their wives and the births of their babies startlingly life-enhancing events. And they may find unexpected satisfaction in the everyday routines of infant care. However, this is not the case in every family. For many men, increased responsibility may be grudgingly undertaken. His feelings may stem from his prior sense of what a man is supposed to do, from his lack of skill in the techniques of child care, or from discomfort that financial pressures have forced his wife back to work. These are complex—and valid—issues that are unlikely to be easily resolved.

To what extent should older children be involved in the birth of the new baby? At some point, it is sensible to let them know about a pregnancy. A very young child will be sufficiently incomprehending that you can easily wait until late in the pregnancy. Telling a 3-year old during the first trimester is pretty much a waste of time. When Mom's girth has grown and the due date is approaching, the news will make more sense to the child, and there will still be plenty of time for explanations. Should the older siblings be present during their mother's labor and delivery? For school age and adolescent children, sharing the family experience of the birth of a new baby can be a remarkable event. Being present when the baby is born, having the opportunity to hold the newborn, and being in the electric atmosphere that surrounds childbirth—all this can be powerful and positive. It can also be frightening and awful. At the least, the siblings need comprehensive instruction about childbirth; it is a noisy and bloody and thoroughly amazing event. Children need to understand what they may witness. There should be an attendant adult whose sole task is to be there for them. Given all this, most families that choose to invite the big kids along have a uniquely powerful and joyous experience.

As a pediatrician who has been present at hundreds of births, I must say I still find it an exciting and moving experience. I think that the phenomenon of emotional bonding that begins between parents and their new baby is given a special impetus when the father is present and the mother is awake and alert during the delivery. We nearly always fall in love with our newborns, and that's surely a good thing, given how much they need us and how much work they are. There are doubtless any number of mechanisms assuring that this occurs: Some are probably hormonal, affecting the mother; some are learned responses, taught by cultural tradition; and perhaps others are wired into our brains through the processes of evolution. Anyway you look at it, bonding to our babies is essential. Intrusive hospital routines, such as separating parents and babies soon after birth and limiting their contact during the hospital stay, can get in the way of this crucial process. Fortunately, most hospital obstetrical services have loosened up these foolish restraints, and babies and parents can now be together immediately after birth and for most of their time in the hospital. Rooming-in of babies with their mothers (and sometimes fathers as well) is surely the best method for letting this happen. Rooming-in does not mean abandoning mother and baby in a room shortly after birth and then kicking them out twenty-four hours later, when the insurance coverage runs out. It works best when experienced nurses have time to help mothers practice the skills of breast feeding and can give the kind of gentle and supportive instruction in newborn care that many novice parents may need.

How Will You Feed Your Baby?

For many American women today, the choice of how to feed the baby is really no choice at all. If you grew up giving baby dolls toy bottles, surrounded by mothers who bottle fed their infants, and advertisments for infant formulas you may never seriously consider nursing your newborn at your breast. Formula feeding is a fascinating phenomenon; it really should be considered a psychological and nutritional experiment of considerable magnitude. Until the early part of this century, the physiologic needs of the baby were so poorly understood, and the safety of cows' milk so dubious, that bottle feeding was a truly dangerous undertaking. If a woman could not or would not nurse her baby, her only safe alternative was to hire a wet nurse who could breast feed in her stead. Nowadays, the availability of palatable and safe infant formula has transformed American infant feeding, and the majority of our babies are formula fed. The immediate health risks of properly prepared formula have much decreased, although bottle fed babies still tend to have more infections, especially ear infections, than breast fed babies. In countries with inadequate sanitation, bottle feeding remains quite hazardous; many formula fed babies die from infections, especially intestinal disorders caused by contaminated formula. The long term effects of formula feeding remain inadequately studied and largely unknown. The companies that manufacture and sell infant formula have generally attempted to produce a product which mimics the natural product of the human breast, but it is not a perfect match. The composition of sugars, fats, and amino acids is different. There are a substantial number of constituents in breast milk which are not in formula. Some of these have known health advantages, like lactoferrin, which increases the absorption of iron from the gut, or immunoglobulins, which help protect the baby from infections. Certain polyunsaturated fatty acids present in generous amounts in breast milk, but not in formula, appear to be needed for the optimum development of the baby's nervous system. Other substances are still being studied, and their functions in infant health and nutrition are not yet understood. Furthermore, I continue to wonder about the wisdom of feeding babies a low cholesterol food like baby formula instead of breast milk which has a strikingly high cholesterol content. Given the very large amount of cholesterol present in the human brain, it seems unwise to assume that milk company chemists know enough about the requirements of the growing infant's nervous system to second guess Mother Nature. In short, I find it impossible to take the usual line in discussions such as this. I know it is fashionable to say that formula feeding is just fine, but I don't see how a responsible pediatrician can pretend to be reassuring about a practice about which none of us have enough information.

Are there any other reasons to prefer breast feeding? There is some evidence suggesting that allergic disease in infancy is less common in breast fed babies. Breast feeding also may have some protective effect against sudden infant death syndrome (SIDS). Otherwise, the significant advantages to breast feeding seem to be in the mother–child relationship. The shared experience and the emotional bond between mother and nursling can hardly be duplicated through the intermediation of a nursing bottle.

If breast feeding is so terrific, why has it fallen out of favor to such an extent? This is by no means an easy question to answer. In part it may be a reflection of the power of the industrial, commercial world in which we live. We all see a lot more ads for baby formula than we do for breasts. In so far as the human breast is the subject of commercial exploitation, it is as a sexual rather than a nurturing object. We have replaced The Madonna, with the child at her breast, with Madonna, whose breasts are otherwise occupied. The practice of bottle feeding also gives mothers freedom from the need to be with their babies 24 hours a day. As women are increasingly drawn to jobs away from home, breast feeding becomes a hindrance to the mobility they must have.

A word should be said about mixed feedings, that is, breast feeding supplemented by bottles of formula or expressed breast milk as needed. The claim is occasionally made that there are some subtle disadvantages to this common practice. On the contrary, I think that mixed feedings make it possible for many women to work away from home and still continue to nurse. The many babies I've seen in my own practice who have been fed in this fashion have done just fine.

If you are going to nurse your baby, give some thought to preparing your nipples for nursing. The breasts of American women lead a remarkably cosseted existence, shielded from sun and wind, and protected from touch and sight, except for the purposes of sexual arousal. The transition from love object to milk conduit can be a shock. You can minimize it by a process of gradual and gentle desensitization which is detailed in the section on preparation for nursing in Chapter 6.

Adoption

Adoption is a remarkably successful adaptation; untold millions of babies and children have been incorporated in this fashion into human families since the beginning of our species. It is one of the glories of humanity that we can become parents in the fullest sense of the word without the benefit of shared genes, without the biological experiences of pregnancy, and often without the opportunity to begin parenthood at the time of the baby's birth. Becoming adoptive parents, like becoming biological parents, is both an act of will and an act expressing our living nature; we humans truly need to be mothers and fathers. There are so many differing scenarios that precede adoption that any simple discussion is likely to be inadequate. Adoptions can be excruciatingly difficult to arrange, or unbelievably easy and rapid. They may cross oceans, races, and social class barriers. They may involve a variety of reasons of health. The adopting family may be a heterosexual couple, a single parent, a gay or lesbian couple, or a family with other children. What all adoptions have in common is biological discontinuity: The mother who adopts has not had nine months to live with the pregnancy. She will enter the status "new mother" with an inevitable abruptness. Some adopting mothers are able to soften the transition if they have had a long and close relationship with the biological mother during her pregnancy. Some adopting mothers attempt to induce lactation so that they can nurse the new baby, and this is sometimes quite successful. There are also biological barriers in the genetic differences between the adoptive family and the newborn. Families do have certain tendencies to physical and intellectual similarity, and sometimes even temperamental patterns can be built in. All this is to say that we should approach adoption with respect for its complexities, and we should not be surprised when special circumstances evoke special problems; it may take some extra work from everyone involved.

Chapter 5

Arrival: The Perinatal Period

For the majority of American women, having a baby means going to a hospital. For the typical young mother this is the first hospital stay she will experience since her own sojourn as a newborn baby. It is especially for this group of mothers, relatively inexperienced in the ways of hospital life, that I wish to write about these peculiar places. Hospitals are complicated institutions which have developed over the last couple of hundred years to meet a variety of human needs. Sometimes these needs coincide with those of a particular group of patients. If you require a magnetic resonance study of some body part or other, the hospital is the likely place in which to find the appropriate machine. If you are seriously ill with a disease amenable to technically complex treatment, the hospital is the place where that can be undertaken. But if what you need is a quiet, supportive, restful place wherein you can deliver your new baby, surrounded by caring and sensitive people attuned to the multiple needs of you and your family, good luck. You may have such a hospital in your community, but a number of factors work against you. Every institution tends to serve its permanent staff at least as much as it serves its clients. The folks behind the counter at the grocery store or the post office have their jobs to do; they are going to be there all day, five days a week. The fact that you happen to be a customer in a hurry does not carry a great deal of weight in the greater scheme of grocery store or post office life. So a rhythm of commercial life develops in every establishment, and we clients fit ourselves in as best we can. Should we be surprised that the same rules hold true in medical institutions? They also respond to the requirements of the people who are there all day (and all night), every day of the week. Of course there are differences. We expect medical professionals to be driven by a sense of service and vocation, and, to a degree, this is the case. But the people who work in hospitals are also simply human. Doctors and nurses can be tired, overworked, distracted by their own concerns, or just grumpy, like anyone else. Furthermore, we as patients are affected by our sense of the specialness of our personal medical situations, and by anxiety about the hazards that attend every medical encounter. Small wonder if there is disharmony between the admitting nurse on the OB unit, meeting the umpteenth woman in labor this evening, and the excited and frightened young mother-to-be, timing her contractions with the assistance of her anxious young husband.

The easy way for the medical institution to deal with this setup for potential conflict is to develop routines which overwhelm the patient with a sense of the power and authority of the hospital and its staff. The unspoken but quite audible message is "We're comfortably in charge here; just relax and let us do what is best for you." This starts at the admissions desk where you are kept waiting long enough to remind you of your relative unimportance. Large numbers of papers are thrust at you to be signed, selling your progeny into slavery and putting a lien on your house as a minimum condition to admission. Next, you are told to wait for an orderly to take you by wheelchair to the obstetrics department; apparently you cannot even be trusted to walk. In the OB unit, you will be ordered to remove your clothes and don the ridiculous garment called a hospital gown. This device allows instant access, visual and otherwise, to every part of your body you were ever taught to be modest about. Then you are ordered to bed. Your reduction to the level of obedient infant is well under way, and you have had a series of little lessons in How To Be A Good Patient. Some of the more humiliating and senseless obstetrical routines of the recent past have been abandoned; you will not be given an enema, nor will your pubic hair be shaved. But your medical attendants will perform a variety of procedures upon you, usually with minimal if any explanation, and surely without asking your assent. You may also have the common experience of doctors and nurses talking over your head about your labor as if you were not a major actor in the process with certain concerns of your own to be addressed. The net effect on most patients confronting this institutional behemoth is to be turned into passive bags of mush. It is quite difficult to keep in mind that the OB unit really, truly exists to meet the needs of women in labor, their new babies, and their families. In all fairness, I should add that most patients bring to this encounter an intense need to be cared for. So it is perfectly understandable to assume a childlike dependency when engulfed in a hospital situation.

Awareness of this uneven struggle and its adverse effects on all the parties concerned has led to major efforts within most hospitals to build welcoming rather than bullying routines into the management of labor. Wear your own clothes, don't stay in bed during labor unless you want to, have your husband and kids with you, ask questions and insist on answers, and come prepared by childbirth instruction rather than terrified by ignorance. This family-centered childbirth is a reality in many hospitals, but it requires continuing effort to keep a patient-oriented point of view when one is not a patient. If you have a choice of local hospitals, it is worthwhile to inquire about the degree to which each attempts to meet the needs of patients for respectful care. Ask your friends who have had babies recently and ask any doctors or nurses you know.

The point of this extended sermon is to remind you that you will enter the hospital environment as an adult with your own needs, fears, hopes, and feelings. When hospital routines fail to provide what you want, it is perfectly appropriate to let your needs be known and honored if possible. Sometimes the exigencies of the medical world will interfere; there really are emergency situations that require nonemergency needs to be put on hold. But you need not check your individuality at the admissions desk, to be picked up later at the time of discharge.

Labor

Quite a lot is known about the natural progression of normal labor, but not all of what we know is automatically applied in modern American hospitals. Generally speaking, labors go best and fastest when the mother has the support of a labor coach or a doula, when her husband can be with her, and when she is able to be up and about, rather than confined to bed. The quite common practice of monitoring labor with sensing devices attached to the mother makes it difficult to be mobile. The information provided by the monitoring machinery can be misused. It is easy to overread the record and decide that the baby is not tolerating labor; this is often the excuse for abandoning a normal labor and delivery in favor of a hurried Caesarean section. The rise of electronic monitoring parallels the astounding increase in the C-section rate, which is currently 20 to 30% in American hospitals. Studies in Ireland, Guatemala, France, and the U.S. have shown that labors attended by human companions rather than electronic machines are vastly more likely to eventuate in successful vaginal births.

C-section rates fall to 5 to 8%. The machines certainly have a *limited* place in the management of problem pregnancies, but that is about all.

Then there is the issue of pain-controlling medications. Even a calm mother, well prepared for the process of childbirth and helped during her labor by skillful attendants, will have a considerable degree of discomfort. The contractions of the uterine muscle and the pressure of pushing a big baby through a small pelvis causes pain. Fortunately, pain-controlling drugs are available; unfortunately, most of them blur the mother's consciousness and sedate the baby. This can cause a substantial interference with the infant's behavior during the first days of life, sometimes with significant consequences. I think that nursing failures are often the result of sedating the baby. From the mother's point of view, it seems a pity to give her drugs which may render her sleepy and confused during the first hours after the birth, when she could otherwise be enjoying the incredible excitement and joy of early contact with her new infant. The ideal situation is one in which mothers have been taught methods for minimizing discomfort by relaxation and breathing techniques, where they are accompanied and supported during labor, and where drugs are available when they are needed.

Early Contact Between Parents and Newborns. Whether we are humans, penguins, apes, or lions, the newly born are a remarkably vulnerable bunch of little beings. It seems so obvious that the infant requires the ministrations of mother in the period immediately after birth that I am always amazed how commonly and casually this relationship has been violated in American hospitals. From early in this century until about 1970, the use of heavy sedation during labor was so common that newborn babies had to be taken from their mothers for many hours after birth simply because the mothers were so groggy or sleepy. With the rise of natural childbirth and the consequent decrease in the use of narcotics during labor, we can study a much more normal, if not entirely "natural," situation. In the hours immediately following birth, babies are typically alert and interested in their surroundings. They fix their gazes on the faces of their caretakers, and they appear to be responsive to the smiles and speech of their parents. Newborn babies held by their mothers during the first minutes and hours are usually calm and peaceful. In contrast, newborns removed from their mothers will cry and complain. Most unsedated infants will nurse within minutes after birth. One recent Swedish study showed that babies placed nude on their mothers' bare abdomens would gradually inch their way up to her breasts and begin to nurse without any adult assistance at all. The skill, coordination, and accuracy of the infant's efforts are amazing and the effect on the mother of experiencing her baby's need for her is powerful. We should not be surprised by this superb matching of infant requirements and infant abilities. Every other mammalian baby knows how to find its mother's nipples, why not us?

Bonding

For the parents (and often for siblings) the first hours after the birth of a baby are a magical time. There is a powerful sense of family, of belonging to one another, and of being tied into a new biological and social unity. Parents and infants seem ready for this experience, waiting to be joined together. This process of psychological connection was termed **bonding** by Drs. Marshall Klaus and John Kennell, two pediatricians who were among the first to draw attention to the phenomenon in the early 1970s. Dr. Klaus now comments wryly that he wishes they had used a word with less mechanical connotations; bonding is on ongoing process, not an instant event like mending a broken plate with Krazy Glue. During the first hours and days immediately after the baby is born, parents are particularly receptive, ready to feel attached, primed biologically or socially or both to take on the roles of mother and father to their new child. When early parent–infant contact is impossible, the same learning takes place, but it often seems slower and sometimes seems less intense. Studies of the effects of early contact suggest that it may be particularly important to the most vulnerable mothers, those with the least developed support systems within their families and communities. But for all parents, the opportunity to be quietly alone with the new baby is surely desirable and nearly always rewarding. Hospital routines which interfere with this quiet time are rarely important enough to be justified; the healthy baby's first measurement or bath or physical examination can wait. The first hours together of Mom and Dad and Baby belong to them, to be shared, if they wish, with other family members, but to be intruded upon as little as possible by the outside world. I would like to stress that bonding is not a set routine that one must somehow accomplish in a prescribed fashion in order to achieve some sort of measurable success. Articles that tell parents "How to bond with your new baby" miss the point. Bonding is simply a description of the first stages of the quite wonderful process of attachment that connects us to our children. It is not a matter of "doing" it correctly, but rather making sure that as little as possible gets in the way of this completely natural and necessary development.

Of course, sometimes things do get in the way. Even in the best run and most baby-friendly hospitals there will be instances where medical problems with the infant or the mother make early contact difficult. Sick or premature babies often require special care which separates them from their parents much of the time. However, even in these situations much can be done to facilitate bonding. It is now a common scene in newborn intensive care nurseries to see parents holding their tiny premies, or mothers sitting with their nearly naked babies held against their breasts. There is widespread understanding among doctors and nurses of the ill effects of unnecessary separation of parents and newborns, and increasing efforts are made to keep parents with even the most fragile infants.

The Postnatal Period

So, your baby has been born, you've already begun to fall in love with the beautiful little being, the first feeding has been accomplished, and the routine examinations by the nurses and your doctor have confirmed that your infant is as remarkable as you had hoped and expected. What now? Shouldn't you just go home? Probably not yet. Most mothers need rest and it is comforting to go to sleep knowing that you have instant access to experienced hands for awhile. It is also a good idea for the mother to be checked for common problems like postpartum bleeding, at least for a day or so. The newborn also may benefit by a modest amount of supervision during the first days. We like to be assured that every system is in working order; the first urination and the first bowel movement are events of particular interest. Nurses or doctors expert in teaching mothers how to nurse can be a big help. When mothers routinely stayed for three or four days after childbirth, there was ample time for instruction in a variety of tasks such as feeding, burping, temperature taking, and washing. This is no longer possible in our era of rapid discharge, which means that some sort of follow-up service for new families is particularly important. Being home alone with your first child can be an anxiety provoking experience. House calls by a nurse or physician a day or two after the baby goes home are a great help. So is the support of friends and family who can fill in with information and with household assistance like shopping, cleaning, laundry, and cooking.

Normal "Physiologic" Jaundice in Newborns. One advantage of sending babies home early is that hospital personnel have less opportunity to get needlessly excited about normal events like the typical jaundice of the 3-day old baby. Many newborns turn somewhat yellow at around this age. The color is due to an excess of pigment which is the normal byproduct of blood cell metabolism; this yellow material (called bilirubin) must be processed by the baby's liver and excreted into the urine and stool. But the baby's liver has been relatively inactive during fetal life; Mom's liver did all the work. After birth, it takes a few days for the baby's liver to gear up for the new task, and during that time, the bilirubin levels increase and the baby develops a pretty golden color. This is first and most easily seen in the whites of the eyes, and then spreads to the face and the body, gradually progressing to the extremities. When the jaundice is moderate in degree, usually not extending past the thighs, and the baby's color is a creamy yellow rather than a deep egg yolk yellow, the concentration of bilirubin is likely to be a matter of no importance at all. Needless to say, observation of infant skin color is not so easy in dark skinned or Asian infants. As the baby eats more and has more frequent stools, and as the liver takes over its intended role, the jaundice gradually disappears. This can take over a week. Third-day jaundice is most likely to be seen in breast fed babies, probably because they get less food in the first few days before their mothers' milk comes in. It is particularly important not to meddle by offering the breast fed baby formula or extra water in an ill-advised and unnecessary attempt to push this normal process forward. Nor is it advisable to treat this kind of newborn jaundice with phototherapy, the bright light treatment which is so helpful in certain other cases of jaundice where dangerously high levels of bilirubin can be found. It is now generally agreed that the normal, mild jaundice of full-term, healthy newborns rarely if ever requires any medical intervention.

Breast Milk Jaundice. This heavily overdiagnosed entity needs to be mentioned here although it is actually not a problem in the immediate new-born period. Some breast fed babies become jaundiced after they have had a few days of mother's milk, say around one week of age; some start with normal physiologic jaundice at age two or three days but don't lose it at the end of a week or so. Most of these infants have breast milk jaundice, a harmless and poorly understood condition which lasts a month or so and then fades away. It is important to make the diagnosis because we do not want to miss other significant causes of baby jaundice such as blood incompatibilities, liver disorders, or infections. Simple lab tests are often in order. If these show no evidence of other disease, a trial of twenty-four hours off breast milk can be done. The bilirubin level will drop and then usually rebound when breast feeding is resumed. Thereafter, the jaundice can be ignored until it disappears spontaneously in a few weeks.

Can Newborn Babies Become Dehydrated? Dehydration in the newborn period is another nonproblem to which unnecessary attention is paid. Full term newborns are nicely designed to wait for their mothers' milk to come in. The fluid volume of colostrum does not really amount to much, although colostrum is useful for the baby as a source of antibodies and a reward for learning to nurse. So the new baby conserves body fluids, urinates very little, and loses some weight during the first several days of life. That is the plan, and we should not consider ourselves wiser than the Designer who set it up this way. So should newborns ever be given a drink of water? Well, yes, if Mom's milk has not come in and the kid is screaming with thirst. Or if the baby is feverish or ill we will want to be sure that fluid requirements are met. But for healthy, full-term infants, the question of hydration during the first several days of life can be ignored.

Eye Infection Prophylaxis. A century ago the most common cause of blindness in children was severe infection of the eyes, occurring at the time of birth, and caused by the gonorrhea bacterium (Neisseria gonorrhoeae). This germ is often present in the cervix and vagina without causing obvious symptoms, and babies can easily pick up the infection during normal, vaginal births. Since the introduction a century ago of silver nitrate eye drops to prevent the infection, this form of devastating eye infection has become a rarity in the United States. Because many babies developed swollen eyelids and watery eyes for a day or two after silver nitrate treatment, alternative methods were sought. Nowadays, erythromycin or tetracycline ointments are generally used instead. This is a truly useful medical intervention. There is really no way of knowing if a mother has exposed her baby to this germ. Furthermore, any of these prophylactic medications is safe. I've never seen any reactions to the ointments, and even the most severe reactions to silver nitrate clear in a few days. The risk that a baby might develop an undiagnosed or improperly treated gonorrheal conjunctivitis is simply too great to take. After the baby has had a good, long visit with Mom and Dad is a good time for eye prophylaxis and the other useful medical routines to be done.

Vitamin K. Vitamin K is a substance needed for normal blood clotting to take place. Newborn babies have low levels of this vitamin for some days, and are therefore occasionally subject to bleeding problems which can be quite severe. Breast fed infants are particularly at risk since vitamin K levels in breast milk are not high. Eventually, K is manufactured within our intestines by bacteria, but this takes some time to get underway. This problem is easily prevented by giving every newborn a small injection of vitamin K. Giving the K by mouth is a tempting but mistaken alternative. The oral method, used in Germany and the United Kingdom, has resulted in many cases of intracranial bleeding even when multiple doses were given. Your baby should receive extra vitamin K in the first day of life, and the safest way is by injection. This routine can also wait until after your first get-acquainted visit, but don't let it be omitted.

Going Home

Parents (and siblings if present) and the new baby all benefit from having quiet time together during the first hours and days after birth. But there are competing needs that get in the way. The hospital routines have to grind their way to completion. Babies are examined, and tests are taken, such as the crucial screening tests on a few drops of the new baby's blood. These tests look for a variety of disorders like thyroid deficiency that require rapid intervention to be successfully treated. Even in this era of brief hospital stays, an attempt is usually made to assure that new families know something about infant care, especially feeding the baby. Meanwhile, every relative and family friend within a 50-mile radius wants to come to see the baby. Any number of times, I've had to shoulder my way into hospital rooms so crowded with visitors that it was difficult to find mother and infant in the melee. This overpowering urge to see the newborn is quite wonderful; there is a sort of primitive wisdom expressing itself here. Unfortunately, it does interfere with snatching a few peaceful hours of privacy.

Once you are back home, the problem with your newborn continues. Friends and neighbors will telephone to say that they will just drop by for a few moments to visit. This is a well meant but flagrant untruth; no one has ever been known to visit a new baby for a few minutes. Minimum visits are about half an hour, and a succession of these will eat up the day quite effectively. Can you as new parents protect your privacy and conserve your energy by limiting visitors? Probably not, but it's worth a try. Scheduling the bulk of these visits a week or two hence is one stratagem. Taking the phone off the hook helps. One mother in my practice who had herself been raised in a military family posted a very official looking, typewritten sign on the front door which said "BY ORDER OF THE ATTENDING PEDIATRICIAN, NO VISITORS UNTIL NEXT WEEK." Like so much of parenthood, dealing with friends and family is a balancing act. Offers

EVERYDAY PEDIATRICS FOR PARENTS

of help, prepared meals, and some expert answers about questions of baby care are always welcome. And I'm sure you would prefer not to alienate touchy relatives by suggesting that their visit would be most welcome in about a month and a half. But you will also find that you need (and will cherish) some peaceful time with the house empty except for yourselves and the new baby.

At the risk of sounding unduly pessimistic I should mention that peaceful time is not always automatic. Some newborns have just miserable first nights at home. They cry, they fret, they won't eat, they won't sleep, and it is difficult to figure out what they want. This is not the same thing as infant colic, the episodic fretfulness of somewhat older infants. The first night's fussiness seems to be related to the process of settling in at home, and might reflect the unease with which inexperienced parents handle the child. Fortunately, everyone gets used to everyone else in a day or two and the fussiness disappears. During this transition period, I think the new baby is learning that Mom and Dad are really nice, competent, and trustworthy people. Meanwhile, Mom and Dad are beginning to believe that they really will be able to take care of the new baby. Whether they know it or not, they have also begun to learn to "read" their newborns cries, expressions, and moods. Part of this learning is due to a conscious effort to figure out what is happening, and part is probably the result of primitive, intuitive processes.

Now that you are finally home, you are ready for **Grossman's First Law of Baby Care: *Keep it simple.*** Human babies really don't need much. Every day they are brought home to environments as diverse as tents, igloos, rain forests, and walk-up apartments. The requirements common to all babies are a place to sleep, plenty to eat, loving care, and appropriate clothing. Everything else is window dressing.

Sleep—101

Initially, where the baby sleeps is simple. Next to Mom has surely been the rule for nearly all of human experience. It's handy for everyone, it's just the right temperature, and it feels good. An otherwise fretful infant may be transformed into a calm little bundle of sleepiness by getting as close to Mom as possible. For babies who don't mind a bit of distance, a bassinet or a cradle, or one end of a child-size crib are also fine. It is worth mentioning that babies are safest on fairly firm surfaces. Very soft materials like sheepskins are comforting, but, unhappily, these have been linked to unexpected infant death (the condition referred to as SIDS). There is also evidence that cases of sudden infant death are more common in babies who sleep on their bellies. The combination of soft, mushy bed surfaces and prone (belly down) sleeping is the most hazardous. Despite the fact that most babies seem to sleep better on their bellies, it is worthwhile to teach them to sleep on their backs. (For more details about SIDS see Chapter 46.) How long a new baby should share the parents' bed is a good question. Mothers and fathers may not see eye to eye on this issue. Mothers' interest in sexual intercourse frequently diminishes during pregnancy. Even after she has fully recovered from childbirth, her energies are usually bound to her new infant. It sometimes seems as though the love that new mothers feel for their infants displaces the sexual love they have had for their husbands. It may be some time before she has any desire to resume an active sex life. The father has probably not experienced any decrease in his sex drive during his wife's pregnancy, but he has very likely experienced a significant decrease in opportunities for intercourse. After the baby arrives, things may get worse. If she is nursing, the baby has taken over his wife's breasts, and besides, there never seems to be enough time. The longer the new baby shares their bed, the longer it is likely to be before a couple returns to anything like their pre-parenthood sexual patterns, a situation containing significant hazards for the health of the marriage.

When the baby is out of the parent's bed and into a crib or a bassinet, is it best to provide a separate bedroom as well? Only within the last century or two, and only among relatively well-to-do families has this become an option. It is clear that human families used to sleep huddled together in fairly close quarters. But now most middle class families in industrialized nations like ours sleep as separately as they can manage. I think this is a reflection of the general loosening of family ties that characterizes our era, and particularly, our country. This is a nation of wide horizons and, for much of our history, open frontiers; we don't stay at home, we leave. Our forebears left their families and their countries to come to America; their children left home and headed west, and the pattern of nuclear families, isolated from the web of family generational support and control, has become the national norm. We begin to teach this expectation of intrafamily distance at an early age. When the new baby is placed down the hall in her own room, or in a bedroom with a sibling, we are teaching the first of many lessons in distance. It is as if we are saying "Get used to it, please; in only eighteen years you will go away to college." Is this a good idea? Well, we Americans cherish our independence and our mobility, but we also bemoan the deterioration of strong family bonds. Separation is surely a two-edged sword. Having said all that, should baby be down the hall or not? For some infants, it seems wholly unimportant; they will sleep peacefully anywhere. If that is your baby's temperament, separate bedrooms may help you to enjoy sounder sleep (and less inhibited sex). Infants' sleep is like that of adults in its variable depth; periods of deep sleep alternate with periods of light sleep and near awakening. Some babies will arouse more easily and completely when they sense the presence of their parents nearby. These babies will often sleep longer stretches at a time when they are sleeping separately. One additional factor to consider is the recent finding that SIDS is less common among babies who share a bedroom (but not a bed) with an adult. The incidence of SIDS is greatest between the ages of 1 month and 7 months after which it is extremely rare.

Eventually, sleeping arrangements will be decided pragmatically in most families. Parents get over some of the anxiety that makes distance seem hazardous, and they become sufficiently sleep deprived by the demands of the newborn that any tactic promising a few more minutes of rest seems awfully desirable. At that point, baby is packed up and moved out.

A Comfortable Environment for the New Baby. I've always loved making house calls on new babies and their families except for one thing: the common tendency to keep the temperature of the house high enough to grow tropical fruit in the living room. It is true that the newborn can become easily chilled, especially in the first day or so of life. But this can be handled with an extra blanket. Keeping the entire family at a temperature suitable for roasting a leg of lamb is unnecessary. Babies will let you know if the surrounding temperature suits them. Excessive cold will make newborns pull themselves into a ball, and their lips, hands, and feet will feel cold. (During the first days most babies have rather bluish hands and feet, anyway; that does not mean anything.) An overheated baby will sleep with arms and legs outstretched, and he will probably look flushed and a bit sweaty. In any case, hot or cold, most babies don't seem to care all that much. The best rule is to keep the house temperature at whatever level the rest of the family prefers; the baby will adapt. I promise.

Safety

It may seem premature to raise the issue of safety at such at early stage in the infant's career. It is true that the major risks of early childhood develop when kids can walk and climb and explore the house. But even new babies can get into hazardous situations. The first is in **automobiles;** there is every reason to insist that your baby be strapped into a safe, infant-sized car seat from the very first day. No exceptions, no excuses. If the baby complains, that is too bad. They simply have to learn that car travel involves a car seat; every baby gets used to it eventually.

At home, the dangers of which you need be aware are relatively few. Scalding **hot water** is available in many households. It is imperative that the water heater thermostat be turned down far enough to ensure that water is never higher than 120° F. This is plenty hot enough for all household purposes and will decrease the risk of accidental burns. Infants also need to be protected against **falls;** even quite young babies will surprise you by turning over. When a baby is on a high surface like a changing table, keep a restraining hand on her, and position her sideways if you can, so that an unexpected flip will find her still on the table and not on the floor.

The other hazards that people worry about are attacks by angry brothers or sisters or **family pets.** Pets are a complicated topic, partly because they do pose some real dangers and partly because we pet owners are a wildly irrational bunch. It is by no means always easy to determine who comes first in families, the pet, the children, or the parents. When a man and a women become a couple, it is quite common for one spouse to bring a pet into the relationship. With any luck at all, and even minimal good sense, the new spouse will take precedence over the old pet in the affections of its original owner. (This transfer of love and power may be slow and painful for all the parties concerned.) A similar situation arises when a couple and their beloved cat or dog is joined by the new baby. To describe the pet as annoyed by this unwelcome intrusion hardly does justice to the depth of feelings involved. Fortunately, millennia of life with human beings have taught the majority of cats and dogs that their adult caretakers will not tolerate any significant show of force directed against newborns. I have never seen anything worse than a dirty look directed against the newcomers. Unfortunately however, serious and sometimes even fatal attacks do occur. Thanks to irresponsible breeding, some dogs have earned reputations for aggressive behavior. Pit Bulls are responsible for more attacks against people than any other breed. Statistics show that Rottweilers and German Shepherds, once trusted working dogs, have also become particularly dangerous. In fact, any dog, large or small, has to be considered to pose a risk to children. It is difficult to think of a good reason for having animals with sharp teeth, bad tempers, and strong muscles anywhere

EVERYDAY PEDIATRICS FOR PARENTS

around kids. A considerable degree of care needs to be taken in households where such pets reside. Ferrets have recently been promoted as family pets, and already there are reports in the medical literature of serious injuries and even deaths of babies caused by these little beasts. They should be considered wholly unsuited to domestic life near children.

The other hazards posed by pets include diseases, most commonly Salmonella infections from turtles, parasites of all sorts from dogs and cats, and respiratory allergy, especially to cats and birds. All of these are problems likely to develop with older children, but worth keeping in mind when you are considering cohabiting with pet animals.

As distinct from the issues posed by pets, those involving **siblings** allow fewer options. It is really not possible to give an angry older brother away. Happily, an older sibling's feelings can be handled with less draconian measures. I think that most parents are aware that jealousy is a normal and even expected response to a new pregnancy. No matter that your firstborn has been importuning you to get him a new brother; when it becomes clear that the new brother is actually on the way, most children will have second thoughts. A moment's reflection will make clear to them that there is only so much parental attention to go around. Do I really want to share my toys, my room, and my parents with a competitor? When the infant arrives, accompanied by joyous outpourings of delight from previously reliable aunts and uncles, a clever child may well decide that ordering up a new baby for the family was a dreadful error. Not infrequently, an older child will endure the presence of the infant for a few days and then suggest that it would be a good idea to take him back to the hospital and leave him there. Sometimes these impulses are expressed directly, but not always. During my house call on the family of a 1-week old girl, her mother reported to me that the 6-year old brother was absolutely delighted with his new sister. As I was about to leave, we heard, through the slightly ajar front door, big brother singing a little song and doing a dance on the door mat. As he stamped up and down, he sang "Good-bye, Baby, Baby go home; Good-bye, Baby, Baby go home." So much for brotherly love.

Recognizing that sibling rivalry exists is one thing; dealing with it is another matter. An immense literature and an even larger folklore provide all sorts of advice regarding the relationships, smooth and otherwise, between sibs. The story of Cain and Abel suggests that this is not a new phenomenon. Be prepared to receive, unasked for, a bewildering variety of well meant pieces of advice on this topic. The range of ideas should suggest to you that there is no foolproof formula; when a tactic really works, people are smart enough to stop looking for alternative methods. I think the reason for the multiplicity of approaches to sibling rivalry is that it is both important and insoluble. Kids are jealous because they want and need so much parental love and attention—and sharing hurts. Perhaps the best we can do is expect it, acknowledge it when it erupts, and set reasonable limits about acceptable forms of expression. Some families begin the process of introducing the newcomer to the older kids quite early in the pregnancy. I suppose the theory here is to give them extra time to assimilate the news, but I'm not convinced it makes much difference. Providing a baby doll "all your own" for the older child during Mom's pregnancy may be useful, especially for an older girl. Perhaps her maternal play with the doll will somehow help the older child come to terms with onrushing siblinghood. I can't see that it is likely to make her any happier to share Mom with a little stranger. Presenting the older child with a new doll at the time baby is born is a variant technique, doubtless appreciated by kids who like dolls, but not necessarily therapeutic for sibling hatred.

In the long run only four strategies make much sense to me. First, be prepared to commiserate with your older kids about how tough it is to share parental attention and to cope with the changes in the household. "Honey, I imagine you're really angry about all the time the baby takes and how often you have to wait your turn." Second, try to find some time for the older kids by themselves; even fifteen minutes of undivided parental attention seems to make a difference. Ask visitors to pay at least a little attention to the older kids when they come to see your newborn. Third, at least initially, avoid casting the older kids in the roles of household slaves in service to the newborn. Eventually, everyone in a family has tasks to do in order to keep the family functioning, and that's fine. But assign responsibilities gradually if you can. It is a lot easier to help take care of your baby sister *after* you have gotten over your initial shock at having been dethroned. And it is easier yet when Baby is 2 or 3 months old and has decided that Sister and Brother are totally charming people whom one meets with a delighted smile and a welcoming gurgle. Fourth, set limits regarding the physical expression of jealousy. It is not helpful for kids to be allowed to hit or bite the baby. The baby won't appreciate it, and the older children will be frightened by their own unchecked aggression. They are clearly having fairly murderous impulses, and being allowed to act them out leaves many children feeling dangerously out of control. "You can be as angry at Baby as you want, but you are not allowed to hurt her at all!" There is no point in pretending that these rules or any others will lead inevitably to happy, loving families, free of competition and resentment. That does not seem to be the nature of human family life, especially in small, nuclear families where two adults must provide for the emotional nurturance of all the children. I suspect that extended families which include other relatives have an easier time with this issue because a child has a larger group of potentially supportive adults.

One final word about sibling rivalry: Children within a family actually do not try to hurt each other in any serious fashion. This may sound like an outrageously optimistic statement, and doubtless there are occasional exceptions, but it is exceedingly unusual to see any substantial physical damage done by siblings to one another. Somehow, we give our children the message that limits must be observed in the expression of the angry impulses that are an inevitable part of family life. A good thing, too.

Patterns of Sleep

When people write about what to expect regarding sleep during infancy they sometimes give the impression that there is a normal pattern to which most babies will eventually adhere. This is a wildly misleading simplification. **Grossman's Law of Infant Sleep: *It's unpredictable.*** About all one can say is that newborns tend to sleep more than the rest of us, that they alternate between deep sleep and lighter sleep states more frequently than older children or adults, and that they wake more frequently to be fed than is usually convenient. The precise pattern will vary depending on a host of factors, some environmental, some intrinsically human, and some individually programmed. Most of our insight comes from studies of other animals. Research suggests that sleeping patterns are linked to eating patterns. In general, comparing one species of animal with another, the richer and more concentrated the mother's milk, the longer the offspring can go between feedings. Human milk is relatively unconcentrated and one would, therefore, expect human infants to wake often in order to nurse. When one observes human behavior in primitive societies, this is precisely what one sees. The new babies are often carried in a cloth sling against the mother's body. At frequent intervals, the infant will stir and awaken, the mother will nurse her baby, and the baby will return to sleep. This sequence may be repeated dozens of times a day. Needless to say, it is unusual for American babies to be cared for in this fashion. More often, our babies will tend to rouse from a deep sleep cycle to light sleep about every hour. They will become fully awake and demand a feeding about 8 to 20 times a day. Since breast milk is more easily and rapidly digested that artificial formulas, the breast fed baby can be expected to need more frequent meals.

In the first few days, frequency of feedings and occurrence of wakeful periods is unrelated to time of day; babies are as likely to be awake at night as during the day. Gradually, they adapt to the adult pattern of longer periods of sleep at night, but this is a slow process for many infants. "Sleeping through" for 6 to 8 hours at a stretch can take anywhere from a few months to a couple of years, although many babies manage it within about half a year. You can make it easier for infants to sleep at night by providing a quiet, dark bedroom so that the hourly change in the depth of sleep is less likely to be converted to full awakening. Furthermore, the episodes of nighttime feedings can be accomplished with a minimum of stimulation; the lesson you are teaching is that it's fine to wake up to be fed, but don't expect playtime. The fiddle factor in all this is the infant herself. She will make it clear within the first few months that she is an individual with a preferred time for play, attention, and feedings. Some placid infants will accept all sorts of imposed regimens. Other, more willful babies decide at an early age that the world had better attend to their needs with alacrity.

From the first days of life, most babies will have some periods of wakefulness either before or after a feeding during which they are alert and interested in their surroundings. These times gradually stretch out into more prolonged and reasonably predictable times for play and socializing. By the end of the first month you will have a pretty good idea when to expect this. Unhappily, it often coincides with the late afternoon witching hours when everyone is tired, the older kids are hungry, and adult energies are not at their highest. At this point, every family needs a resident grandmother or, at the least, a neighborhood teenager to help out. Investing in household assistance can help families survive what can otherwise become a grueling experience of trying to meet too many needs with too few hands.

Intake and Outgo: Food, Urine, and Stools

In the matter of appetite, as in just about everything else you can imagine, babies vary wildly during the first few days of life. Full-term infants are so well prepared to wait for mother's milk to come in that the scant amounts of colostrum are sufficient to keep most of them content for about 3 days. On the other hand, bottle fed infants may take a few ounces every few hours from the very first feeding. Consequently, their production of urine and of feces starts sooner and is decidedly more copious than that of breast fed babies. During this period, the breast fed babies may have so little urine output that their diapers are barely damp; don't worry, they will make up for lost time after your milk comes in. After the first several days, urine production should result in wet diapers every few hours, day and night. In any case, breast fed or bottle fed, expect the first urination during the first two days; the baby who hasn't peed by then may have a problem with either the production or passage of urine. Occasionally, you may notice a small patch of a brickdust reddish stain on the wet part of the diaper; this is a harmless pigment that can develop in concentrated urine in early infancy. The first stools are dark green-black sticky, gooey messes called meconium. The appearance of the very first stool is a matter of some importance; if there is no stool within two days something may be amiss with the infant's digestive system. As the baby begins to take in milk, the stools become lighter green, then brownish yellow and eventually yellow. The stools of babies on soy or predigested formulas may stay green or brown. The stool texture varies depending on the milk and on the efficiency of the baby's gut. Breast feeding results in a looser stool, often bright yellow, like egg yolk mixed with cottage cheese. Sometimes there will be remarkably little residual stool at all, hardly more than a copious yellow stain on the diaper. Breast milk stools smell faintly acidic or fermented. "Humanized" cows' milk formulas (like Enfamil, Similac and Gerber's) typically result in smelly and pastier stools. Soy and predigested formula stools tend to be stinky and unpredictably varied in texture. You may be surprised at the amount of grunting and straining that can accompany the production of a bowel movement. Even quite loose stools are sometimes heralded by an audible amount of infant effort. This phenomenon disappears with time as the baby learns that nothing much in the way of conscious effort is required; the large intestine knows its job. But it is quite another matter if a baby strains and fusses to produce a hard stool. This is often seen in formula fed infants who need some extra carbohydrate (like sugar or molasses) added to their bottles for a time. This is discussed in detail in Chapter 6 on infant feeding.

Clothing Newborn Babies

Dressing your new baby provides an excellent opportunity to engage in conspicuous consumption and exhausting yourself in the attempt. The temptation to cover infants with fancy garments is particularly difficult for grandparents to resist, but the parents, being closer to the problem, may find it easier to keep a grip on reality. Keep in mind that every stitch of clothing you put on the poor child will be spat up on, if not worse, and will need to be removed, washed, and dried innumerable times. Simplicity has a great deal going for it. Standard hospital nursery garb is a useful measure of practicality: A shirt of the wrap-around type rather than a pullover, a diaper, and a cotton receiving blanket is a good combination. Add as many heavier blankets as the weather indicates. After the first few hours of life, hats are rarely needed unless the infant is exposed to excessive cold. For state occasions there may be some excuse for sleepers, dresses, sacks, socks, and others fanciful raiments, but not for everyday life.

The choice of **diapers,** disposable versus washable, vexes every conscientious parent. Consider the problem of dealing with the hundreds of millions of soiled, discarded, disposable diapers every year. But despite their expense and wastefulness, disposables are awfully convenient. Furthermore, the new types with built-in urine absorbing gels require fewer changes. Cotton diapers have an ecological cost as well; it takes a great deal of water and energy to keep them washed and dried. The out-of-pocket expense for cotton diapers laundered at home is the least, but of course, the time and effort is the greatest. Diaper services are no more costly than disposables, and their convenience is much appreciated, especially during the first, hectic months.

Skin Care

Why bathe a baby every day? We Americans worry too much about dirt. Most infants do very well with a bath every few days. Of course, there are exceptions. Some babies have naturally oily skins, and tend to look a bit greasy unless they are washed fairly often. This is strictly a cosmetic question, and how often you wash your baby will depend largely on how you think your baby should look. An occasional baby will get scruffy yellow scale on the face and redness in skin creases unless a daily bath is given. This condition is called seborrhea (see page 232), and it does tend to get worse if unattended. There is no need for expensive soaps or liquid cleansers; any mild soap is fine. "Baby" shampoos are buffered to avoid eye irritation, so it makes sense to use them to wash the infant's head and face. But there are a host of miscellaneous and useless products sold for infant skin care. Baby powder and baby oil seem to be going out of fashion, which is just as well. A number of creams and ointments are promoted for use around the baby's anus and in the diaper area, allegedly to prevent diaper rashes. They don't work. What does work is getting the bottom clean after every stool, either with a wash cloth and water or with a disposable diaper wipe, and changing diapers often enough to keep the diaper area reasonably dry. If a large, loose stool has found its way into every nook and cranny of your daughter's vulva, cleaning will require the gentle use of soap and water on a washcloth or some pieces of absorbent cotton.

One sacrosanct piece of nonsensical advice is to avoid a tub bath until the navel has healed. There is something about navel magic that breeds belief in ritual rules; why, for example, should the diaper be folded to avoid touching the remnant of umbilical cord, and why should rubbing alcohol be placed on or about the poor shriveled little thing? Navels have healed in every mammalian species for some years now without our well-meaning intervention. The advice that applies here is **Grossman's Second Law of Baby Care: *Resist the urge to medicalize normal processes.*** People, even little people, are tough. If human beings needed advanced degrees to be successful parents, the world would not be facing overpopulation.

Chapter 6

Feeding Your New Baby

Breast Feeding

It is unfortuante that there is any necessity for a chapter about breast feeding babies. It seems a bit like giving instruction on how to breath or how to walk. A skill that is so basic to the survival of the human species should be built-in. The need for this discussion is the result of two social trends. The first of these is the popularization of formula feeding, which resulted in several generations of mothers who could not teach their daughters what they themselves did not know. This is a perfect example of the hazards of medicalization: turning the most basic female function into an infrequently chosen and poorly understood alternative to a medically supervised, factory produced, highly advertised, and expensive commercial product. The second factor is the sexualization of the breast, which has become so complete that young women have to relearn and newly experience their bodies as nurturing as well as sexual. The American view appears to be that the breast is generally an object to be shared by consenting adults and hardly the proper place for babies.

Most of the pregnant women I meet at prenatal visits have already made up their minds about nursing. I am happy to say that the majority of them are looking forward to breast feeding their babies. Many are wondering whether they can combine nursing with formula feeding so that they can return to work, or so that the baby's father can share the feeding. It is important to be realistic about these plans. A demanding, full-time job away from home makes it very difficult for a mother to keep her milk supply going. Even if she can express her milk during the workday and bring it back to the baby, the physical stress may be excessive. The idea of sharing the job with the father tends to work in the latter part of the first year when the baby is close to sleeping through the night; in the early months, most mothers have so much milk production in the night that they will want to nurse just for their own comfort.

The other uncertainties I hear are "Can I really nurse the baby?" and "Do I really want to?" These questions may stem simply from lack of experience with other successfully nursing mothers. For the woman who was herself bottle fed, and whose peers have chosen to bottle feed, the lack of role models can be daunting. I think that women who are unsure about whether to nurse should proceed cautiously. There is no sense in being pushed into a decision which may not fit. Nursing undertaken because of family or medical pressure is likely to fail. The wisest course is to try to clarify your options. Your doctor or your local hospital can give you information about classes on breast feeding which may be offered by lactation specialists, nurses, or doctors. The innumerable books on breast feeding are useful, as is help from the nursing mothers' groups La Leche League and The Nursing Mothers' Council. Advocates of nursing, like advocates of whales, handguns, or anything else, sometimes tend to a bit of zealotry; take the advice you get with some caution.

The role of fathers in the decision to nurse and in the subsequent success of nursing is crucial. His wife's first pregnancy is likely to be a challenging time in a man's life. It signifies a major step toward fulfilling the biological destiny of both partners in the family, and for each of them it heralds the beginning of a new, completely adult role, that of parent. This is a prospect both exciting and daunting. For the father-to-be, parenthood signals the absolute end of carefree youth. The new life coming along imposes grownup responsibilities of a new and different order. I recall the bittersweet decision of one of my sons-in-law to give up the hazardous pastimes he loved as he contemplated fatherhood; no more hang gliding, no more motorcycle riding, no more bungee jumping. He had been willing to take chances with his own life, but he would not take chances with the life of the father of his baby. The father-to-be is also faced with giving up certain rights and privileges regarding the body of his wife. It hardly needs to be said that the breasts of women are important sexually as well as nutritionally. The man whose wife nurses her baby may well feel displaced by his son or daughter. Jealousy of this kind may be ignoble and embarrassing but it is real none the less. These feelings are worth discussing before the decision to nurse is made. Later, the continuing support of fathers remains central to nursing success.

Preparation for Nursing. Breasts which have always been protected from wind and weather are ill-suited to withstand the attack of a hungry newborn. Scrubbing the nipples during a shower or vigorously toweling them afterwards does not "toughen them up" (you are not trying to get calluses!) but can reduce sensitivity. Carefully limited sun exposure may also be useful. In the weeks just before delivery, expressing colostrum appears to facilitate the beginning of nursing. A good time to do this is during a warm shower. Press your thumb and forefinger together behind your nipple, and gently attempt to milk out a drop or so of the thick, creamy fluid. Most women are successful after a few days of brief attempts, and many develop a remarkably free flow by the time the baby is born, guaranteeing the happy child an easy meal. However, some mothers discover that this much nipple stimulation causes uterine contractions; if this occurs, stop.

Some women's nipples are quite flat or even slightly inverted. This may change during pregnancy, and the nipples may become protuberant enough for the baby to get a good nursing grip. If this isn't happening by the middle of pregnancy, it is well worth while to wear a doughnut shaped breast shield under your bra; this device will press gently around the nipple and areola, and encourage the nipple to come forward. Gentle nipple manipulation during a shower or during lovemaking may also increase nipple prominence.

Starting to Nurse. After the baby is born, early and frequent nursings help to bring the milk in quickly and may minimize breast engorgement. Rooming-in during the hospital stay will make it easier to nurse on demand. The length of time on the breast will depend in part on your skin color. If you are a white-skinned strawberry blond, you will probably have sensitive nipples; nurse only a few minutes at each breast at first, and take your time about increasing the length of each nursing. If you have dark skin, you can expect less nipple sensitivity and you can nurse for longer periods. Eventually, most American babies nurse 5 to 20 minutes at each breast from 6 to 12 times a day; it may take days or weeks for an infant to have the stamina to take both breasts at a feeding. The whole question of how long a baby nurses at a time becomes difficult to answer because many babies nurse and rest and nurse and rest. Do you count the rest periods or not? It is important not to get too hung up on the statistics. Our expectations of infant feeding have been skewed by the decades of experience with artificially fed babies. The bottle fed infant works much less hard to get a meal, and the big feeding of slowly digested formula stays longer in the stomach. For these infants, 5 to 7 feeds a day are often sufficient and a schedule of a bottle every 3 to 5 hours develops. In contrast, the small meals of rapidly digested, low-protein breast milk are required much more often. In primitive societies where the baby is nearly always next to the mother, feedings of 20 or more times a day are standard.

Giving bottles of anything to normal, full-term newborns is deleterious to nursing. Contrary to hospital nursery mythology, one cannot prevent physiologic jaundice with water or glucose supplements. The only usual indication for extra water or sugar water during the first few days is nipple soreness so severe that nursing time must be limited. Giving bottles of formula to breast fed babies in the first week or so is simply a bad idea. Formula feeds will decrease the baby's appetite and delay the next nursing, and teach the infant that an easily available alternative is as near as the refrigerator.

It is worth remembering that some mothers make vast quantities of milk within a week or two after starting to nurse, but other mothers may take several weeks to reach optimal milk production. It can be difficult to avoid the use of supplemental bottles of formula during this period. Frequent nursings and occasional bottles of sugar water may bridge the gaps.

Nursing Comfort. An important component in nursing comfort is the mother's posture and support. If you are physically tense during nursing, and if you support the baby's weight without assistance, nursing will be a tiring process. But if you can find a comfortable chair whose arms, suitably cushioned, can do the job of propping the baby in place, the nursing period can be one of physical rest and relaxation. Be aware of the posture you assume; your arms and shoulders should look and feel relaxed. Nursing should be a one-armed procedure, leaving your other hand free to hold a book or the telephone or a glass of beer. The reference to the beer is deliberate; many mothers report intense thirst accompanying the act of nursing, especially during the first weeks. (More about beer later.) Mothers sometimes report a shiver or a chill when their

EVERYDAY PEDIATRICS FOR PARENTS

milk lets down; this is harmless and disappears with time. More commonly, mothers will feel a surge of joy during letdown, especially during the early days of nursing. For some women, nursing stimulates powerful sexual feelings as well. Mother nature seems to have made multiple provisions for the encouragement of breast feeding. The last point about nursing technique is to keep clothes and bedding out of the way in the first days of nursing. Your baby needs to feel and smell your breast, and this can be pretty hard to manage if brassiere, sheets, blankets, and nightgowns keep falling over its nose.

Nipple and Breast Discomfort. This brings us to the uncomfortable subject of sore nipples. During the first days of nursing, most mothers experience some nipple pain, especially at the start of a feeding as the baby gets the nipple firmly in its mouth. Holding the infant so that the entire nipple can be in the baby's mouth is important; the baby who chews on the end of the nipple is an inefficient as well as painful nurser. This can be avoided by holding the baby a little above your breast, with your arm well supported by pillows, rather than leaning over the baby with the baby looking up at the breast. The baby-above posture allows the baby's head and mouth to fall into the breast. Some babies automatically open wide and take the entire nipple and much of the surrounding areola deeply into their mouths. This can be helped along by stroking the baby's cheek near the mouth with your finger or your nipple, and putting the nipple and areola into the baby's mouth when it is most generously open. It is practically never necessary to hold your breast away from the baby's nose; they manage to breath nicely even when surrounded by the most pillowy bosoms.

Normal nipple sensitivity can be helped by heat; a hair blow-dryer, a bright lamp or a little sunlight can all be soothing. Exposure to air after nursings is also helpful. Doughnut shaped breast shields keep clothing away from the nipples, but nipple shields (the kind that fit directly over the nipples) should be avoided if at all possible; once used, they are very hard to get rid of because the baby learns to depend on them. The new, very thin models are least objectionable since they allow more normal nursing. A wonderful variety of creams and liquids have been proposed for local application to sore nipples; most of them do little good and some (like alcohol and tincture of benzoin) are actively harmful. Plain hydrous lanolin is moderately helpful for some women. Babies do not object to lanolin despite the fact that it smells a bit like a clean, wet sheep. The best advice is to minimize washing, especially with soap, and forget about nipple creams unless the nipples become excessively red, sore, and cracked. In those instances, use a combination of nonprescription 1% hydrocortisone cream plus an antiyeast cream such as clotrimazole or miconazole. Clotrimazole and miconazole are marketed for use against athlete's foot and vaginal yeast infections, and they work equally well against yeast infections which often contribute to nipple soreness. Apply a little of each cream to your nipples and the surrounding reddened area after each nursing. Don't wash off before your next nursing; your baby won't care and the minute residue is harmless. Very rarely, there will be a component of bacterial infection indicated by tiny pimples or crusting; your doctor will probably treat this with an antibacterial ointment or an oral antibiotic.

Plugged Milk Ducts and Breast Infections. Nursing mothers commonly experience temporary plugging of a milk duct. When this occurs a firm, tender lump is noticeable somewhere in the breast. Usually this is a few inches away from the nipple, and often the overlying skin will be pink or even red. This condition can look a lot like a true breast infection, but plugged ducts are rarely accompanied by fever or chills, and the mother does not feel sick. If you think you may have an infection, see your doctor. Breast infections generally clear up promptly with the help of an oral antibiotic taken by mouth. Nursing during the worst stage of the infection may be somewhat painful, but it may actually help healing to proceed, and it does not hurt the baby. The milk will not be infected and the amount of antibiotic excreted into the milk is no problem, so long as it is one which is safe for babies. The only antibiotics we try to keep away from babies are the tetracyclines and the quinolones (like ciprofloxacin) and, in the case of babies in the first weeks of life, the sulfonamides (like Gantrisin, Septra, Bactrim, etcetera). Ask your doctor if the drug prescribed for your infection is in any of these categories; sometimes we forget that the medicine we give the mother also goes to the nursing baby.

If the swelling is caused by a plugged milk duct, all you need to do is apply warm compresses or use an electric heating pad for 15 or 20 minutes, 3 or 4 times a day, and gently massage the swollen, sore area while you are nursing, pressing in toward the nipple. You may need to take a mild pain reliever like aspirin or acetaminophen as well. Plugged ducts tend to resolve within a very few days.

Breast Milk: Is There Enough and Is It Any Good?

Mothers are often concerned about the quality and quantity of their milk. Quality is a nonissue; breast milk is not a uniform product but it is always adequate in quality for a term infant. Quantity is another matter. In our measurement obsessed society, there is probably a fortune to be made for the inventor of a device which would show the milk capacity of a mother's breast. Certainly the vast majority of women can and do produce enough milk, especially during the first few months, but there is a small group of women who are not good nursers. Some of them have impossible nipples, so flat or inverted that the baby cannot nurse effectively; some just don't make much milk. This should not be a surprise; even mammals bred for milk production vary in ability to make milk.

It is also true that milk production can vary from time to time. You should suspect a decrease in milk production if you have been nursing successfully for weeks or months and then notice that your baby is becoming fretful at the breast, especially in the afternoon or evening when your supply is most likely to be low. Other hints of inadequate milk include decreases in the baby's stools and urine, and an increase in nursing frequency, particularly at night. You may sense that your breasts feel less full and heavy. The least useful tactic for estimating milk production is weighing the baby before and after a nursing. For one thing, baby scales are not very accurate. For another, the mere act of measurement can stimulate enough anxiety to cut off milk flow quite dramatically.

The usual factors leading to a decrease in breast milk are maternal exhaustion, inadequate maternal diet, and infrequent nursing. Resuming the use of birth control pills will often decrease milk production, especially if started in the very first months. This is less of a problem with the low-dose mini-pills. A common scenario is the decrease in milk during the second or third month when most mothers are feeling energetic, are recovered from the work of pregnancy and childbirth, and have dived back into full-time activity. It is easy to find yourself overcommitted and under-rested just when you thought you had earned your SUPERMOM! tee-shirt. Sometimes stressful circumstances can inhibit milk production, such as too many overly critical visitors or other psychological stresses. Depending on the particular causes, some or all of the following ideas may be useful:

1. Increase maternal rest time; fit in an afternoon nap if possible.
2. Hire or beg some help; get someone to do the shopping, cooking, and cleaning for awhile. This may be a relative, a husband, a friend, or a local high school student.
3. Increase the frequency of nursings; even brief nursings help. The more feedings per day, the greater the volume.

4. Eat! Mothers need three meals a day. Fluids, as such, do not need to be stressed; one's natural thirst will ensure fluid intake. Calcium intake is important in the long run for maternal health but does not seem to matter for milk production. Mothers are often under considerable pressure to lose weight in the early post-natal period; a calorie-restricted diet will predictably diminish breast milk.

5. Brewers' yeast is a time honored folk remedy *that works*. Take 1 tablet (or 1 teaspoon of powder mixed into juice) 3 times a day with meals at first and slowly increase to 3 tablets, 3 times a day, if tolerated. Too much yeast causes cramps and gas in some women.

6. For generations, beer has been recommended to increase milk production. Both regular beer and nonalcoholic beer stimulate the pituitary gland at the base of the brain to excrete extra prolactin, a hormone which is crucial in milk production. So, it makes sense to use beer for a boost if the volume of milk is insufficient. It is probably best to take the beer during or after a nursing; if you drink it just before, some of the alcohol will get into the milk and your baby may be slightly sedated and nurse less vigorously. Of course, there may be times when you will not at all mind having a slightly sedated baby. You can also get most of the prolactin-stimulating effect from nonalcoholic beer; 6 to 12 ounces, once or twice a day is an effective amount.

7. Various medications have been proposed as milk stimulants, but the mothers in my practice have not found them useful.

8. Oxytocin is a pituitary hormone which plays a major role in the milk letdown reflex. It is available in a nasal spray which can be used if a mother has difficulty in letting her milk down. This is a very rare problem.

9. Give your baby as little supplemental formula as you can.

10. Get rid of helpful relatives dispensing unsought advice, if possible.

It takes 2 to 3 days to begin to obtain a satisfactory return of adequate breast milk. It is seldom necessary to continue all these measures indefinitely, but recurrent episodes of decreased milk are not unusual.

There are rare cases of infants who somehow fail to indicate to their mothers that they are grossly undernourished. Most often the mother is perfectly able to respond to the baby's needs, but the baby is too quiet and apathetic to get her attention. Monthly well child visits with accurate weighings will quickly reveal this situation.

At the other end of the spectrum is the mother who makes too much milk. This usually evens out within a few weeks as the breasts' supply diminishes to equal demand. Occasionally, a baby will be so overfed that it will spit up impressive amounts after feedings. I once hospitalized an infant for suspected intestinal obstruction whose only problem was overeating. The solution is to nurse at only one breast per feeding, at least until milk production decreases.

Supplemental Bottles. Nearly every breast fed baby is going to get a certain number of bottles. Using an occasional supplemental bottle can give Dad a chance to feed the baby, or Mom a chance to get out of the house on her own. Avoid supplemental bottles if at all possible until nursing is thoroughly established, a matter of a few weeks in most cases. There is no point in confusing your baby. Sometimes these supplements will be bottles of breast milk which have been collected by breast pumping or manual milk expression. Breast milk can be put into nursing bottles and frozen; it remains perfectly safe and nourishing despite weeks or months in the freezer. Whatever amount of milk you have been able to collect at one time can be put in a bottle; later, you can add more freshly expressed milk to the same bottle until you have enough for a feeding. Some writers on this subject advise against this practice, but I cannot see why.

Supplemental bottles of formula are useful if you want to get out to a movie and don't happen to have some extra breast milk in the freezer. This means using a humanized cows' milk formula (Enfamil, Similac, Gerber's, etc.). Special formulas like soy or predigested cow's milk (Nutramigen) are occasionally prescribed. During the first year, it is a good idea to avoid bottles of fresh cows' milk for infant feeding; it is much harder to digest and much more likely to cause allergic reactions than the altered milk formulas specially developed for infants. The other products to avoid are the so-called "soy milks" sold in markets in the dairy case. These are not designed for babies, are much lower in calcium and other nutrients, and far less digestible.

The easiest way to give a supplemental bottle is to use an infant formula in powdered form. These are stable at room temperature, last for months after being opened without the risk of spoiling, and generally cost a bit less than liquid formulas. If you use supplemental bottles rarely, an open can of liquid formula may mold before you would ever use it up. For details on preparing unsterile formula by the simple, single-bottle method, see the following section on formula feeding.

Nursing Twins. The mother of twins has innumerable special issues among which nursing techniques are rather minor. Some mothers of twins have enough milk for both babies without the need to supplement at all. Most mothers will choose to nurse one baby at a time, either one breast per infant plus a supplementary bottle if needed, or giving one baby both breasts and the other baby a bottle at one feeding and alternating at the next. Some mothers are adept at nursing both babies at once but this takes some agility and practice. There is a cleverly designed U-shaped, firm pillow that wraps around the mom's middle and allows each twin to be comfortably supported during joint nursings. If you have twins, the most useful thing you can do is to get in touch with other families with twins; the shared practical experience is invaluable, and maybe someone will lend you a twin stroller. Your doctor or your local hospital may be able to put you in touch with a Parents of Twins group in your area, or get in touch with the National Organization of Mothers of Twins Clubs, Inc., PO Box 23188, Albuquerque, NM, 87192-1188; (800) 243-2276.

Nursing Premies. Nursing premature babies weighing about 4 pounds or more generally pose little difficulty. Smaller babies will need to be started on tube feedings or bottle feedings using special "premie" nipples, with a gradual transition to the breast as the babies gain size and vigor. For very small, low birth-weight premies, there is some evidence that breast milk supplemented by the more concentrated premature formulas is the best feeding method. Of course, in dealing with these complicated situations, the specific advice of experienced nursery nurses and pediatricians will be invaluable.

Expressing Breast Milk. The mother who needs to express her milk may find manual expression tedious and difficult, at least until she has perfected the technique. A number of breast pumps are available, among which electric pumps are clearly most efficient. The little battery operated pumps are not much good. Some models use alternating pressure and suction; this seems the quickest, and most comfortable. The manual devices use suction only and tend to be quite slow. The local chapter of La Leche League or The Nursing Mothers' Council will be a good resource regarding breast pump rentals or purchase.

Maternal Medications Excreted into Breast Milk. A frequent question is the safety of maternal medication. I must say that I don't worry much about this. If the medicines excreted into the breast milk, usually in small amounts, are safe to give an infant, it does not seem worthwhile to interrupt nursing. Some drugs will have noticeable but unimportant effects; maternal cathartics may loosen a baby's stool, codeine may be mildly sedating. Obviously, mothers should not nurse when they are taking medications that come with a known significant risk to the baby; this would include antimetabolites used in cancer chemotherapy and for certain other serious illnesses, radioactive substances, the antibiotics previously noted in the discussion of breast infection, and some psychoactive agents, especially those used for serious mental illnesses. I think one has to balance risks. A depressed mother taking an antidepressant might be so distressed at having to stop nursing that a wiser choice for her might be to continue both the nursing and the medication. As I've already mentioned, oral contraceptives pose a special problem: If taken during the first few months after childbirth, they often greatly inhibit milk production. Use as low a dose as possible and wait as long as you can before starting them.

Stools of Breast Fed Babies. The breast fed baby produces an extensive palette of colors in her bowel movements. Black meconium in the newborn period is followed by greenish transitional stools which are followed by bright golden-yellow stools after the mother's milk comes in. The stools are usually soft and wet, sometimes just a yellow stain with little substance, sometimes a copious mass like eggs scrambled with cottage cheese. There is a little clear mucus in some babies' stools; large amounts of mucus indicate either some intestinal irritation or a bad cold with lots of swallowed nasal mucus. In the first weeks, most breast fed babies have a stool with or after every feeding. This is the result of an active gastrocolic reflex: The stomach fills and the large intestine empties. Later, this reflex becomes less active and the baby has fewer and fewer stools; one or two a day is common but some babies go days between each bowel movement. This is not really constipation because the stools remain quite soft and comfortable. Once in a while, a baby will become fussy for a few hours before finally having one of these delayed stools. You can stimulate an increase in stool frequency by giving the infant a little extra carbohydrate. White or brown sugar (about ½ to 1 teaspoon) or molasses (¼ to ½ teaspoon) in 1or 2 ounces of water once or twice a day usually suffices.

Breast Milk Jaundice. See pages 30-31 for discussion of this topic.

Menstruation and Fertility. Mothers whose babies are exclusively or largely breast fed will not usually experience the resumption of menses for several months. When their first periods begin, some mothers report that the baby seems unhappy with nursing for day or two; this is not related to any apparent change in milk volume but presumably there is a change in smell or taste. The phenomenon is transient and usually does not recur with the succeeding menstrual periods. It needs to be noted that fertility is diminished but not absent when mothers are nursing. Even during the first few months before periods have resumed, there is a small but real chance of becoming pregnant.

Distractible Nursers. A common problem in the middle of the first year of nursing is distractibility. An active and responsive baby may become so interested in his environment that he pulls away from the nipple every time the dog walks into the room or the phone rings. Even worse, some babies will turn away from the breast without letting go of the nipple. For these infants, nursing may need to be accomplished in a quiet and darkened room. Distractible babies often decide at an early age that nursing is too confining, and may wean themselves to the bottle or the cup if given the option.

How Long Should You Nurse?

This is a wonderfully complex issue. I remember our first child's pediatrician telling us that babies should be weaned from breast or bottle early in the second year "to avoid oral dependency." We were impressed at the time but soon recovered our skepticism when we realized that the data to support this rule were probably nonexistent. Weaning age is basically socially determined. A New Guinea tribe with a prohibition against sexual intercourse while the mother is nursing tends to wean it's young by the middle of the first year, at the latest. At the other extreme, traditional Sioux Indians weaned their children at age 5 or 6 years. Every group has its own rules.

The baby also has something to say about this. Some infants really love to nurse and will give up the breast only with coercion. Others, especially very active babies, lose interest in nursing and wean themselves sometime in the first year. Fathers play a role as well. The nursing mother and her baby form a close bond that may exclude the father. He may feel sexual jealousy as well. The net effect is that some men put considerable pressure on their wives to give up nursing.

I think the mother's feelings should be the defining factor. Every mother's experience of nursing is different. Some women love the whole process; they enjoy the physical sensations of the baby at the breast, and they feel fulfilled as women in a powerful way. Giving up nursing for such a women is a real loss. One mother of four children sat in my office and wept as she related that her 7-month old son had abruptly weaned himself. "He is the last baby I'll ever nurse; now that I've gotten really good at being the mother of an infant, I'll never do it again and it seems such a waste." For other mothers, nursing is fine for feeding babies but means much less to them; it's easy to stop. And for a few women nursing is an uncomfortable chore which they undertake dutifully but without joy; they tend to wean quite early. Nursing can also be perceived as a considerable physical strain; only after weaning do some mothers regain their sense of prepregnancy energy.

How to Wean

Weaning is a straightforward process. Babies less than 1-year old should be weaned to an infant formula to minimize the risk of an allergic reaction; over 1 year, it is fine to wean to fresh cows' milk, either whole milk or part-skimmed 2%. Neither part-skimmed 1% nor completely skimmed milk have enough calories to meet the needs of fast growing infants. (There is more discussion on this subject later in this chapter on weaning bottle fed infants and in Chapter 20— Food and Nutrition.) Most American babies are weaned to the bottle or a combination of bottle plus cup, however, if the baby is older than 12 to 18 months, it may be possible to wean directly to the cup, skipping the bottle stage altogether. I don't see any advantage to this. If the baby still enjoys the act of sucking, why push him into precocious maturity? (More comments about this issue can be found later in this chapter in the section on weaning from the bottle.) A gradual replacement of breast milk with cows' milk is usually easiest for everyone; a rapid change is likely to cause constipation, sore breasts, and hard feelings. Substitute a bottle or cup for the least important nursing and every week or so drop another nursing. Often the nursing that feels most important to mother or baby will be retained for additional weeks.

If the weaning process goes on for months, someone involved may need assistance in letting go. If it is the child, you may need help in feeling free to give your baby a boost over a developmental hurdle. This is a perfect example of a situation that can recur many times in a child's life; some tasks look very difficult, and it is hard for parents to muster the calm assurance that the child can master change and growth. The rule that applies here is **Grossman's Law of Coping:** ***If other children have managed this challenge, your child can manage it as well.*** On the other hand, if it is the mother that can't let go, it may be worthwhile for her to explore the reasons. The simple act of expressing her feelings in words with a close friend, her husband, or her doctor may be enough to clarify her choices and let her make the change.

Formula Feeding

One may as well give credit where credit is due. The formula feeding of human infants is a massive nutritional experiment which appears to be working out reasonably well. Considering that neither Holsteins nor soybeans were actually evolved to provide the nourishment for our babies, their suitably altered products turn out to do a pretty good job; not perfect, but not all that bad, either.

This was not always the case. The first attempts to use cows' milk as a baby food were hampered by a host of problems including difficulty in digesting unaltered milk protein, deficiencies of iron and vitamin C, and a tendency to develop severe allergic reactions to the stuff. In addition were the problems of insuring freshness and freedom from a variety of nasty bacterial contaminants. But contemporary cows' milk based infant formulas have overcome most of these disadvantages. The protein is rendered much more digestible and less allergenic by heating and other changes, iron and vitamin C have been added, and the canned preparations are reliably sterile. The evaporated milk formulas of an earlier era tended to make babies smell rancid and become constipated. The "humanized" formulas used today avoid most of these problems, although constipation can still be troublesome. The supermarket shelves carry a large selection of practically identical cows' milk products which differ in trivial ways. They may have a variety of carbohydrate sources and a differing mix of protein types, but babies rarely notice which brand you give them. Enfamil, Similac, Gerber's, and Carnation are virtually interchangeable. Some of these come in low iron formulations which don't make much sense; babies need iron. The argument has been made that the regular iron formulas can cause digestive upsets, but careful studies have never demonstrated such a connection. The choices of powdered, concentrated liquid, or ready-to-use liquid differ in cost; the powders are often somewhat cheaper, the ready-to-use always more expensive. Powdered formula is a bit messier to mix, but, conveniently, does not require refrigeration.

An alternative to cows' milk based formula is soybean based formula. The soybean is an excellent protein source, but turning it into a digestible and nourishing product for babies has been difficult. The first such preparations caused endless digestive upsets as human infants struggled to cope with soy proteins. The modern soy formulas containing soy protein isolates are a different story. They are reasonably close facsimiles of human milk, thanks to the work of food chemists, and babies tolerate them most of the time. There remains a tendency for the stools of soy fed babies to look greenish-brown and smell peculiar. The reasons to choose a soy formula are allergy to cows' milk formula or a family history of severe allergy of any kind. Unfortunately, a fair number of babies with cows' milk allergy develop allergy to soy as well, so the switch is not always successful. There is very little evidence that using soy formula reduces the risk of the development of allergy in early childhood.

Other formulas on the market are tailored to special needs. The only type of much interest is a predigested cows' milk based formula, of which Nutramigen brand is the best known. This preparation uses proteins which have been broken down into their component parts; these fragments retain all their nutritional value but are nearly free of the risk of inducing allergy. The only disadvantages are the high cost and the production of unpleasantly smelly stools.

One possible defect common to all these infant formulas is the difference in fat content between them and mothers' milk. As I mentioned in Chapter 4 on deciding whether to nurse, mothers' milk has higher cholesterol and a different set of fatty acids than its competitors. There is increasing evidence that some of these differences may effect the development of infant nervous systems. Some studies have suggested that breast fed babies actually become smarter people. However, this story is by no means finished; stay tuned.

Making baby's formula used to be a time consuming, daily ritual of bottle and nipple washing, formula mixing and sterilization. This was a necessity when the water supply was of dubious safety and fresh milk was used. Today, however, American municipal water supplies are generally free from significant germs and the canned formulas are sterile, so it is usually possible to skip sterilization. However, in areas where tap water is thought to be subject to microbial contamination, it is prudent to use boiled water. When in doubt, call your local water company or department of public health.

How to Make Unsterile, Single Bottle Formula. Your baby's formula need not be sterilized if the milk is safe, the water is obtained from a reliable water supply (or boiled water), and the preparation is used promptly after it is mixed. It *must* be sterilized if unboiled water from unsafe sources is used.

The rules for unsterile formula are:

1. Keep clean, dry bottles in a cupboard, ready to use ; nipples and caps can be kept on the bottles or in a covered jar. After a can of liquid formula is opened, cover it with plastic or foil and keep it refrigerated. Dry, powdered formula does not require refrigeration.

2. Make a bottle of formula just before using it. If you use powdered formula concentrate, put the desired amount of warm water in a clean bottle, add 1 measure (which equals 1 tablespoon) of the formula powder for every 2

ounces of water, shake it thoroughly and give it to the baby. (Adding the formula powder after putting in the water minimizes the formation of lumps which may plug the nipple.) If you use a liquid formula concentrate, mix it with an equal amount of hot water in the bottle.

3. If an unrefrigerated bottle is not used within two hours after mixing, throw it away or give it to the cat. Germs (bacteria) will begin to grow in warm or room temperature formula after about two hours; this will not trouble the cat.

4. If you must take a bottle with you away from home, put powdered formula in the dry bottle, and add the water later when the baby is ready to be fed. Ready-to-use formula in bottles or cans costs more but is even more convenient.

5. Some household water supplies can be contaminated with lead if you have soft water and old pipes. Your local water department or health department can tell you if there is a risk in your household. If lead levels are high, run the water for a minute or so before using it in formula. Cold water is less likely to leach out lead from the water system than hot, so you may wish to avoid water from the hot water tap. You can do this by heating cold water in a pan on the stove before mixing it with the formula powder or concentrate, or heating the prepared formula bottle in a pan of water on the stove.

6. *Do not heat bottles in a microwave!* This method is unsafe because of uneven heating.

7. Teaching your baby to accept room temperature formula is an alternative. Oddly enough, babies don't really seem to care whether their bottles are nicely warmed, room temperature, or even cold.

8. If you give your baby cold formula, you can prepare the whole day's supply at once and refrigerate the bottles until needed. If you are using warm formula, it is fastest to make it up one bottle at a time with warm water, rather than having to wait endlessly for the cold bottle to heat while the baby is screaming at you in the middle of the night.

Bottles and Nipples. Selling nursing bottles and nipples is a lot like selling gasoline: The differences between brands are largely a matter of advertising claims with little relation to reality. Despite what the ads in the baby magazines say, I have no reason to believe that any particular bottle or nipple will decrease the risk of infant colic or air swallowing and lead to a general increase in family happiness. The bottles with disposable plastic bag liners cost more but save the effort of bottle washing. Since bottle sterilization is not usually needed, this is a rather trivial difference. Plastic bottles are lighter and therefore easier for babies to hold when they are old enough to want to. Nipples are nipples; babies don't care. Claims for orthodontic miracles resulting from the use of particular brands of nipples should be assessed with the skepticism reserved for judging miracles of all kinds.

Stools of Formula Fed Babies. Most bottle babies consume a fair amount from the first days of life, so their stools make the transition from black meconium to green to yellow within a few days. The consistency of their stools varies from mustardy to pasty; if a young infant passes dry, formed stools it is likely that constipation is near at hand. As with breast fed babies, stool frequency tends to diminish with time. Within weeks, many babies have only 1 or 2 stools a day. Unlike breast fed babies, who very rarely produce hard or dry stools, some bottle babies get severely constipated if their stool frequency falls below once a day. Stool that is retained in the baby's large intestine for too long is subject to a process of water recycling; the large intestine dries it out and the resulting hard stool is painful for the infant to pass. Adding some extra carbohydrate to the formula is nearly always sufficient to reverse this process. You can use white or brown sugar (½ to 1 teaspoon per bottle), or molasses (¼ to ½ teaspoon per bottle). The darker grades of molasses, especially "blackstrap", seem to be a bit more potent. Malt soup extract (isn't that a great name?) works almost as well, but it requires a much larger dose and costs about ten times as much; no advantages except for the manufacturer. When the stools have become more frequent, softer, and painless, gradually decrease the amount of added carbohydrate. It is often possible to omit it completely after a week or two, but the problem may recur.

Formula Versus Fresh Cows' Milk. When should your baby be introduced to fresh milk? I have mentioned several deficiencies of fresh milk in the feeding of young infants. The problem of digesting fresh cows' milk protein is largely overcome late in the first year as stomach function improves. The risk of inducing allergy by early exposure to fresh cows' milk has also diminished by this age, in part because the baby's intestine does a more thorough job of digesting proteins overall. The deficiency of iron in fresh milk means that some other source must be present in the baby's diet if formula is to be abandoned. Meats, eggs, and iron-fortified baby cereal are all excellent sources, and are all usually available to babies by the end of the first year. Vitamin C is easily found in the mixed diet of most 1-year olds. It can come from oranges, orange juice, summer fruits generally, and many green vegetables, as well as the ubiquitous and overused infant juice preparations to which it is added.

All of these factors imply that age 1 is a reasonable time to begin substituting fresh milk for formula. The transition should be made gradually for two reasons; an abrupt change will induce horrendous constipation in many babies, and the change in taste may be upsetting. Start by substituting 1 ounce of fresh milk for 1 ounce of the formula. After a week or so, substitute an additional ounce, and increase the proportion of fresh milk as the child tolerates the change. It can take a month or two.

There is some disagreement concerning the use of whole versus lowfat milk for babies of this age. As part of the trend towards a moderate restriction of saturated fats in our diets, many families use nonfat or lowfat milk as the family milk. This is nutritionally reasonable for older children, but it can pose problems for babies. Nonfat milk is really not appropriate until the child is taking a varied diet with other sources of nutritionally necessary fats. Furthermore, milk makes up such as substantial part of the toddler's diet that the use of nonfat milk with only 11 calories per ounce can really deprive the child of enough calories for growth. Using 1% lowfat milk with 13 calories per ounce is not much better. On the other hand, there is little difference between the nutritional contribution of 2% lowfat milk (also called 2-10 milk because it has 10% protein) and regular whole milk. The 2% milk has about 18 calories per ounce, whole milk about 20. If you want to use 2% because that is what the rest of the family drinks, that's fine. If you want to use whole milk until age 2 or 3, that's okay too.

Weaning to the Cup. The question of when to wean from bottle to cup is a lot like the question of weaning from the breast. Both are very largely matters of social custom rather than medical science, and therefore opinions about weaning are held with a nearly insane degree of vigor. Why do we care so much about the proper vehicle for the ingestion of milk? In part because we are a society wedded to the notions of independence and progress. In so many ways we Americans act as if we wanted our babies to race immediately from the cradle to career. We dress them in pretend adult clothes (I will never forget some diaper covers made out of denim and decorated like Levi's blue jeans), we push them into competitive sports, we want them to learn academic material in nursery school, and we take them off the bottle and the breast as early as we can manage it. Patience with the normal processes of growth and development, with a leavening of gentleness, might not be wholly out of place.

Of course, your baby will have his or her own point of view. In the latter part of the first year some babies decide that bottles are beneath them and rapidly learn to use the cup. Other children contentedly stay with bottles until kindergarten age, if given the chance. It seems to me that holding on to the bottle is a lot like clinging to a favorite blanket, a pacifier, or a beloved stuffed animal. All are aids in the slow transition from the dependent status of infancy to the larger world of adult life. If the child is moving along at a reasonable rate, is there really any urgency in pressing for more rapid change?

The technique of weaning can be made overly complex. Cups with spouts or built-in straws can be offered but are not particularly helpful. The skill one really wants to teach is the use of a plain, ordinary cup. The simplest method is to offer a small, unbreakable cup to the baby who is old enough to sit up unassisted while he is in his bath. Encourage experimentation with drinking water at the beginning of the bath when the water is not soapy. Spills will not matter and the baby can begin to learn to refill the cup. After a few weeks of playful practice, try it away from the bath. Stay with water until the skill is fairly well established; spilled juice or milk is much messier. The switch will be gradual; most babies move to complete use of the cup during the second or third year, although bedtime bottles may be much appreciated for longer.

If bedtime or midnight bottles are part of your child's routine, there is a real potential for tooth decay. If the bottles stay in the crib and the child takes a nip repeatedly throughout the night, the recurrent flow of milk, with its considerable sugar content, stimulates rapid decay, especially of the front teeth. (The same process can occur in breast fed babies who sleep with their mothers and nurse intermittently during the night.) The solution is straightforward: Abandon midnight bottles as soon as possible, and take the bedtime bottle out of the crib as soon as your baby is asleep.

Vitamins. Giving vitamin supplements to babies has been a sign of modern mothering ever since bottle feeding became popular. For our first few million years, human infants were always breast fed and obtained their vitamins in breast milk, with some additional vitamin D being derived from sunlight. With the popularization of formula feedings based on cows' milk, scurvy (vitamin C deficiency) and rickets (vitamin D deficiency) became real risks. Orange juice initially became the popular supplemental source of vitamin C, but has been superseded by pure vitamin C (ascorbic acid) which is now added to all prepared infant formulas. Neither orange juice nor vitamin C supplements are required by babies who take prepared infant formulas or who are breast fed.

Babies fed formulas based on evaporated milk and water do need supplemental vitamin C, 30 mg daily. Rickets is a disorder of bone growth which is very rare in breast fed babies. There is some vitamin D in breast milk unless the mother herself is profoundly deficient in the vitamin, which can occur if she has little or no exposure to sunlight. Even modest amounts of sun exposure provide adequate vitamin D, but a mother who protects her skin completely from the sun can manage to deplete her own levels and thereby produce D deficient milk. Fresh cows' milk is deficient in vitamin D, but cod liver oil, which is rich in D, was found to prevent rickets even before the vitamin itself had been discovered. Later, ultraviolet irradiation of milk was used to increase vitamin D content. Today all prepared infant formulas are fortified with adequate D. Supplemental doses are required only for some premature infants. Excessive doses of this vitamin should be avoided because it can inhibit growth and cause a variety of other symptoms, some of them quite unpleasant. Should breast feeding mothers who have adequate exposure to the sun give their babies extra vitamin D? If the babies themselves also have some sun exposure, the risk of rickets is infinitessimal. However, the current fad of slathering sunscreen lotions on our babies and ourselves to provide protection at all costs from even minimal sun exposure will probably produce a crop of vitamin D deficient kids. If you refuse to let the rays of our beneficent nearest star touch your skin or that of your infant, some other vitamin D source (400 units daily) is not a bad idea. A better idea is to let everyone, babies included, enjoy a modest amount of unprotected sun exposure. That is part of the Great Vitamin Maker's design, and She presumably understood what She was doing.

If you read the nutritional information on food packages you may have noted that fresh cows' milk comes fortified with extra vitamin A, and you may also have noted that vitamin A is commonly added to infant vitamin drops. Cows' milk already has a generous amount of this vitamin in it as it comes from the cow; it is a fat soluble substance that is present in the butterfat. There is plenty of A in human milk as well. So, why is extra A added? Because the former source of vitamin D in the feeding of American infants and children was cod liver oil, and cod liver oil contains both D and A. Then milk irradiation became the preferred method of obtaining D, and cod liver oil was abandoned. Unfortunately, the habit of supplementing A continued even though there was never any need for it. Similarly with the A in vitamin drops, it is an irrational practice. Skim milk is now widely used in the preparation of infant formulas, and since it is free of vitamin A, supplementation of these formulas with A is always done by the manufacturer. Fresh skim and part-skim cows' milk is supplemented to restore the vitamin A levels present in whole cows' milk; this is a sensible practice.

For more details on other vitamins, see Chapter 20—Food and Nutrition.

Minerals. The growing baby requires a substantial amount of **iron** to make new blood, muscle, and various enzymes. Breast milk includes a protein, lactoferrin, which increases the ability of the infant's intestine to absorb iron, so the relatively small amounts of iron in breast milk are adequate, at least for the first half year or so. Cows' milk has little iron and no lactoferrin, so iron supplementation is necessary. This is provided in prepared infant formulas. If your baby is fed an evaporated milk formula, additional iron is needed, either as iron drops (6 to 10 mg daily), or later in the first year in iron fortified infant cereal, meat, or egg yolk.

Fluoride is an important component of the mineral structure in tooth enamel and, in the proper amount, increases the resistance of teeth to decay. The tooth enamel begins to form during the fourth month of pregnancy. If the mother drinks fluoridated water or takes a fluoride supplement during pregnancy, her babies are born with some decay protection already built in. Thereafter, until the teeth have finished calcifying in the midteens, the child should drink fluoridated water or take a fluoride supplement. Unlike fluoride toothpaste, which adds fluoride mostly to the surface of the tooth, ingested fluoride is built right into the substance of the tooth from the inside. Should breast feeding mothers give additional fluoride if they drink fluoridated water? Most studies have shown that little fluoride is likely to be present in breast milk, and it was previously advised that a supplement was desirable until the baby is taking a substantial volume of fluoridated water. This never made a lot of sense because population studies of children raised in areas with naturally fluoridated water showed excellent decay prevention without any early supplimenation. I don't believe that giving extra fluoride in this situation is necessary. Formula fed infants in fluoridated areas get plenty of fluoride if their bottles are made with tap water, but the ready-to-use formulas do not contain fluoride. In areas without fluoride, start 0.25 mg fluoride daily. The dose is increased to 0.50 mg at 3 years, and 1.0 mg at 6 years. (There is some disagreement concerning when to begin fluoride supplements in early infancy; see the discussion in Chapter 20.) Better yet, work to get fluoridation in your area water supply, and forget the supplements.

Another fad which can have unexpected nutritional effects is the new popularity of bottled waters and home filtering devices. The area in which I have practiced has had fluoridation for decades, so I rarely see much dental decay in children from hereabouts. When I do, it is often the case that the family uses bottled water or has a home filter capable of removing fluoride from the water. Water fluoridation is a true public health advance which has brought better dental health to tens of millions of children and adults. It is a terrible shame to throw it away because health hucksters have convinced the unwary consumers that the public water supply is unsafe, or that a bottled product is somehow superior or more fashionable.

Water. Does your breast fed or bottle fed baby need any extra water? No. Breast milk and formula each contain about 86 to 90% water; that is plenty. I suppose a baby may occasionally get thirsty enough to enjoy some extra water on a very hot day when everyone else is exceptionally thirsty. But generally speaking, ordinary nursing or bottle feedings are more than adequate for babies in good health.

Introduction

Well Babies and Well Children: The Next 18 Years

The chapters that follow deal with a range of topics bearing on the growth and development of well children; every age gets its own chapter. These are the issues that parents have wanted to discuss during well child visits with me; and, some are issues I've raised with them.

The organization, such as it is, reflects my experience with what has seemed important in the lives of the children and families I've met during four decades of pediatric practice. I have not tried to cover every possible area of interest to parents; that would require an encyclopedia rather than a book. Fortunately, bookstores are crammed with volumes addressing all sorts of specific topics, so no one need go without information or advice.

You will probably notice a degree of vagueness in my descriptions of typical behavior and development. This is deliberate. I know how important it is for parents to see that their children are developing at just the right clip, and having seemingly precise milestones would certainly give the illusion of knowledge. But kids vary so much that averages mean less than one might think. You'll hear about the "Terrible Twos" because there is a modest degree of uniformity of psychological development at that age; by late childhood and the early teens the range of typical or "normal" behavior is so broad that only the most general statements can be made.

There are two quite different ways to use Part II. Most parents are so busy with and focused on the daily realities of their own kids that it is truly difficult to think about or read about children of any other age. Dealing with a 6-month old leaves very little emotional or intellectual energy for thinking about 6-year olds or 16-year olds. So most of you will probably use this book as a guide to what to expect *right now*, or perhaps next month. That's fine, but you may also want to use it as an overview. Reading *Everyday Pediatrics for Parents* cover to cover, if you can make the time, will draw your attention to a host of issues that you won't necessarily have to grapple with right now. And it will probably introduce you to some topics that, with any luck, may never apply to your children. My hope is that it will give you a sense of the larger journey on which you and your family have embarked.

Chapter 7

Early Infancy

The Unpredictability of Infants

Now that you're all home and more or less settled in, what's next? The answer to that excellent question is that nobody knows. Babies are an amazingly variable lot, and they exhibit correspondingly variable patterns of behavior. Take eating; some infants rapidly develop fairly predictable schedules. A common example: every three hours all day, with increasing frequency in the evening, and then longer intervals during the night. Other infants are wildly erratic giving you hardly a clue from one day to the next. Sleeping patterns are also variable during early infancy. Most babies sleep nearly equal amounts of time during the day and night. Gradually, their biological clocks begin to function, and nighttime sleep increases. This is aided by social cues; the house is quieter and darker at night, and parents are less inclined to want to play at 3 o'clock in the morning. The intervals between evening feedings may start to lengthen sometime during the first months, but not by much. Don't expect to get a good night's uninterrupted sleep.

It is obviously easier to cope with a regular schedule, and a natural impulse is to attempt to train the baby to conform to some sort of livable system. This can often be accomplished, but the attendant effort and misery may not be worth it. Sometimes it is just best to wait for the baby to discover her own most comfortable rhythm. Here is an excellent example of that recurrent dilemma of child raising: When do you push your child to change, and when do you sit back and await developments instead? There is no correct or easy answer; it depends on a variety of factors.

What parts of this equation can you realistically solve? First, consider the circumstances in which the behavior takes place. Some households have enough flexibility to cope with the unpredictable infant. If there are no other children to feed or get off to school, if plenty of adult hands are available to do everyday chores, and if there are no authoritative voices pushing for early conformity, then it may be easy to watch and wait. But what if you have twins, or a 40-hour-a-week job with a 10-hour weekly commute? You may well decide that conformity is an absolute necessity for survival. I recall a mother of eight who raised them pretty much on her own, describing for me the kind of family discipline she found essential. Every child had prescribed duties every day, and that was that. Her listening 6-year old commented, "But sometimes the big kids will help the 2-year old take out the garbage."

The second part of the equation is your view of how family life is *supposed* to be lived. We each bring to the cribside of our firstborn a largely unspoken and usually unconscious set of expectations. This is our legacy from the families in which we were raised: "That is how it was done in my parents' house and that is how I will do it." It is painfully obvious that if Mom's family and Dad's family happened to do things in different ways, the stage is set for some major debates. There is also a variation on this theme: "That's how it was done in my family and I *hated* it!"

In addition to the previously learned family patterns are the individual styles we all bring to any interpersonal encounter. These may include powerful differences between the gut reactions of mothers and fathers. I know this is sweeping generalization, but it seems to me that most mothers will quite automatically react in a softer and more accommodating fashion to their babies' demands; a substantial number of fathers will react with an urge to control. (This is not the last time I'll raise the issue of differences in male and female behavior. Some readers may prefer a unisex interpretation of human psychology, with its implicit assumption that men and women are interchangeable parts. However, that has not been my experience. I hope you will keep an open mind on the subject since I want to convince you of the wisdom of my view!)

What approach is most likely to be successful in devising family patterns that work? Surely it is the one most explicitly informed by an understanding of the needs and feelings of everyone concerned. This understanding is neither innate nor automatic. It can only be achieved by discussions between parents and within the family.

I know you are eager to understand your new baby, and that includes developing a sense of what sort of child has been deposited in your midst. Unfortunately, the behavior of the very newly born is not much help. Circumstances of birth may quite overshadow even powerfully delineated personality types. The quiet newborn may be a bit groggy from drugs used to ease his mother's discomfort during labor; the fussy one may be reporting that he has a headache from pushing his way through a tight birth canal. Therefore, the wise observer will suspend judgment for a few days at least. Soon enough the real persons will be manifest. I have always found it astounding that such small people, so newly come into the world, can be so definite in their preferences and so different in their reactions. They can be phlegmatic or explosive, easily calmed or not, responsive to adults or indifferent, cuddly and relaxed or tense and squirmy. Early in my career as a doctor when I first began to focus serious attention on babies and children, this variability came as a surprise. The dominant theory for many years was that **nurture** (the environment of the child) was much more important than **nature** (the child's own inherited patterns of development). My own experiences as a pediatrician, a parent, and a grandparent have converted me to a firm belief in the importance of what is built in to the child.

The implication is that babies are not infinitely malleable; our preconceived notions of how we want our babies to act and who we want them to be must be measured against reality. Once in a while there can be dramatic mismatches, and the family's expectations and the actual infant don't mesh very well. Calm parents presented with an excitable infant may well wonder if their baby was switched in the hospital nursery. Probably not; there are plenty of people who don't seem to have inherited their families most treasured traits. The advice that applies here is **Grossman's Law of Expectations:** *You have to raise the one you got, not the one you thought you wanted.*

Colic

One universal mismatch is a colicky baby with any kind of family. What is it, anyway? A Supreme Court justice said about pornography that he couldn't define it but he knew it when he saw it. It is much the same with colic. Colic is probably best described as excessive, intense, and prolonged infant fussiness. The age range is a few weeks to 3 or 4 months old. She may be fairly easy and reasonable much of the day but her evenings and sometimes her nights are spent in what is clearly some sort of discomfort. She acts as if she hurts, sometimes intermittently, and sometimes for hours. We label this "colic" because it reminds us of the behavior associated with intestinal cramps, but actually we don't know what hurts. Colicky babies often have distended bellies and noisy bowel sounds, but this could be due to the air swallowing that accompanies their crying.

We are unclear about colic because parents will differ in the amount of infant fussiness they consider to be normal and more or less acceptable. This is partly a matter of experience; new parents may be alarmed about a volume of crying that would hardly be noticed in a family with several children. It is also a matter of culture. Colicky behavior seems to be less common in societies where infants are held or carried most of the time and breast fed on demand.

What to do about it? First and foremost: Stop blaming yourselves. It is all too easy for outside observers, like friends, grandparents, and pediatricians, to say "No wonder they have such a fussy baby, they are such tense and anxious people." Well, tense and anxious parents can have colicky kids, but so can serene ones. So ignore the snippy comments and instead learn all the little tricks that can help convert a screaming child into a welcome member of his family. Though by no means always successful, you never know what will work and all are worth a try.

Holding and cuddling may seem obvious, but some babies seem to need a remarkable amount of loving human contact. Don't worry—you won't become physically attached to your child for years to come, nor are you teaching him to expect too much attention. All over the world, babies are carried in cloth slings on the hips or backs or across the fronts on their mothers. Continuous, close body contact like this keeps the baby content and still lets the mother get on with her life. Share this task with every able-bodied human in the household who is strong enough to hold a baby.

Swaddling a baby by wrapping her firmly and comfortably in a blanket can be magic. The Russians are great believers in this technique; their books on child care give wonderfully explicit directions with pages of pictures on exactly how to achieve the proper mummified result. I wonder if the swaddled baby is reminded of the good old days in the womb when she was firmly confined. The addition of a warm water bottle next to the baby's belly is sometimes also welcome.

Pacifiers can be the colicky baby's second best friend. Widely condemned in our macho society as reminders of infant dependency, pacifiers have had a hard time gaining respect. Do not expect the lady in the supermarket checkout line to restrain her disapproval when she sees the disgusting rubber object attached to your baby's mouth. Just keep in mind that it's her problem, not yours. Besides the little matter of public image, it is true that pacifiers have some limitations and problems. They wear out, get lost, and fall under the crib. I think they can be overused, especially in older infants, as an easy substitute for more definitive attention. And getting rid of the habit when it becomes a social liability in kindergarten can be challenging. None of these objections need keep you from using pacifiers to help ease colic.

Motion and noise, separately or together, are the bases for a number of colic treatments. Of course, just walking with the baby cuddled against you is the simplest and often the most effective strategy. Rocking in a cradle or a rocking chair, or swinging in a mechanical swing also helps. Some babies are soothed by riding in the car, others by a device that attaches to the crib, vibrates it gently, and produces an automobile-like purr. A similar effect may be obtained by holding the baby on top of a clothes dryer. (Be careful if you do this, and do not leave the baby unattended *even for a second*; it would be a hard fall from such a high place.) Even running a vacuum cleaner has been known to have a quieting effect.

Music and other soothing sounds are another approach. Babies learn while still unborn in the mother's womb. They can hear remarkably well during the latter part of pregnancy, and sounds are transmitted through the mother's body. If a particular piece of music is part of her environment, her baby will learn to recognize it. If it is played in his hearing after he is born, he may become quiet and attentive. Another part of the unborn baby's sound environment is the rhythmic noise made by the flow of blood through the uterus. Tape recordings of uterine sounds can be obtained and played for the fretful infant; the commercial version is called "Mother Nature's Lullaby." There is even a Teddy bear on the market with a uterine sounds tape tucked inside. This sounds hokey, but it often works.

Changing the formula given to bottle fed infants is always tried and rarely helps. Infant formulas are complex foods, and are easily altered. One can change the sugar source from lactose to dextri-maltose to sucrose, the protein from cows' milk to goats' milk to soy to predigested protein to whey. Even the fat content can be altered, given enough ingenuity. Unhappily, only a tiny minority of bottle fed babies will care. Food allergy is rather rare at this age, and when it does occur is usually manifested by an itchy rash called eczema rather than by the development of colic. If both parents have major allergies such as hay fever or asthma, the chance of the baby becoming allergic is greater. In that instance, a trial on predigested cows' milk formula (Nutramigen) or a soy formula is probably worth doing, but the chances of curing the colic are not high.

Omitting cows' milk from the diet of the breast feeding mother actually does help some babies. Great claims were made for this treatment by its Scandinavian originators over a decade ago. They found that most cases of colic disappeared when the nursing mothers abstained from all cows' milk products, including cheese, yogurt, and even butter. I recall reading their report and feeling chagrined and embarrassed that I had failed to discover this connection by myself. When nursing mothers in my practice stopped cows' milk the results were decidedly less dramatic. About one colicky baby out of four really improved, but the other three did not. A few mothers whose babies got better found that they could eat a modest amount of cheese or goats' milk products without causing more colic. It takes about three or four days on a strict milk-free diet before one can judge any effect. Apparently the colic in these children is due to traces in the mother's blood and in her milk of undigested cows' milk protein. After a few months of abstinence from cows' milk these mothers can resume consuming it without further problems. The babies whom I have followed have not shown any signs of cows' milk allergy later in life.

Many **medicines** have been used against colic with generally disappointing results. On the theory that air swallowing is somehow involved with the production of cramps and pain, the defoaming or moistening agent simethicone is often tried. This is supposed to allow trapped air to escape with greater ease. It seems to help once in a while, and since it is inexpensive, available without a prescription, and easy to administer, why not try it? My only concern is that some of the simethicone is absorbed into the child's body, and we are not certain of its possible long-term effects. Intestinal antispasmodics have been used for years; in small doses they can help occasionally, but some have proved hazardous if used to excess. A sedative or tranquilizer is the last resort for a truly miserable baby and her distraught parents. Before you dismiss this option as too bizarre to contemplate, consider just how stressful a prolonged episode of severe colic can be. It is sobering to remember that a fair number of babies have been battered for less compelling reasons. A senior professor of mine told me the formula passed on to him by one of the first pediatricians to practice in San Francisco. "In the middle of the night when all else fails, remember that half a teaspoon of bourbon and a teaspoon of sugar in an ounce of water can make all the difference." It has always seemed to me that this dose might be too large for the baby and was certainly too small for the parents.

The last item that helps is **accurate information.** Have your baby examined by your doctor to reassure you that the problem is really colic and not a serious illness. And it helps to know that this, too, shall pass. Colic really does go away all by itself, for reasons not the least understood. Usually between the ages of 3 and 4 months, nearly always before the end of the first half year, the colicky infant becomes a normal, happy baby. I've been impressed that these babies seem to be an unusually alert and interesting bunch. They are often precocious in their social and intellectual development, and tend to develop into a quite lively lot of children. This may be scant comfort when you are walking your unhappy infant in the middle of the night, but it's nice to have something positive to look forward to.

The Baby's Day. Besides the time spent eating, pooping, sleeping, and crying, how do babies spend their days? The short answer is "learning." They are information sponges. The senses of newborns are remarkably well developed at the time of birth. Hearing is excellent, and touch, taste, and smell are all in working order. It was once believed that vision was blurry in the early weeks of life, but more accurate tests have shown that babies have imprecise but quite useful near-vision. Watch your baby when she is awake and alert and you will often find her observing and listening to you and her other caretakers. Very young infants will even appear to mimic the facial expressions of those around them. It is a little unnerving to realize how closely you are being studied. Within a matter of days, a new baby recognizes its mother by voice, sight, and smell. Within a few weeks, babies seem to recognize and give differing responses to the familiar people in their lives.

Babies also observe the inanimate environment in which they live. In the first months of life they learn about the shapes and sizes of objects around them. This ability has been exploited by the makers of infant "learning" toys who have produced a variety of devices alleged to be aids in the force feeding of the infant mind. The notion is that since babies watch certain shapes and colors more than others, one should display these supposedly stimulating objects and thus encourage baby brain cells to grow faster and bigger and stronger. I think this is simply nonsense based on a complete lack of faith in the natural ability of the baby to collect information according to his own needs and desires. An entire industry, lubricated by commercial greed, feeds on the anxiety of parents. The message is "Buy my brand of learning toy or your baby will never make it to Harvard."

What babies *do* need in their environments are loving adults and interested children who care about them, talk to them, and are available to play with them. Colorful mobiles and pretty pictures on the bedroom walls are all very nice, but the human race has managed to evolve for several million years without either.

Spoiling

But, isn't it possible to care about them *too much*? If we give our infants too much attention, don't we run the risk of spoiling them? This question is a prime example of the danger of mislabeling an issue. First of all, look at the verb we use to describe our concern: "Spoiling" is a loaded word which carries the connotation of irremediable damage. After all, when food is spoiled, we call it "garbage" and throw it out. Restating the issue without talking about spoiling leads to a more accurately focused question. For example: "If we give them too much attention, don't we run the risk of encouraging unreasonable expectations?" I think the answer is sure we do, but that is manageable. Babies learn what to expect in a remarkably short period of time. When a baby is very young, parents want to keep the baby as happy and content as possible. If she is hungry, you feed her; if she is uncomfortable, you are anxious to discover the source of her discomfort and remedy it promptly; if she is lonely and needs to be cuddled, you want to hold her. These are appropriate needs for the infant and appropriate responses for the parents. By recognizing the needs of your infant and satisfying them, you are teaching her that she is cared for and loved. Those are pretty nice lessons at any age and are probably especially important in the early months of life. On the other hand, failure to alter your behavior as your baby grows would surely teach expectations which you would eventually regret. It is all very well to meet infant needs as expeditiously as you can, but when older babies begin to fuss because dinner is not on the table promptly at 5 o'clock, it is time to begin to teach them that life also involves a certain amount of delayed gratification. In short, you should meet the urgently voiced needs of the new baby in an urgent fashion, knowing that, over time, you will slowly teach the developing child that he does not always come first, that sometimes he must wait, and that other people also have needs to be met. If he has a secure base of care and nurturing, he will probably feel more comfortable about the amount of waiting required by the real world as he gets older. This is one of the virtues of being born into a family with older brothers and sisters. There are lots of helping hands available, and baby's needs can be met with reasonable promptitude. But after a few months, the press of family responsibilities means that even the most charming or vocal new baby must learn to wait once in a while. This is a pretty sound combination of lessons for raising civilized people. Parents of an only child or a first child may need to keep an eye on the issue of appropriateness of expectations. When power in the family is concentrated too exclusively in the tiny hands and lungs of its youngest member, it is time to adjust his expectations. Once again, you will be struck by how quickly your baby learns what the new rules are.

And What About the Rest of the Family? The early months of the new baby's life at home may be a joyous time but it is not likely to be an easy time. Everyone is tired, sleep is still disturbed, mealtimes are chaos, schedules are upset, noses are out of joint. The older children, if any, have probably recovered completely from the initial excitement of siblinghood and are contemplating long years of penal servitude in thrall to the newborn's needs. The baby has probably not yet decided that his siblings are fascinating and amusing folks, so there is little, if any, positive feedback from that direction. The parents are now sufficiently sleep deprived that absolutely nothing in life looks more desirable than 10 hours of uninterrupted rest. Mothers are under steadily increasing pressure to return to "work." The supporting cast of family and friends who brought casseroles and loving attention during the first weeks has gone home. It can be a hard adjustment and a lonely time, especially for a socially isolated new mother. You may feel alone, but this is a common dilemma. What can you do to lighten your life? Find a mother-and-baby group for mutual support. Let your friends know that you still exist. Hire every bit of help you can afford. When all is said and done, human beings are truly tribal animals, and our current fashion for living in nuclear family groups shows its greatest weakness during periods of stress like births and deaths. When the great baseball player Ty Cobb was dying he said "If I could do it all over again, I'd have more friends". Excellent advice for us all.

Chapter 8

Age 2 to 4 Months

Family Life—Settling Down?

By now, most families are getting a fairly clear sense of the baby's temperament and behavior patterns. Many infants are starting to sleep for longer stretches, at least in the evening if not during the night. Feedings are more predictable and a bit less frequent. And new parents are less likely to find themselves looking at the baby in his crib and wondering "What do I do now?" By this time, they pretty well know.

First time parents are also nearly always amazed by the sheer amount of time required for the care of their infants. You wouldn't think that such a small being could absorb such endless hours. Feeding, cleaning, changing diapers, holding and comforting, and playing with one little baby can take every waking minute of the day. It is understandable to try to impose some sort of schedule, at least on eating and sleeping. This is often the first clash of wills between baby and parents. It is hard to know what is reasonable and wise, and the patterns that emerge will depend as much on everyone's personal style as on theories of what babies need. A parent with an authoritarian streak may try to forge a predictable daily schedule; a laissez-faire parent may decide to trust the baby to work out his own pattern of eating and sleeping. It is the fortunate family where both parents and baby happen to have the same general approach to life. When that is not the case, expect a possibly fruitless struggle.

This is often an uncomfortable time for fathers. A great many men find very young infants a generally unrewarding and uninteresting bunch, even when the infant is their own. Unhappily, the current social wisdom demands that parenting tasks should be shared equally, from earning the family income to changing the family diapers. If this popular notion fails to resonate in the new father's psyche, as is frequently the case, Mom is deeply disappointed, and Dad is guilty and angry. Added to this conflict is the reality that first parenthood, in particular, signals a great divide in the life experience and self-image of a young father. If he has been a sower of wild oats, a hanger-out with the boys, an ardent devotee of Monday night football, and, in his own view, a free spirit, these attributes and behaviors have become suddenly out of date and undesirable. The new self-image of hard working family man may seem foreign and quite unwelcome.

All this reality may be clearly understood by the new mother, but do not be surprised if she fails to sympathize. She has problems of her own. She is still chronically exhausted, her weight and figure have not returned to normal, her interest in sex is usually nonexistent, her concerns about the family finances have not disappeared. She and her husband have probably not had 10 minutes of quiet, peaceful, adult conversation in months. At this point it may be helpful to start *scheduling* some time for the marriage. A babysitter armed with a bottle makes it possible to have at least a few hours respite from the baby and some time to focus on each other. The applicable rule is **Grossman's Law of Marital Success: *Marriages are living entities that require care and feeding. Ignore them and they wither.***

Older brothers and sisters have some issues as well. The arrival of the new baby heralds a change in status for an older sibling. If he has been the only child, his privileged position is abruptly lost. Karl Marx said that no ruling class gives up power without a revolution; this tends to hold for families as well as larger political entities. The older child may respond by adopting infant ways with a vengeance, and the varieties of regression are limited only by the child's imagination. This can be countered by a combination of expressed sympathy for the victim of expulsion from Eden, plus the institution of rewards signaling his elevated place in the family constellation. "Now that you are the big brother in the family, we think it is time for you to stay up 15 minutes later at night" (or get an extra bedtime story, or have a special trip to the store with Daddy once a week or whatever).

When there are two older kids, the oldest may form an instant alliance with the new baby against the middle child. In this situation, the second child has the worst of all worlds. She loses her babyhood and has to share her older sib as well as her parents. Finding a little separate time for her can be exceedingly difficult but is also extremely important.

Sometimes the best strategy is a little commiseration. "I'll bet its hard for you when Baby Jane gets so much attention these days." Acknowledging your child's feelings is a wonderful way to show her that you understand and care about how she feels. The very act of naming and describing emotional states in an accepting way teaches her that emotions are okay, to be experienced, expressed, and even talked about. I think it is best to avoid putting your comments in the form of a question. "Are you angry and jealous about the baby?" practically demands the answer "No, of course not." None of us is likely to want to admit such nasty and unacceptable feelings.

EVERYDAY PEDIATRICS FOR PARENTS

I should add that not every parent finds this style of communication easy. If it is unlike the way you were talked to by your parents when you were a child, it may seem foreign and forced. However, you may find that a little experimentation helps.

The good news for older children is that babies of this age smile and laugh and coo, and they tend to bestow these rewards most freely on their big sisters and big brothers. Acting toward one's older siblings as though they were delightful playmates and thoroughly charming people rather than potential infanticides must have had considerable survival value during the descent of the human species. A soft answer turneth away wrath, and there is nothing softer than a baby's smile.

Growth and Development

By now, babies are usually smiling quite a bit, either spontaneously, at times of contentment, or socially, in response to interactions with their caretakers. The first brief smiles are often dismissed as "gas", although why anyone would smile in response to such an intestinal stimulus is hard to fathom. The applicable rule is **Grossman's Law of Facial Expressions: *If it looks like a smile, it is a smile.*** After smiling comes cooing and laughing. Babies are becoming better able to control their heads and bodies. By 4 months of age a few babies can turn over, usually from belly to back. Once again, the key word is variability; there is an immense range within which normal development can express itself. Every infant has her own timetable. It is interesting that racial patterns of physical development begin to become obvious in early infancy. Black children tend to show more physical activity and more rapid acquisition of motor skills than white or Asian children, even at this early stage.

Toys and Play. Absolutely everything in the world is new and fascinating to a baby. They stare at everything, reaching out visually to the environment. Then they start reaching with their hands, clumsily at first, and gradually with more and more precision. At this age babies are developing their whole hand grasp; it will be a while before they can appose thumb and fingers in a pincer movement. When an object is grasped, the next move is directly to the mouth. The lips and tongue are the preferred sense organs. After careful mouthing, tasting, and chewing, babies may hold the object up for further visual inspection, but it will probably then be returned to the mouth for more information gathering. This pattern should provide some hints regarding the choice of toys. If a baby can look at it, grab it, and chew it, it will be a hit. They don't need anything very complicated: rattles, soft balls, simple stuffed animals or dolls, objects with a variety of colors and textures. Mobiles are great at this age; depending on their design, they can be watched, kicked, grabbed, or batted at. A sturdy mobile suspended near enough the baby's chest so that he can play with it will be very welcome. But be sure that he will not get dangerously tangled in the mobile's supporting struts.

Feeding

The breast fed infant is still nursing more often than her formula fed cousin. Her stools have probably decreased in frequency, often to a few times a week. Her mother may be experiencing the decrease in breast milk production that accompanies overworking and undersleeping. The methods for increasing milk noted in Chapter 6 can be instituted, or increased formula supplements may be needed. These are typically well tolerated by the baby, but occasionally an infant may learn to prefer the easily obtained bottle to the slower and perhaps less copiously flowing breast.

The formula fed infant is probably taking about 2½ ounces of formula per pound of body weight per day. How much you should offer at a feeding? When a baby is draining every bottle fairly regularly, increase the volume by about 1 ounce and see what happens. There is no point leaving a child hungry.

Somewhere around this age, there is a regrettable tendency to begin to push fluids other than milk and even to start baby on solid foods. This is an innovation peculiar to the twentieth century. Before, mothers were content to feed babies at the breast without recourse to other substances. When the first successful formula feedings were developed nearly a century ago, one had also to give orange juice to prevent scurvy, a vitamin C deficiency disease. As formula feeding became the hallmark of the modern mother, orange juice became a sacrament of good health and up-to-date parenting practices. It was a short step from "orange juice is good for babies" to "any juice is good for babies." In any case, the need for orange juice as a vitamin C source was obviated by the addition of vitamin C to prepared formula or its administration as a pure substance, ascorbic acid, in vitamin drops. The distinct disadvantage of orange juice is its tendency to cause small infants to develop eczema, a nasty allergic rash.

The other disadvantage of juices is that they are not useful additions to a diet of either breast milk or properly made formula. Although they supply nearly as many calories per ounce as milk, they lack all nutrients except sugar and, in some cases, extra unnecessary vitamin C. Their combination of sugar and acidity makes them exceedingly efficient at initiating cavities in baby teeth, and they quickly teach the lesson that thirst can and should be quenched with a sweet drink, rather than with water. Giving a baby a bottle of apple or grape juice is marginally healthier than giving a bottle of Coke, but not by much.

The introduction of baby solids during the first several months of life became popular forty or fifty years ago. It stands as a prime example of the victory of commercial values over sound nutrition and good sense. During that benighted period, an astonishing variety of substances were shoveled into the mouths of spluttering infants. The pertinent but misconceived rule should probably be called Gerbers' Law: If we can bottle it, you should give it to your baby. The disadvantages included the frequent induction of allergic rashes, especially by cereal products and egg white, and the displacement of nutritionally complete and well-balanced breast milk or formula by less nourishing solid foods. A common occurrence was severe constipation, when the infant gut, overwhelmed by the onslaught of hard-to-digest gruels, simply ground to a halt. I am pleased to report that this idiocy has finally been recognized as such. More and more parents omit infant solids until about the middle of the first year when babies easily learn to take foods from a spoon and are better able to digest them.

In all fairness to the baby food companies, the foolish practice of giving early solids would never have amounted to anything without the support of both parents and physicians. I think it is a perfect example of our discomfort with the dependency of infants. It is as if we find the sight of the suckling baby a displeasing reminder that the kid is not yet standing on his own two feet, as a proper, tough, independent American should. We often seem to lose sight of the maxim that to every thing there is a season, and a time to every purpose under the heaven. Folks, they grow up soon enough; don't rush them.

Being Alone and Being Together. Another aspect of this frontier mentality can be seen in the popularity of enforced solitude as a molder of American character. This subject has already been touched upon in Chapter 5 regarding sleeping quarters for the new baby. What about company for the baby during her waking hours? It is clear that babies thrive with lots of human attention. The company of people who cuddle them, talk to them, and play with them teaches them to be normal human beings. In fact, with little or no human interaction they stop growing and die. So, can there be too much of a good thing? Babies also enjoy watching their worlds, exploring with their eyes, ears, and other senses. After all, absolutely everything is fresh and new. Watch a 3-month old in his basket placed under a tree. He observes the leaves, listens to the birds and the passing traffic, and has a fine time. I think that a modest amount of alone time awake is completely appropriate for our babies. They have lots to learn about the world, some of which they must really learn on their own, and they also begin to learn that life can be sustained without constant adult supervision. The playpen is a device that can make this process both smoother and safer. A playpen can be used to concentrate and display a variety of interesting objects for observation and manipulation by the infant. It can also be a relatively safe haven from the incursions of older siblings or pets. A few 15 to 30-minute playpen periods a day are beneficial for both parents and child. If you are going to use a playpen, start early, during the first few months. Attempting to introduce one later in the first year after she has already begun to roll or creep to a goal may lead to furious resistance at the impingement on her newfound mobility. In any case, by 12 to 18 months, you can expect your baby to perceive her playpen as a jail, and you will regretfully put it into the back of the closet to await its next occupant.

Safety

This is the last time in your baby's career that safety concerns are easily met. You need to make sure that he does not turn over abruptly and fall from the bed or sofa or changing table. Make the assumption that he may have acquired this skill *before* he unexpectedly manifests it. Of course he must be securely fastened into an infant car seat whenever he is in a car. This can be a considerable bother especially when you are traveling by air and have to drag the bulky thing along. Do it anyway; ***car seats save lives.***

There will be many aspects of infant safety to consider when he is a bit older and much more mobile. Stairs, heaters, poisons, and excessively hot tap water, to list a few. For a preview of what is to come, see page 91.

Day Care

This is a difficult subject for me to discuss because I feel so strongly about it, and because families have so little control over the choices that face them. The financial reality of American life today is that most two parent families have become accustomed to living on two incomes. This is in part due to the loss of real income among working class and much of middle class America. Inflation has outstripped wages; industrial and corporate downsizing has drastically reduced high wage employment. But many of us got used to living pretty high on the hog during the last several decades. We still love our electronic gadgets and toys, and we still want the money to buy them. Add soaring health costs, the sky-rocketing cost of housing, and the decay of public schools that makes private education seem so necessary to many families. Unless you are wealthy, the only option seems to be for Mom to become (or resume being) a wage earner. For single parent families, the pressures are correspondingly greater and the choices narrower. For most single mothers, it's work or welfare.

Another factor is that we have raised a generation of young women who *want* to be out in the work world. To these women, being stuck at home, isolated in a single family dwelling, away from peers and friends, dealing day in and day out with the limited human rewards of raising little kids and keeping house—resembles the American nightmare rather than the American dream. A few generations of American women tried living that way, and it did not work out very well. For a woman who has had experience in a decent job, staying home with the kids may look a lot like solitary confinement.

The solution that has evolved is the mess called day care. Of course, some day care situations are great. A loving family member or a skillful mother who can take care of one more child along with her own is an ideal set up. Or well-trained professionals in well-staffed and organized small day care centers can provide a stimulating and nurturing environment for children. But many day care situations are appalling. Untold numbers of babies and children are warehoused in large centers with inadequate facilities staffed by poorly trained, overworked, and badly paid helpers. For 8 to 10 hours of a baby's day, the adults in her life are interchangeable parts who come and go. A television set instead of a human being is companion to far too many American kids, far too much of the time. The lessons we teach a child in a loving, caring, and safe setting are that she is loved, cared about, and valued. The lessons learned by the child in the usual impersonal, noisy, chaotic day care center is that she is unimportant, not cared about, and hardly worth noticing. The destructive results are not exactly astonishing. I recall a psychologist's sad but insightful comment concerning a day care child referred to her for evaluation: "There's not enough ego there."

Day care kids tend to be sick kids, especially during the first few years. In any group care setting with children in diapers, there is a great deal of sharing of stool with its usual content of interesting viruses, bacteria, and parasites. A day care worker changes Baby A's dirty diaper, and immediately goes to Baby B, carrying some stool and germs on her fingers. She is rushed and overworked, and she has no time to wash her hands. Baby C, whose hands are not so clean either, transfers a bit of fecal material to a toy which goes into the mouth of

Baby D. Respiratory germs also abound. Baby E awakens with a cold. His parents, both of whom need to go to work, decide it is just a touch of allergy, so off he goes to day care where he generously shares his viruses with Baby F and Baby G. In our pediatric practice my partners and I found that the introduction of day care vastly increased the number of infants with ear infections and other complications of common respiratory disease. Severe and sometimes chronic intestinal infections used to be unusual in our babies. But among those in day care, they became commonplace. One particular parasite called Giardia went from being a great rarity, found mostly in Sierra back packers who drank contaminated mountain water, to an everyday part of the lives of infants and their adult caretakers. Our office records revealed that babies had 14 times as many illness visits in recent years since day care became the rule, compared to the 1950s and 1960s when day care of infants was practically unheard of.

Are there any advantages for the child in early exposure to day care? Well, there is a premature kind of independence in many of the kids who have survived day care. I suppose if you want to raise your baby to be a commodities trader or a policeman, early day care may be as good a place as any to start teaching the lesson that it's a jungle out there.

The best solutions are by no means easy to find. Even for the mother who stays at home for the first 2 or 3 years of her babies' lives, some kind of support system is a necessity. She needs time away from the house and the kids, time with her friends, time on her own. Some husbands do manage to share the household tasks; some women have friends or family who will help. Shared child care with another family can work very well, especially for babies past early infancy: Tuesday and Thursday mornings the kids are at your house, Wednesday and Friday they are at mine.

Working part time is an excellent compromise and job-sharing is slowly catching on. Then one can often get along with less day care. Finding another mother who can take care of your child part time may work well for both families.

In any case, the smaller the setting the better, especially for the youngest kids. Family day care, where a skilled and experienced mother or a well-trained child care worker with a few children at her home is usually satisfactory. The problems with these settings is that 3 to 6 kids can be too much for anyone to handle by herself. Larger centers may be able to afford more equipment and more generous play spaces, but the limiting factors are always human: too many children and not enough knowledgeable, loving adults.

When we as a nation begin to value our babies and our children, perhaps we will seriously address the inadequacies I have described. Until then, parents will have to scrabble for solutions.

Chapter 9

Age 4 to 6 Months

They Are Not All Chips Off the Old Block

Physical growth is very rapid during the new baby's first half year. By 6 months of age, the infant will generally have doubled its birth weight and grown somewhere in the neighborhood of 6 inches. As the middle of the first year approaches, physical growth has begun to slow down a bit, but this deceleration is only noticeable if you are diligently recording carefully measured weights and lengths every month. In contrast, the development of new physical skills remains obvious. By this time, babies are usually rolling over, at least from belly to back, some are sitting up without support, and most are able to sit at least briefly with a little help. They are increasingly interested in reaching for and manipulating their environment. They bat at mobiles, hold toys, grab for bottles, and try to mouth and chew every interesting object. For many babies, sensing the world through their mouths continues to be at least as important and useful as sensing it through their eyes and hands. Their ability to move towards a goal is wildly variable. Some squirm and wriggle their way in pursuit of a desirable toy or some interesting household hazard, others creep effectively on their bellies, and a few have learned to crawl on hands and knees. There are also infants who have absolutely no apparent interest in ambulation. They sit or lie wherever they are placed and watch the world go by. All these patterns of activity or the lack of it are completely normal.

In a few instances, you will probably discern something of the activity levels to be expected in the future. Some babies are in constant motion, sleeping all over the crib, scooting and rolling all over the room, and moving from toy to toy within seconds. Wait a few years and these are likely to be the kids who fidget during circle time in nursery school and can't wait to get outside to roar around the playground. At the other extreme, babies who will become focused problem solvers may already be engaged in the endless analysis of every new toy. There are limits to this crystal ball-gazing approach to the study of temperament and personal style, but it can be helpful to see your children's behavior in a larger and longer perspective. Also, keep in mind that some behaviors are simply age and stage-related. The stranger shyness that develops in the middle of the first year predicts nothing at all; it is simply the usual response of the child to the realization that the human world is divided into "family" and "not family." Among American children from nuclear families, stranger anxiety is pretty much the rule. During the 1960s when my partners and I in pediatric practice saw a large number of commune-reared children, we noted that stranger anxiety was sometimes almost totally absent. The babies seemed to define adults as pretty much interchangeable parts. I think that babies who see very few adults during the first few months are somewhat more likely to be stranger anxious later in infancy. A fairly brisk traffic in family, friends, and babysitters may make the eventual recognition of the category "stranger" a bit less threatening. In any event, stranger anxiety is expected and natural, and with few exceptions it goes away without any special parental effort.

Sleep

By the middle of the first year, most American babies are sleeping for long stretches at night; many are asleep for 8 to 10 hours straight. All American parents are ready for their babies to sleep at least this long, and longer would be even better. Thus, the stage is set for one of the first examples of discordance between the needs of the generations. As I have already commented in Chapter 5, this is best thought about in terms of the history of the race contrasted to the present day realities and expectations of adults. It seems clear that infants and mothers have slept side by side throughout the first few million years of human existence. It is also clear that older children slept next to their parents as a matter of course. The invention of separate beds and separate bedrooms is a fairly recent innovation, and the practice of sleeping away from one's children was probably limited to the very rich until the last few hundred years. In America today, separate sleeping is expected to be mastered within months, and it is treasured thereafter. Not only does it make possible uninterrupted parental sleep and less inhibited and noisier parental sex, but it serves as a paradigm for the desired growth of the child's independence. Everyone involved benefits, although this will be less obvious to the child who cannot be expected to understand the advantage he reaps in solitary strength. In any event, sometime during the middle of the first year "She doesn't sleep through the night" becomes the most common topic of conversation between parents. The age at which steps can be taken to alter this state of affairs depends largely on your views of the propriety of letting small infants cry for hours, plus your fantasies about the effect of the experience on the baby. Some years ago, a German mother told me that the practice in her country was to let the babies cry it out in the very first weeks of life; she assured me that German infants slept through thereafter, secure in the knowledge that awakening and crying to be fed was a complete waste of time. This seems to me to be an awful thing to impose on a newborn, both physiologically and emotionally, let alone the problem for the mother who would awaken bursting with milk by midnight.

So, when do you ask a baby to sleep for, say, an 8-hour stretch? A few pragmatic points may be noted. First, at least 50% of all American babies sleep this long spontaneously by 4 to 6 months of age, so it must be reasonably physiological. Second, most parents are becoming increasingly strung out after half a year of night-waking. A sleep-deprived mother is no great joy to anyone, and her baby will be well advised to sleep through in order to be rewarded with a smiling and rested mother in the morning. Third, it is amazingly easy to train the vast majority of 6-month olds not to awaken in the night, and they appear not to hold a grudge. If it strikes you that these arguments are slender reeds to support a decision of this importance, you are certainly correct. But that's life: lots of gray space, little black and white.

Grossman's First Sleep Stratagem: *The time to teach the baby to sleep through is when both parents are in complete agreement about its necessity.* It is too easy for one parent to sabotage the whole process unless both have suffered enough to face a few nights of misery.

Grossman's Second Sleep Stratagem: *The key to learning to sleep through is learning that night—waking is utterly unrewarding; nothing good happens.* This means that the baby who awakens is neither cuddled nor fed nor changed.

Grossman's Third Sleep Stratagem: *When the baby awakens in the night, let her know that she has not been abandoned to the wolves.* After a few minutes of crying (the baby's, and sometimes the mother's as well), one parent should go to the infant and tell her frankly and firmly that she should go back to sleep. This will presumably reassure the baby that her parents may be mean, but at least they are still at home. It is not only possible but likely that the periods of crying, punctuated by very brief parental appearances, will persist for a remarkably long time. About an hour is usual on the first night, but two or three sets of one hour each are not unusual. The second night is easier, less than an hour of piteous screams being about par. The third night is likely to be nearly quiet. Exceptionally, the process may take as much as two weeks.

Grossman's Fourth Sleep Stratagem: *Keep firmly in mind that babies subjected to this program awaken quite happy, even after the most horrendous nights of crying.* They are clearly as pleased as ever to see Mom and Dad, and in my experience there are no traces of upset behavior either during the entirety of the training procedure or later. I am aware that some writers on this subject consider this method an unconscionable form of child abuse. This seems to me to show a lack of faith in the ability of babies to adapt to the realistic requirements of family life. Babies are remarkably fast learners. It is important for parents not to underestimate their ability to understand and adapt

While we are on the subject of sleep, let's mention the fascinating notion that babies must somehow *learn* to fall asleep by themselves. It has become commonplace to read the advice that you should never allow a baby to go to sleep at the breast, or while being held during a bottle feeding, or in general in the company of an adult. The idea is that the baby somehow must master the esoteric art of losing consciousness in solitude. Every other young animal seems to be able to go to sleep without tutoring in the technique; are human infants so unskilled in basic body functions that they require instruction in the acquisition and giving up of wakefulness? Somehow it seems rather unlikely. Where is the evidence behind the theory of Learning to Fall Asleep? Have carefully designed experiments or long-term studies been conducted which demonstrate the dire effects of being in adult company when drowsing off? How have we managed all these millennia without noticing the problem?

One reason this piece of nonsense so annoys me is that it is an example of the mine field of informational garbage through which parents must navigate. Absolutely everyone seems to want to tell us mothers and fathers how to raise our kids, and a substantial portion of those purveyors of pretty theories are ill-informed zealots with an axe to grind or a product to sell. I recommend applying **Grossman's First and Second Laws on Advice: 1)** *Advice offered as gospel truth of world-saving importance is particularly suspect; the more heat, the less light.* Wisdom is usually incremental, not earth shattering. When someone tells you that the *only* way to proceed is his way, you can be reasonably sure that you are in the presence of a nut. **2)** *Be particularly*

***skeptical of ideas which do not seem to mesh with your prior under-
standing of the world.*** A really far-out notion needs a great deal of supporting evidence to be taken seriously. If your response to a statement is
"Unbelievable!" you're right, it is.

Feeding

Every time I browse the shelves of our local bookstores, I am startled by the
number of volumes dedicated to the subject of how and what to feed babies.
Whole books! Am I missing something here? Is it really so complicated a subject that hundreds of pages of text are required? I suppose books like this can
be useful in so far as they provide general nutritional information regarding
what we all need to thrive and grow. But it's a shame if they give the impression that infant feeding is some sort of academic discipline requiring advanced,
graduate study. What follows is my version of Infant Feeding 1A. The upper
division course can be found in Chapter 20 - Foods and Nutrition and Chapter
21 - Eating Problems.

Solid Foods. Introducing solid foods earlier than the middle of the first year
is ordinarily the result of external pressure. The exhortations of friends and
family ("Haven't you started to feed her yet?") and the blandishments of the
advertisements will often be enough to initiate the process. There are also some
very large and very hungry infants whose mothers tell me "I can't fill him up
with milk." My usual advice that more milk will indeed fill him up is not always
convincing. However, by 5 or 6 months some of the pressure to start solids may
begin to come from the baby. The infant who sits on your lap during the family dinner, salivating and watching each forkful of food travel from plate to
mouth, and grabbing every scrap that comes close is making a pretty clear
statement of readiness to be fed something other than breast milk or formula.
The baby's judgment may be wrong but it will doubtless get something to eat,
and the venture will probably be successful. Most infants of this age learn easily to deal with spoon-fed, pureed foods; digestive problems are fairly rare,
although an occasional baby gets completely constipated from baby cereal. The
main risk is the induction of allergy from wheat, corn, egg white, orange, chocolate, peanut, fish, and shellfish. Introduce these foods cautiously—and later. If
either parent has a major allergy like hay fever or asthma it is probably wise to
start these allergy-triggering foods even more slowly. We know that the propen-
sity to develop allergic disease is inherited, and we think that waiting until late
in the first year or early in the second year before exposing the baby to these

foods will decrease the likelihood of allergies in early childhood. However, we don't know if it will make any difference in the long run.

Parents vary marvelously in their approach to solid feedings. You may be surprised by your initial enthusiasm, especially with your firstborn; feeding your babies speaks to something deep and primitive within the parental animal. The thrill does wear off a bit with subsequent children as you become aware that the first solid foods are a messy chore as well as an exciting rite of passage. But the inner voice still whispers, "I feed, therefore I am." This is important; it leads us to nourish our young, an absolute necessity, but it gets in our way when the child begins to want control of his food, and you may find it quite difficult to let this happen.

What do you feed a baby? I recall the rigid lists we were given in medical school by our professor of pediatrics; so and so many teaspoons of this and that vegetable, fruit, and cereal, all dependent on some esoteric formula of weight, height, and barometric pressure. I probably still have my lecture notes somewhere. In truth, the issue is not that complicated. First, look at the baby's milk feeding; if it is breast milk or iron-fortified formula, the initial solid feeds are really nutritionally unimportant. Other factors can determine the choices. If it is a low-iron formula, the first feeds should be rich in iron, which means commercially prepared baby rice or barley cereal. The iron which has been added to that uninteresting looking powder is a special formulation which is very well absorbed. Babies usually like infant cereal, especially if it is mixed with formula, breast milk, or pureed fruit. Bananas or applesauce are usually chosen because they are easily accepted and practically never allergenic. If the cereal proves to be constipating, use less, and mix in more fruit, especially summer fruits like peaches and plums, either raw or cooked. Other iron sources are meats, which most babies don't much care for at first, and egg yolk, which is something of a mess. For the baby who is already getting some iron (from breast milk or iron-fortified formula), it is still usually a good idea to start with cereal and fruit—because it works. An occasional infant prefers vegetables, and that's fine. Try offering a teaspoon of whatever food is chosen, first once, then twice a day. Increase the volume slowly as the baby's interest and gastrointestinal tract allow. Within a few weeks most babies are taking 2 to 3 ounces twice a day. Add new foods one at a time, for the first few months. This makes it easier to determine if any given food is causing trouble. If you give vanilla custard pudding (which has 6 to 8 ingredients in it) on Thursday and your baby breaks out in a rash on Friday, how can you tell which one of the pudding's several constituents is to blame? Another factor in choosing infant foods is availability. In the American diet, wheat (which includes white flour products) is ubiquitous, and in the form of breads, crackers, cereals, and pasta, it is easily eaten by older infants who have started to finger feed. Because it is also highly allergenic, you might like to delay its use until about the end of the first year when the infant's maturing gut can do a better job of breaking it down to a sufficiently digested (and therefore hypo-allergenic) form. However, it is basically impossible to keep wheat out of the hands and mouths of American babies.

So, an average baby will start rice or barley cereal and fruit at 5 to 6 months, vegetables (with or without meat) at 7 to 8 months, wheat at 8 or more months, and the other allergenic foods slowly thereafter. If your infant shows any food intolerance—slow down; there is no hurry. If there are no apparent problems, most babies can be on a nearly complete family diet by 12 to 14 months. Children whose parents have major allergies may take 16 to 18 months to reach that point.

The pureed foods can be either homemade or commercially prepared baby food. The only commercial food which is really superior to homemade is baby cereal because of its excellent iron fortification. There is no way for us to duplicate this in our kitchens and no particular reason to try. Despite their rather dismal appearance and bland taste, rice cereal and barley cereal are very good choices. (There is no reason to use "high protein" cereals, since babies get so much protein from milk, and both the corn and the wheat cereals should be avoided until late in the first year because they are allergenic.)

Any parent who has a food processor, a blender, or a baby food grinder can prepare superior pureed fruits, vegetables, and meats at a fraction of the cost and with much better taste than the commercially prepared products. Canning foods inevitably degrades flavors, and baby foods have been made even less palatable since the baby food companies no longer flavor foods with appropriate amounts of salt. Can you imagine anyone wanting to eat pureed, salt-free, canned green beans? The notion that it is important to give infants salt-free and sugar-free foods for the few months before they are introduced to the sweetened and salted family diet seems hard to justify; after all, the baby will eventually eat whatever the family eats. The alternative is simple pureeing of food already prepared for the family—salt, seasonings, and all. There is no reason to avoid strong flavors in baby foods; babies all over the world are rapidly introduced to garlic and spices and herbs in the family diet. The only exceptions are bitter or peppery flavors which seem to be more slowly acquired tastes. Save time by pouring the pureed fruit or vegetables or vegetable-meat mixture into an ice cube tray and freezing it; this provides a number of easily prepared servings.

Finger Feeding. As the baby develops her ability to reach and grasp, she will usually become interested in starting to feed herself. The variations on this theme are considerable. Some infants are not only excited by finger feeding, but they want to take over the entire process of obtaining food. They grab utensils from the ministering adult and may refuse any proffered food under adult control. At the other extreme are babies who enjoy being fed and have no interest whatsoever in taking charge. First finger foods are those which can be managed with the infant's whole-hand grasp; puffy rice crackers, graham crackers, toast, celery, meat bones (like chicken drum sticks), and large pieces of soft fruit are all good examples.

During the first several months of finger feeding, you will occasionally have to retrieve a chunk of food from your baby's mouth. It is always scary when a baby splutters and chokes, usually on a large piece which is too big to swallow. The risk that it will actually go down his windpipe is minimal with these foods. ***The dangerous foods which are best avoided for the first two years are raw carrots, nuts, popcorn, large chunks of wieners and other meats, and whole grapes.*** It is a very good idea to know how to clear an obstructed airway. The old method of administering a series of sharp blows with the heel of the hand to the infant's upper back while he is held head down over your lap is easy to learn and quite reassuring to have available, even though you will probably never have to use it. Alternative methods include chest compressions or abdominal thrusts (the Heimlich maneuver). Learning to carry out these maneuvers effectively requires specific instruction. Call your local Red Cross for information on infant and child safety classes, or ask your doctor to teach you.

As the thumb-finger pincer grip is mastered at about 7 to 10 months, smaller pieces of food may be offered. These can include dry cereals like Cheerios and Rice Chex, pasta, cooked vegetables, cooked and raw fruits, soft meats (such as poultry), and lumpy scrambled eggs. The defining rules are:

1. Milk is still the mainstay of the baby's diet.
2. There is no magic amount of solid food the baby must ingest.
3. The whole undertaking is designed as a transition to the self-fed, mostly solid food diet of the toddler. This is not a training ground for a Food Olympics with prizes for the largest intake of the most foods.

Safety

Toward the end of the first half year babies are becoming substantially more mobile, so this is the time when you need to study your home environment for health hazards. The idea is to find them before your baby does. Initially, the major risks to a baby's safety are likely to be at floor level. Soon, however, an infant can pull to standing, and then a whole new group of hazards becomes accessible. Later, when your baby can climb, yet another set of challenges awaits you. You may as well deal with all of these areas at once. It takes some time and effort—and it is worth it.

Poisons. *Any household chemicals and cleaning substances should be considered dangerous.* Some are too toxic to have at all and should be thrown away. A good example of useless but dangerous chemicals are the so-called household disinfectants like Lysol and Hexol; I can think of no situations where you need anything stronger than soap or detergent and water to deal with germs around the house. An even nastier group of potential poisons are liquid polishes and waxes that include hydrocarbon solvents; these are capable of causing particularly unpleasant cases of lung damage if consumed. Use foam or paste waxes if you want gleaming furniture. If you really need very dangerous substances like lye, drain openers, acetone, or paint thinner, they must literally be locked up. Have a fail-safe system with dangerous chemicals up and out or reach, and also behind a latched door. Safety latches are available in hardware stores; they are a bother for the adults, and they don't work all that well, but they are better than nothing.

Every household must have **syrup of ipecac** available in a designated place known to all of the adult caretakers. It can't help if it's hidden. Syrup of ipecac causes vomiting. It should *not* be given if the child has taken a hydrocarbon like paint thinner or turpentine, or a caustic such as lye. For other poisons, give 1 to 2 teaspoons per dose for babies under 1 year, a tablespoon for small children; a second dose can be given if vomiting has not occurred within 15 or 20 minutes. Activated charcoal is an antidote commonly used in emergency rooms. It works by adsorbing poisons in the stomach and then carrying them through the gut in a harmless form. Unfortunately, it is not a really practical material for home use; the stuff looks like dirt, and children are, not surprisingly, resistant to drinking it.

It is absolutely essential to know ahead of time how you will handle a possible poisoning. Talk to your doctor about this: Does she want you to call her first, or after you have given ipecac? Or should you call the local poison control center or the hospital emergency room? Who gets called if your doctor is not available? This is a situation where you need prompt and knowledgeable advice available 24 hours a day.

Dangerous Small Objects. Everything goes into the mouths of babies, and some of what goes in can plug up the airway. Keeping hazardous objects out of their reach is no small task. The rule of the Consumer Products Safety Act is a good place to look for guidance. Recent studies have shown that even larger objects can sometimes cause fatal choking. ***Avoid any objects smaller than 1³⁄₄ inches in diameter and shorter than 3 inches.*** Ball-shaped objects are more dangerous than irregular shapes. **Balloons** are probably the most hazardous of all children's toys, not only for small babies but for toddlers and older children. A piece of balloon is easily inhaled and will block the child's airway.

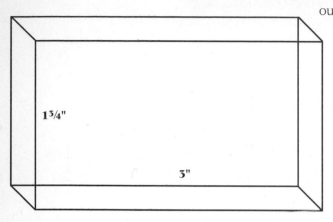

1³⁄₄"

3"

Get used to keeping a sharp eye out for all sorts of household objects; toys, marbles, little balls, and whatever else finds its way into the paths of crawlers and toddlers. Please take the time to bend over, pick them up, and put these potential killers out of reach.

Electrical Hazards. The risk of an electric burn from wall sockets is really quite small, unless you provide him with a slender metal probe to make contact. Even baby fingers are too large to push into those tiny slots, which is a good thing because the little plastic wall socket covers are largely useless; babies love to remove them. The real threat in most houses is the **electric cord** which can be picked up and chewed. The resultant mouth and lip destruction is serious. Electric cords within reach of babies and small children should be attached flush to adjacent walls or baseboards; use insulated electrician's staples or heavy tape.

Breakables. The safest approach is to store breakables out of the child's reach. An inexperienced and optimistic parent or a parent trying to hold on to a semblance of a prechild, civilized ambiance may believe that careful supervision of the baby will suffice. "Why, I never let her out of my sight!" This approach fails.

EVERYDAY PEDIATRICS FOR PARENTS

Stairs. Automatic door closers are easily installed. Install them. Sturdy gates are life saving. Use them. Make sure that the baby can't fall through the banisters.

Windows and Doors. Safety glass or tempered glass should be installed in any window or glass door that could be fallen against or run into. This is expensive, but it can avoid some even more expensive lacerations. Sometimes furniture can be positioned to minimize the risk of collisions with dangerous glass, but this is a less certain measure. Children can be protected from falling out of windows by simple devices that limit the size of the window opening.

Hot Water. Turn the heater control as low as possible to minimize the danger of scalds. The temperature should be 120° F maximum. This sometimes means that the household runs out of hot water, but it avoids potentially devastating burns.

Heating System. Free standing stoves and heaters may need a protective fence. Hardware or building supply stores are good sources of fencing material. Floor furnaces are a hazard in older houses. The illustration shows how to construct a simple wooden cage to keep the baby from stepping or falling on the hot metal grid.

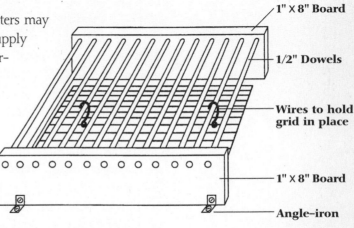

1" X 8" Board

1/2" Dowels

Wires to hold grid in place

1" X 8" Board

Angle–iron

Outside. Gardens need to be free of attractive pelleted snail poison; all garden poisons should be stored in a safe place. The presence of poisonous plants will vary depending on where you live. Your local county agricultural agent and local plant nurseries are good sources of information. A secure fence and gate makes outside play possible with less adult supervision.

Making the household environment safe is a major undertaking and a continuing problem. Kids get increasingly adept at finding the dangerous places and objects in the house. Even in very cautious families, hazards will creep back in as the first child gets older and more trustworthy. You have to start from scratch with each new baby.

Chapter 10

Age 6 to 9 Months

Growth and Development

As the baby enters the second half of his first year, rapid changes are evident in every developmental area. Most are welcome and wonderful, but a few are not. These include stranger anxiety, increased clinginess alternating with increased independence, and sleep fighting.

In the preceding chapter I mentioned that many children begin to be shy with strangers late in their first half year. It is even more likely to appear during the second half year, although an occasional baby does not show any shyness until about age 1½ years. It is remarkable that this is nearly always limited to adults; the delight and fascination with which infants view children and adolescents hardly wavers during the period when most babies are quite cautious with unfamiliar grownups. Some infants are selective and may be shy only with men or people with dark skin or deep voices. There are a few babies who reject all human contact except with their mothers during the height of this phase. This can lead to hurt feelings on the part of fathers and grandparents for a few weeks or even months.

At about the same time, you will see the ambivalence with which the newly mobile infant explores her world. She crawls daringly away, discovers that the adults are no longer in sight, and either retreats or wails. She may be brave enough to move out of the room, away from her adult caretaker, but she will object if the adult leaves her for an instant. This phase passes, just as the stranger shyness will pass, but it can get pretty wearing until the baby grows into the next, braver period.

Sleep fighting seems like a different matter. These are the babies who decide that if they go down for a nap or go to sleep at night they will miss something interesting. They yawn and rub their eyes and try to stay awake by main force. When they are put down, they scream in what sounds like rage, rather than fear or loneliness. If you recognize this as an example of infant bad judgment, and enforce the naps and the usual evening bedtime, your baby will rapidly agree to abide by the house rules. Unfortunately, in many families the baby stays up as late as the adults; everyone has an infant-centered evening, and the mother and father never have a peaceful, adult minute together. A few years like this can be tough on a marriage.

EVERYDAY PEDIATRICS FOR PARENTS

Physical skills are moving along rapidly. This is the age when most babies learn to sit up without support. They can turn over both ways, belly to back and back to belly, creep or roll towards a goal, manipulate objects with both hands, and play with their feet. Many babies are pulling to standing, and some are cruising around furniture with a side-stepping motion. Some are crawling and a few are actually walking.

A few comments are in order concerning crawling. There is no precise timetable for the acquisition of this skill, nor is there a specific, approved technique which must be used. Some infants crawl neatly and rapidly on hands and knees by age 4 or 5 months. Other babies discover alternative methods of transportation and never really bother to crawl at all. My oldest daughter learned to move efficiently around our rug-free apartment on her bottom, using a wonderful one-legged method as if she were propelling a scooter without wheels. We hardly ever saw her crawl, and she graduated directly to normal walking. I mention this because of the cockamamie notion of the importance of what is termed cross-patterned crawling: right arm and left leg forward at the same time, followed by left arm and right leg together. Some years ago, someone promulgated the theory that failure to crawl in this fashion would make it difficult for the child to learn to read and write. Like other bits of pseudoscientific folklore, it stuck in our collective consciousness like a fish bone in the throat: hard to swallow but equally hard to get rid of.

Toys and Playmates. The exploration of her world continues to top every baby's agenda. She can now explore more distant parts of her environment and she does so with enthusiasm. This includes chewing on fallen leaves and the dog's tail, finger painting with her pureed fruit, studying the interesting sounds obtained by banging toys on hard objects, and a host of other simple but necessary tactics which will help her learn about the physical nature of her surroundings.

Toys have a rather small role in all this. Balls, rattles, and other simple toys are of some interest, but babies don't require complicated devices deliberately designed for "play." Despite this inexpensive reality, the toy industry spews out a vast variety of playthings allegedly made for this age group. Many of these objects are labeled as "learning toys," and this claim is just as suspect as it was regarding the toys offered for younger infants. This mass of plastic junk is probably not actively harmful for infant development. An argument might even be made that it is a useful and effective introduction to the television world which will engulf most slightly older American babies. Like television, junk toys are bright, noisy, and generally useless. Also like television, the toy industry's products will tend to replace more valuable and spontaneous experiences which the child could structure for herself.

Playmates of similar ages are obviously a major part of the lives of older children. For most 6 to 9-month old infants this is not yet the case. Babies pay remarkably little attention to other babies, even when they share the same crib or playpen. Observing my two sets of identical twin granddaughters has been instructive to me in this regard. Sophie would crawl right over Reta on the way to a desired toy without seeming to take notice of the difference between her sister and any other impediment to locomotion. Kate would play peacefully alongside of Emma even when Emma was crying piteously about some obscure personal problem. Later in the first year babies begin to be more interested in their age mates, but before then not much social interaction is visible.

Language. As is true for so many areas of development, the acquisition of language is another wonderfully variable process. The sequence is certainly predictable; cooing and other random sounding noises, then babbling and screeching in a kind of experimental mode. Later come single syllables of no particular meaning, jabbering in what almost sounds like a private language, then imitating and using simple words. Most infants have at least one reasonably clear word by 1 year of age; it is most often "dada," or the name of a family pet, or a word indicating breast or bottle. Interestingly, "mama" is only rarely the first word. My own theory about the frequent choice of "dada" is that it has had survival value for infants as evidence to generations of fathers of their specific paternity. "Listen to that! He knows me!" Mothers, in contrast, already have adequate information concerning their biological links with their babies and do not stand in need of reassurance about the fact.

The variability in language is mostly in the speed with which this process unfolds. Some babies are actually speaking sentences before age 1; others have no understandable speech at all until late in the second year. Both of these patterns can be completely normal. A distinction needs to be drawn between what the baby understands and the language the baby uses. Some infants understand a great deal but say next to nothing. Nor is it always easy to determine how much a baby actually hears since they pick up a great deal of information from cues other than words; they read our gestures, tone of voice, and the social context as well as the words themselves. This can be remarkably misleading. I recall a family of two profoundly deaf parents who were unaware that one of their children was hard-of-hearing because he could understand and respond so accurately to his environment. What follows from all of this is that speech acquisition deserves experienced observation. An important aspect of well child care at your doctor's office is the evaluation of your baby's ability to hear, understand, and use language.

Teething

Like everything else in physical growth, the timing of the tooth eruption is inconstant. The first baby teeth may already have erupted at the time of birth; fortunately for the comfort of nursing mothers this is a great rarity. Generally, the first teeth come through the gums at around 6 months of age. The lower central front teeth, the central incisors, are usually first, and the rest of the teeth follow slowly. By the end of the first year most kids have all 8 incisors and perhaps a lower molar or two.

One of the abiding controversies among parents, pediatricians, and other observers of early childhood is whether teething causes uncomfortable symptoms for the child. This may seem to be a truly stupid question to the parent whose child has been miserable or feverish every time a new tooth is about to appear. However, the reluctance of some physicians to attribute symptoms to teething has respectable roots. In an earlier age, doctors as well as everyone else blamed teething for a wide variety of ills now clearly understood to have other causes. In the nineteenth century it was commonplace to describe "teething convulsions" and even to list teething as a cause of death. Most of us would prefer not to repeat this kind of error. More importantly, we don't want other symptoms to be overlooked by parents because they are assumed to be teething related. Having said all that, it is appropriate to aver that teething can certainly cause discomfort. There is sometimes quite evident local tenderness around the nearly but not quite erupted tooth. Some children have a runny nose for a few days before every new tooth, others have a touch of loose stools, and a few actually run a degree or two of measurable fever. Many kids are just nonspecifically grumpy.

It is not always easy to be sure that a tooth *is* about to erupt. If you watch the gums of babies at this age you may see a definite swelling appear where the tooth will eventually break through. When the tooth nears the inner surface of the gum you may be able to see that the ridge on the biting edge of the gum has begun to disappear; it is as if it is being erased from the inside. Sometimes a red or purple discoloration will appear where a few drops of blood escape into the tissues of the gum. None of this means much, and none of it predicts how soon a tooth will actually come through. They appear in their own good time without any assistance.

Treatment for the miscellaneous miseries of teething should be tailored to the patient. If there is significant fussiness or fever, acetaminophen by mouth is remarkably helpful. For some reason, tooth discomfort seems to worsen at night. A dose of acetaminophen at bedtime and perhaps again every 4 hours if your baby awakens is often a good idea. Don't bother rubbing acetaminophen on the gums; it has no local anesthetic effect. In fact, local applications like teething lotions are rarely much help because all they do is numb the outer surface of the gum; the discomfort is caused by pressure from the inside. Counter pressure from a teething ring or a little gentle massage of the area around the tooth seems to calm some infants. Any teething-associated drippy noses or loose stools will not amount to much and do not require any treatment. Interestingly, teething symptoms tend to become less troublesome as children get older. Most of the teeth erupting after the first year come in unheralded by any complaint.

Feeding

The infant's diet is gradually expanding to include most if not all of the adult family diet. Most babies accept a broad range of foods with interest and enthusiasm, which helps set the stage for parental concern in the second or third year when preferences tend to narrow. A major change is the increasing proportion of finger-fed food as the baby masters the thumb-fingers pincer grasp. At this point a fascinating process begins which is important as a paradigm for much larger issues. Until now the feeding relationship between infant and adult has been characterized by the baby providing cues regarding his needs which the adult attempts to identify and satisfy. As he begins to graduate to self feeding, the baby begins to make a different set of choices and give a new and variable set of cues. It is no longer a matter of "I'm hungry, please feed me." Now it is sometimes "I'm hungry, but I prefer to feed myself." He may show this by turning his head away from the spoonful of food, or by grabbing it in midair, or by burying both hands in the bowl of cereal. Of course, the simple and appropriate adult response is to increase the availability of finger foods, and gradually phase out adult controlled spoon feeding. For a few months, until he can use a spoon himself, the infant can do very nicely with finger foods as the sole solids.

Unfortunately but understandably, many parents react with a combination of resentment and discomfort. Your roles are being transformed; you are no longer wholly in charge. Not only is it hard to give up control to the baby, but it is natural to be concerned that finger feeding will be inadequate to your child's nutritional needs. "If he feeds himself, it all goes on the floor" is a common theme and this is often the case. No question about it, self-feeding is a real mess in its early stages, and total caloric intake may dip for a few weeks. Still, the most important issue is the beginning of the transfer of power. Here begins the process of our children's inevitable growth towards independence, and so begins the concern it evokes in us. What applies here is **Grossman's Law of Childhood Autonomy: *We parents have only 18 or so years to turn over full responsibility to a child.*** The transition to self feeding is an excellent place to start weaning ourselves from full control of the child's life.

This is also the age when babies are introduced to the cup; a variety of lipped, beaked, and covered cups have been devised to make the learning process less messy. Years ago, a wise mother taught me an alternative strategy that bypasses these transitional devices: Give the baby a small, unbreakable cup to use at the beginning of his bath. He can practice drinking clean bath water to his heart's content without anyone being concerned about spills. (I know, I already mentioned this in Chapter 6 - Feeding Your Baby, but some readers may have forgotten or worse—maybe some of you skipped it.)

Safety. I'm sorry to have to mention this again, but it's time. Have you instituted the safety measures I suggested in the preceding chapter? What, they haven't been completed? You haven't bought the syrup of ipecac yet? Why not?

And What About the Rest of the Family? For many families, the chaos of the early months of the baby's first year has settled down to a busy but tolerable routine. The older kids have figured out reasonable methods of adaptation to the newcomer, and the parents may be getting a glimmer of normal adult existence from time to time. If your family is still in turmoil it may be time to figure out why and do something about it. Parents' groups can be a big help in finding solutions to everyday problems. So can family doctors, pediatricians, and therapists of one kind or another. No matter what the nature of the difficulty you and your family are facing, remember that other families have faced something quite similar—and survived. None of us are required to reinvent the wheel.

Chapter 11

Age 9 to 12 Months

Growth and Development

Somewhere around the end of the first year, a qualitative leap from baby to toddler occurs. You might have noted a similar though less dramatic change a few months earlier, when increased social responsiveness and physical skills transformed him from an infant to an older baby. This may sound a little nonsensical but it is significant. These seemingly abrupt developmental changes continue to occur all through childhood, and through adult life as well, for that matter. We codify these differing levels of personal organization as "stages," and they help us to understand and predict a variety of behavioral changes. The risk of thinking in these terms is that we become so pleased with the concept that we try to fit each child and her behaviors into the age-appropriate stage, instead of observing the ways in which she may not fit the stage at all. It should be obvious that general descriptive statements will not do justice to the variability of human beings. Having sounded this warning against an incautious use of the idea of stages, I must say that I find them useful. They remind me that development is, to an extent, predictable, that certain patterns of family struggle can be expected to arise and to subside, and that changes from one stage to the next seem to occur as discrete events. We see this when we watch our kids acquire a new skill; the child changes in one day from the status of nonswimmer to that of swimmer; the nonreader suddenly gets the idea and becomes a reader. To the observer it seems that a reorganization has happened, rather than an incremental process. It is just the same with stages; the baby is all of a sudden a child; the child is all of a sudden a "Terrible Two." When we become aware that baby has disappeared, having been replaced by small child, we need to reformulate our expectations and start to deal with the new set of challenges and opportunities provided by the new person.

Changes in speech and understanding can be dramatic at the end of the first year. Many toddlers have a few words, and many more have considerable understanding, both of words and of nonverbal forms of communication. Although their attention span is not very long, most children this age enjoy being read to from baby books. Physical skills are also changing; they generally sit solidly, pull to standing, and cruise around furniture. Crawling up stairs and climbing furniture are popular although sometimes hazardous pastimes. Many

EVERYDAY PEDIATRICS FOR PARENTS

10 to 12-month olds are trying to walk, and a fair number have already mastered the skill. A few are already running.

Setting Limits

With this age group comes the necessity of setting limits to the activities of our increasingly mobile and infinitely curious children. The task of teaching children the rules for survival in the home and in society must be met in every culture. For the parents of an intrusive 9 to 12-month old, this generally translates into saying "NO!" about ninety times a day. It also means providing a safe environment, which will somewhat decrease the number of "no's." But there will be some situations where *enforcing* a limit is imperative.

Parents must decide what limits to set with each child. Typically, the rules are most stringent with the firstborn. This is largely because inexperienced parents suffer from unrealistic goals, and have no idea how hard it is to keep kids in line. "You never let me get away with that!" is the accurate complaint of every eldest child as she watches her little sister's mischief go unchecked. Every family develops its own set of house rules regarding the limits of acceptable behavior. Not infrequently, there are actually two sets of rules, Dad's and Mom's. This makes life decidedly more complicated for everyone and is certainly worth avoiding if you can. But the rules by which we would like our families to live are clear expressions of who we are as human beings. It is not easy to tailor your views to anyone else's expectations, even when the other person is your spouse. Try to set rules which honestly reflect your individual and particular values, patterns and prejudices. If this means that your family has two sets of nonidentical rules, your children will learn to navigate among them, one way or another.

The Usefulness of Temper Tantrums. When the first limits are set, the first temper tantrum is not far behind. Temper tantrums are the least appreciated and, I believe, potentially among the most valuable learning experiences of early childhood. When a child wants something forbidden, a sequence of events may develop which carry considerable pedagogical impact. A sample scenario: I want to play with the nice, shiny knife. My mother removes it from my reach. I get furious and scream. My mother comments that she is sorry that I'm angry, but knives are not for babies to play with. I get even angrier, throw myself to the floor and scream louder. Nothing happens! I don't get the knife, no one seems terribly upset that I am so mad, and I get over my anger and find something else to do. If I'm really upset, I may go over to Mom for a hug. And

I begin to learn that 1) there are limits in my world, some things I cannot do; 2) Mom is still in charge; 3) when I'm frustrated I get very angry, express my anger and get over it; 4) expressing my feelings is safe, even feelings that are powerful and unpleasant. Well, this ideal sequence is my fantasy of what can be learned through a few years of temper tantrums. I don't mean to suggest that you need go out of your way to provoke unnecessary tantrums in your children; there will be plenty of opportunities without advance planning. But when a tantrum erupts, it can be allowed to run its course rather than cut short by punishment or placating parental intervention.

I've dwelt on this at length because tantrums are usually discussed as if they were somehow undesirable for the child to experience. They are certainly experienced by parents as unnerving and often embarrassing. The glares of the lady in the grocery store clearly convey her judgment: "Can't that woman control her spoiled little brat?" I'm afraid there is no protection from the opinions of the grocery store public. Still, I continue to wonder why those who want parents to avoid or control temper tantrums fail to appreciate their valuable aspects. I can't imagine a better place to start dealing with the subject of frustration and anger than in the family, as a small child. If not then, when?

Learning About Limits. Setting limits for children at this age involves teaching the child that certain actions are forbidden on pain of parental disapproval. Some babies are wonderfully responsive to these lessons; a mild sharpness of tone or a small scowl will occasionally convince a girl (much more rarely, a boy) that a limit must be recognized and obeyed. At the other end of the spectrum are the fairly numerous children who never really seem to internalize rules; I presume that they end up mugging pedestrians or selling junk bonds to widows and orphans. For most kids it takes 3 or 4 years to build a moderately reliable inner voice that says "I can't do that." Your best tools in this undertaking are verbal—a good, sharp "NO!"—and physical removal (separating child from the forbidden object or person). This presents an excellent opportunity to practice acknowledging your child's feelings. "You really want to pull the control knobs off the TV, but Daddy doesn't want you to, and you can't." He won't understand the words, but he'll hear the music. The next step is isolation; children truly hate this, so it works. Fritz Redl, the Viennese psychologist who pioneered psychotherapy with delinquent youth, put it succinctly: To set a limit or punish a child you must get his attention. If he is not somewhat shaken up (psychologically, not physically), he will not notice. Does this sound unduly harsh? After all, we are talking about charming little toddlers.

EVERYDAY PEDIATRICS FOR PARENTS

I think that the underlying theory is the same at any age: Get the kid's attention, make it clear that the behavior is unacceptable and the consequences unpleasant. There are remarkably few alternatives to this method.

The practice of hitting children is often tempting for the parent, especially during the witching hours of late afternoon when everyone is likely to be tired, overwrought, and hungry. In the very short run, hitting works; it does get the child's attention. But in the longer run, the disadvantages of corporal punishment outweigh its attractions. Unhappily, it teaches the lesson that big people hit little people and get away with it, not a lesson that you really want to inculcate in your children. Furthermore, repeated physical punishment, short of real child abuse, loses its importance; the usual swat on the bottom comes to be discounted by the recipient. Professor Edwards Park is said to have remarked that in order to be effective, a spanking had to be in the nature of a treat; that is to say, something unexpected and rare. The only other alternative is reasoned discourse, but you will discover that very small children cannot be convinced by logical arguments alone. Sometime after age 3 years, explanations may help a parent to enforce the family rules. If the words are kept simple and reinforced with the old methods of removal and isolation, talking is worth a try. Until then, such attempts are generally useless.

Learning and Play. Toward the end of the first year, the hints of personality pattern which were noted in early infancy are becoming powerfully evident. This is nowhere more visible than in the baby's play. By this age each child has his own personal approach to the world. Clear preferences are becoming evident in choices of toys, style of approach to the household environment, attention span for an activity, response to frustration when an object fails to do whatever the infant had in mind for it, and need for adult attention. The best reason to categorize children along these or other dimensions is because it may help us to perceive and appreciate the wonderful differences our children express. Many of us begin the process of parenthood with strongly held notions of how we want our children to develop. The feedback provided by the baby can make clear that there are limits set by the child's innate disposition to the achievement of the parental fantasy. I began to understand this when my wife and I gave toy cars and trucks to our firstborn daughter; she was perfectly pleasant about rejecting them, but reject them she did. When little boys of the same age were given her toys, they not only played with the vehicles, they accompanied their play with automotive sound effects. After seeing this in a few dozen babies, I became open to the possibility of sexually determined differences in infant behavior. This was a hard lesson for me to learn as a parent because it failed to confirm my former prejudice that most differences between boys and girls were culturally imposed. Other parents will have other prejudices and may also find it difficult to accept the disparity between expectation and reality.

Feeding

As the end of the first year approaches, most infants are increasingly self fed; their fine motor coordination allows enough thumb and finger use for them to eat small pieces of soft table foods. A very few girls will already be using spoons. (Most girls are reasonably adept with utensils by 1½ years, boys a bit later.) At this age growth is proceeding at a slower pace, and consequently the baby actually needs fewer calories per pound of body weight. The parent who has been watching the baby eat more and more may abruptly notice him eating less and less; at least that may appear to be the case. Furthermore, the baby now has quite pronounced food preferences and may vigorously reject what he had previously accepted. He also increasingly demands total physical control of the meal, which automatically excludes all the pureed foods you were accustomed to feeding him, and large amounts of his finger food end up in his bib and on the floor. The net effect of these trends is a quantum jump in parental anxiety about food. It is clear to the parent that, left to his own devices, the baby will never get enough to eat. This is when the following rules may apply. **Grossman's First Law of Toddler Feeding:** *Little children are at least as smart as puppies and, like puppies, will not starve themselves to death.*

Grossman's Second Law of Toddler Feeding: *The acquisition of self-feeding skills is a model for the gradual shift of power from parents to child.* It is a safe time and place for you to practice giving some responsibility to the baby, and it is good for everyone. If you prize neatness at the table you will have a particularly hard time with this transitional process. Tuna fish on the cheeks and cottage cheese used as a hair mousse are unattractive at best, but this is not the age to worry about table manners. **Grossman's Third Law of Toddler Feeding:** *The best antidote to parental feeding anxiety is an adequate repertoire of finger foods.* Foods which require a spoon must temporarily be abandoned. Happily, there is a substantial list of alternatives. Finger-feeding babies do best with raw or cooked fruits, soft cooked vegetables, small pieces of soft meats such as chicken, hamburger, ham, sausage, and fish, lumpy scrambled eggs, cheeses, all kinds of pasta, cooked dry legumes, soybean curd, dry cereals like Cheerios or Chex, and all kinds of breads or crackers. Small sandwiches made with avocado, nut butters, liverwurst, or anything else that will stick to the bread are usually happily consumed. Reheating leftover meat and vegetables from last night's adult dinner is a good idea since most infants will have their last meal before the grownups are ready to eat theirs. From this generous list the baby will develop a modestly sized group of favorite foods; it may appear unduly restricted in terms of adult preferences, but it works fine for the baby. In the diet of the American toddler, the only nutrients likely to be deficient are vitamin C and iron, both of which are present in breast milk and modern infant formulas but absent from fresh milk. These are easily supplied: vitamin C from oranges, tomatoes, potatoes, melons, berries, leafy greens, and other green vegetables; iron from meats, eggs, cereals and cereal-based foods, legumes, nuts and nut butters, and a little from leafy greens. It is exceptional to need a supplemental chemical source unless the diet is restricted for medical or other reasons.

Chapter 12

Age 1 to 2 Years

Growth and Development

During the first year of life babies acquire their new physical skills at their own individual rates. Babies all have their own timetables, and by the beginning of the second year the rate of development of each child's physical skills has become apparent. The range of variation among children is striking. Some is familial: Certain families seem to have powerful patterns of slow or fast acquisition of skills. Some is pathological: Slow development is occasionally a symptom of some underlying disorder. But mostly the variation is random, without real significance except as a source of parental pride or worry. In our competitive society it is easy and natural to enroll our infants in an imagined Baby Olympics. We inevitably compare our own children with each other, as well as with all the other children we know. Comparing kids is hard to avoid, but I think it is useless and often harmful. Kids get the message that their worth is somehow measured only in comparison with others. We must not become so focused on rank-ordering our children that we lose sight of the individuality and value of each child.

Each of these skills has its own wide and rather fuzzy range of normal. Most babies turn over (at least from belly to back) by about age 6 months, but some soft, fat infants don't manage this until 8 or 9 months. Sitting alone can vary from younger than 5 months to as old as 10 months. Crawling on hands and knees (or hands and feet) can start by 5 months but 6 to 9 months is usual. Pulling to standing is another skill which may be mastered as early as 6 months, or it may not appear until the second year. The skill to which most of us parents pay the closest attention is walking; it can be seen at 6 months, is usually happening somewhere around 12 to 14 months, but can be delayed in normal children up to 18 months or more. What is most important about all this is the *whole* pattern of development, physical, social, and intellectual. The baby who is slow in all areas becomes a cause for concern, whereas the baby who is slow only in physical skills is quite likely to be a normal variant.

Language

Most infants have some *passive* language late in the first year; they are likely to understand the names of important people, pets, and objects. Infants begin to use speech *actively* a bit later; first words may appear as early as 6 to 8 months but more commonly just before 1 year. During the second year most speech is in the form of single words; phrases and sentences appear later that year or not until age 2. During this time the child's passive vocabulary is expanding rapidly; even without the help of nonverbal information, the child understands a great deal of what is heard. Stop and consider the common practice of speaking "over the heads" of our toddlers and young children. We all get in the habit of talking in the presence of our babies as if they were not there, and it is easy to ignore the changing reality that their understanding is increasing by leaps and bounds. Sometime during the second year, and probably much earlier for verbally proficient children, this assumption becomes quite mistaken. When I hear a darling little 18-month old say "Oh, shit!" I assume that some important adult in her life has ignored the ease and avidity of her acquisition of new words. An interesting corollary of this is seen in the bilingual or trilingual family. Kids initially manage two languages quite well; they will often ignore a third language. Eventually one usually sees the child preferring the language of its peers. Many children in foreign language-speaking families will refuse to speak their mother tongue after a few years, although they continue to hear and understand it at home.

In recent years there has been an upsurge of interest in the nature of human speech and the way in which children acquire language. It is becoming evident that our brains are cunningly and effectively designed for the understanding and production of speech. Given a reasonable amount of input—that is, people in the vicinity who talk to each other and to the child— kids master language automatically. Because it matters to them that they understand, they attend to their environments, and by golly, they learn to talk! Thus, parents who do not have to have an advanced degree in linguistics still manage to produce verbally proficient children. So, doubtless it is wise to talk to them, even before they *seem* to pay much attention. And it is certainly sensible to pay attention to their verbal productions, even when you are unsure of their meaning. However, you are not required to provide a complex curriculum of language learning opportunities.

Individuation. The child's sense of separateness usually becomes apparent in the latter months of the first year. Of course, it's impossible to know what is going on within the minds of small infants, but there does seem to be a necessary progression between the first reality of the fetus's unity with the mother to the later reality of the child's existence apart from her. Watch a baby touching the mother's face or breast, and later, examining his own hands and feet. He sometimes looks as if he were trying to figure out where he begins and she leaves off. As he develops this sense of self, he seems to experiment with the use of his will. Deliberate limit testing is typical. The baby crawls over to the television, puts a hand on the controls and smiles wickedly back at the watching parent as if to say "Are you really going to keep me from playing with this?"

In the second year, many toddlers have come to terms, at least temporarily, with the idea of limits, and some of them appear to be having second thoughts about the wisdom of separateness in general. You will see this in 18-month clinginess, a common although not universal phenomenon. This is a passing phase about which you need do nothing at all except live through it. However, it is worth mentioning that a small number of children take many years to come to terms with separateness. These are the shy babies who stay shy. Their stranger shyness in middle infancy is prolonged, painful, and close to universal. They may be terribly well behaved because they are too frightened to test limits at all. More often than not, the shy child learns to cope with society and moves out into the world with increasing ease. If this does not happen, medical and psychological evaluation is a wise idea.

Playmates

Watching babies during the first year, one gets the impression that they pretty much ignore one another. They are nearly always intensely interested in older children and in adults, but regard their age mates as if they are saying to themselves "There's nothing this little baby can teach me." By the end of the first year some babies will engage in parallel play: two or more infants each independently involved in a common play situation. Even in these situations, infants often treat each other as just another inanimate object of no special importance. Sometime during the second year this begins to change. There are several factors determining the development of peer relationships. Foremost is the individual child's own social style. An outgoing, ebullient, fearless toddler will approach another child with obvious interest or with the clear intent to appropriate a desirable toy. The second factor is turf: I'm a lot braver in my own home. I will protect my toys from foreign incursion, but I may tolerate or even enjoy the presence of a another toddler, as long as he keeps a respectful distance from my favorite teddy bear and my blankie. The last factor is familiarity. If toddlers see each other at least every week there is a real possibility of developing continuing relationships and play patterns. Two or three times a week is even better. Some of the early students of child development thought that real play between children did not start until age 2 or 3 years. I suspect this misapprehension was caused by watching children who were strangers to each other in unfamiliar settings.

When real interactive play develops, it quickly leads to real interactive fighting, pushing, shoving, and biting. It takes a considerable time for the young of our species to figure out that peace is wonderful. This should come as no surprise; the evidence from human history suggests that many of the older members of Homo sapiens have yet to gain this insight. Can we adults speed the process for our children? Yes, but it is tricky. There is no point in expecting mature patterns of sweetly collaborative play in early childhood. Children can learn to share and take turns, but these are painful lessons, reluctantly absorbed. Cooperative behavior techniques developed in the former Soviet Union many years ago might make an interesting experiment. In Soviet nursery schools some of the toys were constructed so that they were usable only if a group of kids pooled their efforts to move the toy train or manipulate the dump truck. The theory was that children would generalize the lesson that cooperation was a good idea. I have no idea whether this attempt succeeded. When competition and aggression rear their ugly heads, the question faced by the adult overseers is whether to intervene with soft words and firm separation, or to let the kids work it out themselves with teeth, fists, and screams. The answer may depend, to a degree, on circumstances. I recall a mother in my practice who told me what had happened to her 3-year old daughter. The child came into the house one morning, crying bitterly because an older girl had hit her and taken her ball. Her mother said "I shoved her back out the door and told her not to come home until she had beaten up the other kid and gotten her ball back. She stood on the stoop and screamed and cried a while, and then she went on up the street, found the other girl, hit her good, and took back her ball." I suppose my amazement and dismay showed pretty clearly on my face, because she went on to explain that in the rough part of town where they lived, one such defeat for a child would have marked her as a permanent victim. It was, she knew, a harsh lesson, but it was a necessary one. Solutions of this type may not be needed for families whose living situations are less difficult. However, there is something to be said for letting kids experience the rough edges of interpersonal behavior without instant adult intervention.

Is there any particular advantage to a child in providing him with companions of his own age during the first years? I don't see that it makes much difference. The child raised with other children certainly becomes acculturated into the life of his peers earlier than the child raised only among adults, but what's the hurry? Kids learn soon enough the rules of interchild activity. Furthermore, the child raised among many children will inevitably have less adult attention, and it is from adults that the small child has the most to learn about the larger world. I suppose if one is attempting to raise a child with the most sharply honed peer-relationship skills, then early and intense peer contact makes sense. Otherwise, the amount of time with other infants and toddlers is an issue of no great weight.

Sleep

The good Lord in His wisdom has decreed that toddlers still need naps, thereby assuring their caretakers some time to brush their hair, or go the toilet, or even eat a delayed breakfast. Unhappily, the timing and number of the naps at this age is becoming somewhat unpredictable. The transition between 2 naps and 1 nap per day has probably already taken place, but when the child is on the cusp and can't seem to settle on one pattern or the other, the family will experience a few weeks or months of temporal confusion. I don't believe that there is any way of hurrying this process along. Some parents truly need consistent structure in family life and if their children happen to be reasonably malleable, they will successfully impose a solution that works for them. "It's 1 o'clock; therefore, you are tired, and I am going to put you down for a nice nap." But even households where the kids fall asleep at odd and unusual hours, whether it suits the adults or not, a pattern emerges eventually.

As is often the case, the worst problems arise when the needs of parents and kids are not well matched. Sometimes the parents who crave order are blessed with a vigorously independent and not very tired toddler. These folks may find themselves engaged in a fruitless battle if they try to impose a nap when it is neither wanted nor needed. On the other hand, more laid-back parents may be so solicitous of their child's wishes and whims that they fail to see the clear signs of exhaustion that signal the need for some peace and quiet. It is important to recognize when our kids are making a ritual complaint of no real significance. The child who always cries piteously when it is clearly time for a nap will generally stop in a few minutes after being put to bed. His tears should be seen as a mild and unsuccessful attempt at manipulation, one of the favorite and most successful pastimes of the young.

Of course, nap times are not the only possible battlegrounds pertaining to sleep. Bedtime at night may still (or again) be an issue during the second year. Several factors can intersect around the question of when and how a child goes to sleep. Family expectations vary widely depending on ethnic and cultural patterns, socioeconomic class, degree of family organization, number of adults available to help, and the psychological needs and beliefs of the parents. Some cultures make no hard and fast distinction between the generations in regard to participation in "adult" activities. The children are expected to be present at all kinds of events from which middle class Americans would doubtless exempt them. This is partly a matter of space: If you live in one room, your children will be present, awake or asleep, a very great deal of the time. The phenomenon of two overworked parents also bears on the question of hours of sleep. Parents who are away from their children 10 or 12 or 14 hours a day are torn by their own conflicting needs. They want quiet time for themselves, time to renew acquaintance with their spouses, time to do the necessary household chores, and also time to be with the kids they are working so long and hard to support. It's hard to be firm about your child's bedtime when you have barely seen her all day. The combination of exhaustion, guilt, and deprivation of the opportunity to be a real, present-for-the-child mommy or daddy can be unutterably painful. The result is a parent who gives the child wildly ambivalent messages about sleep. If you say "I guess it's time for you to go to bed, okay, honey?" your child will accurately note the unsureness of "I guess" and the question "Okay, honey?" Given that information, most kids will decide that they would rather stay up. If you say " It's time to go to bed," you may or may not get an argument, but at least you will not have invited one.

Even when you are quite sure about the necessity of bedtime and present the child with a united front, the child may demur. With her newly found ability to climb out of bed and wander back to the more interesting precincts of family life, the toddler poses new problems of control. For the majority of kids, the simple act of returning them to bed a few times will suffice. They get the message that bedtime is really bedtime; there is no point in engaging in a struggle about it, so they may as well go to sleep when they are told to. Parents often inadvertantly sabotage this process by granting one more story or offering compromises that reward the resistant behavior. If the child is reasonably sure that Mom or Dad will accompany him back to bed, and keep him company while he falls asleep, why not give it a try? This can become a major area of disagreement between parents, which most kids will exploit with great vigor.

What about the child whose stubborn insistence on fighting bedtime is *not* reversed by the usual routines of being returned to bed without rewards of any sort? The temptation to inflict some sort of punishment is by no means unusual; tired adults can get pretty cranky. But effective punishment of toddlers is a rather limited business. After all, what can you do? Inflicting harsh words or worse seems a poor way to end the child's day. About the only effective method is to provide a physical barrier to egress from the child's bedroom. The idea of locking a small child in her room at bedtime will strike many parents as cruel and will undoubtedly be experienced by many children as terrifying. The compromise that often works well is a stout gate or a Dutch half-door with a sturdy latch. This allows the child to understand that she has not been abandoned, and that her complaints can still be heard by the grownups, even though she has to remain in her room. I think this kind of barrier works because it is a palpable symbol of parental control. We parents sometimes forget how much our children need to have the sense that we are in charge, with the obvious implications that we know what is best for them, and that we will protect them when we must from their own immature impulses. There are many instances in the course of rearing children when your parental role will require that you set limits against which our children will rail. I think being a responsible parent *requires* you to undertake this role. It may strain your sense of faith in your own good judgment, it will not increase your short-term popularity with your kids, and it will force you to believe in their ability to cope with the real world, but setting limits is simply part of the package called being mothers and fathers.

Toilet Training

Every era has its favorite child-rearing problems; in the 1930s and 1940s the central issues were infant feeding and toilet training. Now the popular topic seems to be sleeping through the night. Why have American families become more relaxed about toilet behavior? I think that mastery of the toilet began to be less important when automatic washers and dryers became part of most American homes. As long as she had to rinse, wash, rinse again, wring out, hang up, and dry every single diaper, Mom had plenty of motivation to teach the baby to use the toilet. Now, the pressure is off both baby and parent. With the availability of disposable diapers, diaper services, and home laundries, we can afford to let the child develop the physical control and psychological readiness needed for toileting. This new pattern of patience is by no means uniform. The Chinese grandmothers in my practice still begin toilet training their grandchildren by the middle of the first year and usually have produced perfect stool control by about age 1. Very impressive. I see similar efforts on the part of black grandmothers from the deep South; their methods are different but they also aim for very early control and often attain it. Early training demands intense vigilance; the baby is scooped up and rushed to the toilet at the first hint of an imminent stool. If the infant is resistant, a titanic battle of wills develops with unpredictable results. I think a substantial number of chronically constipated adults are still fighting Grandma when they feel the urge to eliminate.

At the other end of this spectrum are the adults whose message to the child is that it doesn't matter when mature toilet patterns are mastered. This does not seem wise; children need clarity about family expectations in an area where baby behavior is different from adult behavior. Otherwise the implicit message is "We think that you are still a baby."

It is noteworthy that girls are often more interested in toilet training than boys. If one provides her with a floor-based potty chair, the 18-month old may train herself promptly and easily. Then again, she may not, in which case renewed interest may reappear by 2 or 2½ years. Boys are sometimes quite interested in peeing like Daddy, standing up next to the toilet; they enjoy experimenting with urination outside on a lawn or in the dirt. But their enthusiasm

EVERYDAY PEDIATRICS FOR PARENTS

for going in the potty chair may be quite limited; some boys seem clearly to be afraid of the act. One way or another, both boys and girls are usually day-trained for urine by the age of 3; consistent use of the potty for stool often takes a bit longer. Staying dry at night is really a different skill; lots of 4 and 5-year olds are still wet at night, at least part of the time.

So, how are you supposed to toilet train your child? Let me count the ways. Method #1: Train the Kid in 1 Day! This is a truly strange notion. Is there any other developmental skill which we would try to impose and expect to be mastered in 24 hours? I can see the attractiveness of instant training to completely exhausted, overextended parents. If this method seriously tempts you, it might be wisest to take it as a sign that you are too busy by half. Method #2: Do nothing and hope that he will eventually notice that wet and soiled diapers are uncomfortable. As I have already noted, one problem with laissez-faire toilet training is the message "We don't expect age-appropriate behavior from you." Any child who has a reasonable amount of contact with his peers knows who uses the toilet and who does not. If these facts are not apparent to him directly, the other children of his acquaintance will clue him in, usually in a brutally honest fashion. The result of this peer pressure may be self training, but don't count on it. Method #3: Let the other children train the youngest. This method is common in cultures where children of varying ages spend a great deal of time together. It can work very well in large families where the child rearing tasks are shared between parents and elder siblings. Method # 4: Watch for signs that your child is becoming aware of the processes of elimination. It is probably helpful to have talked to your baby about defecating and urinating while you have been cleaning and changing him during the preceding months. His familiarity with the toilet practices of the others in the family will also help. Basically, you are teaching him that there is a sequence of:
1. urge to defecate or urinate,
2. trip to the toilet,
3. the act or acts themselves,
4. a visible and flushable product.

You are also teaching him that this is a desirable set of skills to acquire, and that he will graduate to the exalted status of the Toilet-Trained in due time. Easy access to a potty chair on the floor allows him to become familiar with the requisite machinery. Use it for dry runs, sitting on the pot fully clothed, and for doll or stuffed animal play. When he has become comfortable with the whole idea, seating him on the pot when you sense an imminent act of elimination will often start the ball rolling. Of course, this is easiest for the kids whose elimination has some predictable regularity. For most children, the inner reward of mastery plus the obvious pleasure of the parents at every attempt provide sufficient motivation. But when the process languishes and stalls a set of supplemental, external rewards may be useful. One animal cracker for any attempt whatsoever, two for serious efforts, three for success, for example. This method may be objected to on the grounds that bribery has no place in child rearing, but I think such a puritanical opinion misses the essential difference between a bribe (bad!) and a reward (good!). A bribe, after all, is given to encourage behavior which is really not in the best interests of the recipient, to pervert his behavior, or corrupt his judgment, as the dictionary puts it. A reward, in contrast, is objective evidence of one's otherwise rather abstract approbation; the cookie reinforces the words of praise. When the process of toilet training is completed, the animal crackers are no longer needed.

Unhappily for this pat little story, there are a sizable group of kids who decide that toilet training is part of a plot by the oppressive adult power structure, and they refuse to be co-opted. This kind of decision is likeliest among the most rambunctious and negative Terrible Two population. If this happens in your family, you are probably having so many problems that toilet training may seem like a relatively unimportant question; day to day survival (his and yours) is uppermost in your minds. These children do eventually learn to be housebroken. Peer pressure may do it, or intervention by an adult other than a parent. The child's message in that situation is "I'll do it for my teacher but not for Mommy and Daddy." That's okay, too.

Food

The decrease in appetite which you have probably noted before your child's first birthday has not gone away. Despite his gradually increasing size, the toddler's food requirements hardly increase at all during the second year. Somewhere around 1000 calories per day will nicely meet the needs of most children of this age. By the end of the second year, they may need another couple of hundred calories, which is not a very impressive amount. Furthermore, the 1-year old's appetite often becomes less predictable. Days of heavy eating are sometimes followed by days when he never finishes a meal. Many children begin to exhibit the common pattern of a big breakfast, a fair lunch, and a small or nonexistent dinner. This is actually a reasonable pattern in terms of energy requirements, but it dramatically contrasts with the typical American view that breakfast is a small and unimportant meal, while dinner is, nutritionally speaking, the main event. When the toddler and small child stay out of step with the rest of the family in this fashion, their preferences induce parental anxiety and culinary frustration. If any meal during the day requires significant planning, shopping, and preparation, it is likely to be dinner, and that is likely to be the meal in which toddlers have the least interest. So, expect your young children to eat small dinners, and whenever possible, plan to offer dinner-type food at breakfast or lunch, when it will be more warmly welcomed. This is a remarkably hard lesson for many parents to learn. After all the trouble to which we go to provide a luscious lamb chop, attended by an appropriate sidedish, the kid doesn't touch it and we are justifiably annoyed. A better plan is to save it for next day's lunch, and let him have bread and peanut butter for dinner, instead.

One-year old babies are commonly omnivorous. The rule seems to be "If it doesn't crawl too fast for me, I'll eat it." Early in the second year this satisfying state of affairs is frequently replaced by a fastidious concern for just the right food. First to disappear is the vegetable. The sole effect of nutritional education in American schools appears to be that every parent believes life is dependent largely on three servings daily of leafy greens. It is therefore unfortunate that normal, healthy, and thriving toddlers tend increasingly to exclude vegetables from their diets. They usually continue to consume large volumes of milk and juices, and they develop an impressive fondness for cereal-based foods of all kinds, including breads, crackers, and pasta. They also eat eggs and soft meats and most of them continue to enjoy fruits, but fewer and fewer vegetables pass their lips. Apply **Grossman's First Law of Vegetables: *Vegetables are not magic wands for growth.*** For practical purposes, the combination of fruits plus cereals provide the same general group of nutrients that the child previously obtained from vegetables. These include carbohydrates, fiber, a variety of minerals, vitamin A, most of the B-complex vitamins, and vitamin C.

An equally important rule is **Grossman's Second Law of Vegetables: *Limit the volume of milk and juice so that the toddler will have some appetite left for solids.*** This advice seems self-evident but it needs to be stated; many people consider milk and juices to be "beverages," presumably devoid of caloric content, and therefore without effect on the child's eating. Since the child's appetite is closely controlled by a calorie-sensitive center in the brain, the contribution of calories from milk or juice has the same effect on total food intake as the calories from solids. Whole milk has about 20 calories per ounce, orange juice about 14. If your 1-year old drinks 16 ounces of milk and

4 ounces of orange juice, he has already taken in about 370 of the 1000 he needs every day. That leaves only 630 calories to be divided up among three meals plus a small snack or two. Anyone who has ever been on a restricted calorie diet knows how little food that represents. If your 1-year old is drinking a quart of milk (640 calories) and 8 ounces of juice (112 calories), the resulting 752 calories provided by liquids doesn't leave a lot of room for much else. Obviously, the major candidate for rationing in your toddler's diet is fruit juice; it carries a load of calories and little else. Good old natural apple juice, the babies' favorite tipple, is nearly devoid of vitamins and minerals; for all practical purposes it is just sugar water. Orange juice at least has vitamin C; 3 ounces a day provides the 45 mg the toddler requires. Limiting toddlers to 16 ounces of milk a day makes sense. That volume will provide more than enough calcium, plus 16 grams of excellent protein. If you give him "2-10" milk, which is 2% partly skimmed milk fortified with nonfat milk powder, he will actually get nearly 20 grams of protein, plus a bonus of an extra 100 mg of calcium. (There is a more complete discussion regarding whole milk and lowfat milk in Chapter 20 – Food and Nutrition.) How you arrive at this desirable volume of milk will depend on how much milk, either formula or breast milk, your child is used to taking. Most breast fed American babies are nursing less often at this age. Of course, there is no easy way of measuring breast milk intake, but it is reasonably accurate to assume feedings of 3 to 5 ounces each. As nursings are dropped, plan on replacing them with the equivalent milk by cup or bottle. Bottle fed infants should be on a similar path, with fewer and smaller bottles, aiming for about 16 ounces a day sometime during the second year. There is no big hurry about this transition. If your daughter has been accustomed to 4 or 5 bottles a day of 8 ounces each, she may need a number of months to settle down to a volume more suited to her advancing age.

Sometime during the second year, the subject of weaning will arise. I've already talked about this in Chapter 6 – Feeding Your New Baby. The only point I'd like to add concerns social pressure. From a developmental and social point of view, every culture has its rules about the timing of weaning; the child who continues on the bottle for much longer than the local norm is likely to hear some caustic comments about prolonged babyhood from peers and random, ambient adults. It is, after all, every American's birthright to correct unacceptable variations in the child-rearing practices of others. If the bottle-toting toddler is tough enough, she may simply ignore the pressure. If she is sensitive to her environment, she may decide that she is still being treated like a baby and wonder why Mommy and Daddy don't expect her to grow up like all the other kids. I can't offer a neat, concise Grossman's Law of Weaning. The wisest course seems to be to set a goal that respects the individual child's needs, gives her a clear sense of what is expected, and gently channels her progress towards the next, more mature phase. Have faith; I have yet to see a college freshman who has not managed to switch to the cup.

Teeth

I have not mentioned much about teeth so far because baby teeth generally require little parental attention. You are fortunate if you live in an area with fluoridated water because that simple method of increasing the fluoride content of tooth enamel decreases the incidence of tooth decay by about one half. If your tap water is not fluoridated I hope you have been giving your child fluoride drops or chewable tablets; they are more trouble than fluoridated water, but they work just as well. Tooth cleaning in infancy can pretty much be ignored. Unless the child is eating sticky sweets, his first few teeth are practically self cleaning. Later, when he has a mouth full of teeth and the spaces between teeth can capture food particles, some tooth brushing is in order. This is best approached with considerable delicacy; you really do not want to make tooth care a ritual struggle. Most often, children want to mimic their parents tooth cleaning practices. They can start with a brief and mostly symbolic bit of play with a small, soft toothbrush. When they have decided that toothbrushing is fun, you can add a *small* amount of fluoridated toothpaste. Really large volumes of fluoridated toothpaste will be swallowed and the extra fluoride may cause faint white streaking on the developing teeth, so keep the amount quite small.

If you and your child's doctor are content with the appearance of the baby teeth there is no great urgency for the first dental visit. Sometime during the first few years should be soon enough. Dentists who limit their practices to children typically have offices with a child-oriented flavor which may be particularly helpful for a shy child. However, some general dentists are great with kids and enjoy having them as patients. One way to introduce children to dentistry is to arrange for your child to accompany you to a routine dental visit. The whole scene may seem less foreign and threatening if she can watch Daddy in the dental chair. One the other hand, if you are personally terrified of dentists, you may not be the best person for dental show and tell.

Safety

The increasing ability of the 1-year old to move rapidly and unpredictably makes safety an increasingly complex issue. Not only does he have the run of the house at floor level, but he can now stand up and reach dangerous objects on table tops, and he can climb onto the furniture and up the stairs. Outside, he can use his newfound ability to walk and run by dashing away from you and into the street. What to do? Well, first of all, do not expect to be able to control his dangerous behavior with words. One-year old children cannot be expected to obey, and your shouted "No!" is likely to be ignored. There are two ways to keep toddlers safe: Give them a safe environment, or, if that is impossible, keep them under your physical control. In the house this means continued awareness about what is in reach; keep in mind the risks of a full cup of hot coffee at the edge of the breakfast room table, a sharp metal tool within reach, a stairway unprotected by gates at the top and the bottom, or small pieces of toys on the floor. Outside the house it means a fenced and gated yard for play, and it means the closest possible attention during exploratory strolls along the sidewalk. *If she is not in reach, she isn't safe.*

I'm sorry to keep nagging you about safety, but it is important because the changes in children's abilities changes the spectrum of children's potential for accidents. Thomas Jefferson said "Eternal vigilance is the price of liberty." If he were writing a book for parents, he might have said "Eternal vigilance is the price of keeping bones unbroken and skin intact." Less poetic, but equally true.

Chapter 13

Age 2 to 3 Years

Behavior and Development

There is absolutely nothing else during childhood to match the explosive development of the first year of life. The speed and complexity of change from what one of my daughters called baby blobs into complicated little people at age 1 year is barely believable. The second year is no slouch either. Physical, intellectual, and social growth continue at a great rate, and infancy becomes a vague memory. I used to have difficulty remembering what my own children had been like even a few months before; the vivid reality of the present made the recent past invisible. By the beginning of the third year, the rate of change seems to slow down a bit, and early childhood begins to unfold. This is not to say that less is happening at this age; it is just that so much development has already taken place. Baby's first word is inevitably more noteworthy than his two hundred and first; his first step is more likely to be recorded than his first hop, skip, or jump.

Look at any group of 2-year olds and you will continue to be impressed by their variability. Most are verbally adept enough to understand the bulk of simple adult conversation, often more than the parents would like to have overheard. The 2-year old's active speech will usually be in phrases and some sentences, but a few children of this age will be fully conversational, their discourse complete with sentences and paragraphs. Play will be increasingly complex, with fantasy productions involving toys, dolls, and stuffed animals. The boys especially will be involved in cars and trucks. Picture books are favorites, with or without an adult to interpret. Outdoor play will involve dirt, sand, water, and wheel toys. By this age, clear differences are evident in styles of play and activity in general. Some 2-year olds are intensely physical, running and climbing and exploring. These active children move fast and often with unexpected grace and skill. It is not unusual to see a physically adept toddler throw and catch a ball with real precision. Others are much more interested in social interaction; they are most content with an adult to mimic or follow, or another child to involve in play. Still others like quiet and solitary play; they look at books or play with household objects or toys. They will watch the other children at the park but rarely approach them; they don't head instantly for the slides and climbing structures. This variability seems to be a built-in characteristic. I don't mean to imply that opportunities for and examples of desirable activities have no influence on a child's development. If you happen to be born into a family of soccer players, you will be out there kicking a ball at an early age, in part because that is what everyone else is doing. However, the skill with which you kick it and the amount of pleasure you have in the endeavor are heavily influenced by the mind and body you to bring to the soccer field. This can cause concern for a parent whose child fails to fit unspoken and often unconscious parental expectations or desires. One little boy in my practice had the good fortune to be born with remarkable artistic ability which became apparent even before his third birthday. Unhappily, his father was a physical education teacher whose vision of little boyhood included bats and balls rather than crayons and paper. The resultant mismatch between parental dreams and the reality of his son's interests and talents was painful to everyone.

Safety. Here is another topic where the personal style of your child makes all the difference. Of course, a certain level of protection from hazards is required for every child: car seats, poisons kept out of reach, hot water heaters set for 120°- 130° F, just to remind you of a few safety details. But some kids have an uncanny ability to ferret out hidden and forgotten perils, and their lives tend to be punctuated with emergency room visits and calls to the poison control center. These are usually vigorous, intrusive, and endlessly curious children, not easily dissuaded by adult limit setting. If your first child was mild and easily controlled and your second child is one of these bombshells, you will need to revise your views about what constitutes adequate safety practices.

Power

This is the big issue of this age group. Sometime during this year, usually at about 2½, the "TERRIBLE TWOS" erupt. Here is a piece of folk wisdom which is *absolutely real;* the struggles for authority over the lives of these toddlers are predictable and bloody. These battles are also *absolutely necessary,* at least for the vast majority of American children.

The process which seems to be central is the child's dawning sense of his own strength and separateness. It is as though the child has to fight the parents to define his own boundaries. I have often had the image of an assertive and contrary 30-month old child dissecting himself away from his mother and father, trying to discern who he is, as distinct from his prior sense of immersion and identity with them. Perhaps that is why the fight is nearly always most intense with the mother; after all, the child has been, quite literally, a part of her body and her being. However, the fight with father can be just as fierce, especially when the father has played a large part in the child's care.

When your child becomes involved in this struggle you will find that she is endlessly and inventively pushing to discover the reach of her power. She will be annoyingly negative, seeking to prove what she can do by telling you what she will *not* do. This behavior is nearly always limited to the immediate family setting. At day care or nursery school, or at play in the home of a friend, the Terrible Two isn't terrible at all. It is as if the child says, "Why should I bother to fight my friend's mother or my nursery school teacher? I know that I am separate from them, and I don't have to prove anything."

Your response to this onslaught of aggression will largely determine the flavor of the ensuing months. A common pattern for the loving and inexperienced parents of a first child is to retreat, giving in to demands, no matter how bizarre, and placating every whim. The predictable effect is an exponential increase in trouble; having pushed her parents to discover the limits of her power, and finding no clear boundary, the child pushes further. The analogy of an invading army sending out scouting parties to reconnoiter the enemy's defenses comes to mind.

Parental placating can all too easily become a way of life. There can be a number of reasons for this. You may not realize that the child can understand and accept rules. You may fear the loss of the child's love: "If I don't let him come to bed with us in the night, he'll hate me." You may lack a model from your own childhood of loving but firm limit setting: "When I was a child, the only way they set limits was to hit me." With particularly vigorous limit pushers, the problem becomes parental exhaustion: "It is just easier to say yes." In any case, the 2-year old for whom limits are not set becomes more and more demanding and difficult; there is sometimes a frantic quality to the ensuing behavior. It is as if the child is saying "My God, who is in charge around here? I'm only two-years old and I don't know how to run this family!"

At the other extreme are the parents who respond to the child with anger and rigidity, without considering that perhaps it is time to build a little more power into his family role. I hope you have not already forgotten **Grossman's Law of Childhood Autonomy:** *Parents have only 18 or so years to turn over full responsibility to a child.* A punitive and unyielding parental position sets the stage for a long and nasty fight. The struggle at age 2 is only one engagement in a long series of battles for personal independence. There will be another predictable phase at around age 4, usually a little less intense than age 2, but tough enough. And again in late childhood, there are the fights about reporting in to Mom, about where bike riding is allowed, when and how to do the chores, who is in charge of television, and so on. The process only escalates in adolescence; the family which fears and attempts to hobble the teenager's thrust for power will have a tough 5 or 6 years.

So, what is the best way to cope with the 2-year old on the march? There isn't a "best way," and that is the crux of it. Understanding the process as one of necessary and healthy individuation, can help you see the negativism and limit-pushing with at least a modicum of sympathy. If you can allow an increase in the child's control of her life in some areas, her independence needs may be sufficiently satisfied for awhile. This may enable you to maintain firm limits and rules elsewhere with less effort and more success. Where those lines are drawn and how they are enforced must be a matter for you to discover for yourselves; one family's reasonable rules may be another family's chaos. The tactics will also vary depending on the particular child. Confrontations can occasionally be avoided by giving prior notice that an event is coming up. "We'll be leaving in a few minutes" may be easier for a child to agree to, whereas "We're going now" without a prior warning, is reason enough for a struggle. I've already mentioned the virtues of acknowledging his feelings out loud. If you have gotten into the habit of doing this when emotions seem to be running at high tide, keep up the good work, but don't expect too much in the way of a positive response from a 2-year old under the sway of a massive will to power. A time-honored method of limited utility is distraction, the attempt to deflect the child's attention in a more desirable direction. Unhappily, this is so transparent a ruse that it often fails. Some kids really make it easy; a clear statement, or even a raised eyebrow will be enough to tell a timid child that he has reached the edge of his authority. But another child will all but spit in Mom's eye rather than submit. With the tough ones, it is usually necessary to pick your battles with care. These kids are so willing to fight about everything that life can become an endless series of time-outs. Very few parents can tolerate such campaigns of attrition. Most parents decide to cede power in a number of nonlethal areas. Okay, you can wear your party dress to nursery school, nap on the floor instead of your bed, and bathe only once a fortnight. But the crucial areas of control had better be kept and effective methods must be devised in order to convince Terrible Twos that they have to live by Mom and Dad's dicta.

Toilet Training

It is a shame that the physiologic readiness to use a toilet develops during this year as it coincides with the psychologic readiness to fight Mom and Dad about everything. The feisty 2-year old soon understands that his parents really want him to give up diapers in favor of the toilet, and all too often he says to himself "The hell with it; there's nothing in it for me!" If the use of the toilet can be taught by other children, which happens in some societies, or if it is learned in the relatively neutral setting of a child care center, the child may be able to perceive the act as an interesting opportunity to develop mastery. At home, however, he often sees it as the parents' game, pure and simple.

EVERYDAY PEDIATRICS FOR PARENTS

One way out of this quagmire is behavior modification, using the system of rewards (not bribes) I described in the preceding chapter. Older children can work toward a goal with more abstract markers: star charts, points that add up to a prize, that sort of thing. But not 2-year olds; they need instant gratification. For some kids, the parents noisy and heartfelt approval is sufficient. That is fine when it works, but don't be surprised by failure. An interesting aspect of the use of behavior modifying rewards in general is that the need for the reward rapidly disappears as soon as the task is mastered or the new behavior is established. Somehow the act becomes satisfying in itself.

There are, of course, children who quickly decide that the use of a potty chair or a toilet is wholly incompatible with their chosen life-style. They may hide from the adults as soon as they sense an oncoming stool, or they may remain brazenly in view, squirming and straining as they pit their anal sphincters against the smooth muscle of their colons. The child who presses his buttocks to the floor, or crosses his legs, turning a nice shade of blue in the process, is giving dramatic evidence that he does not want to graduate to the use of the toilet. The best tactic in this situation is to tell the child that he appears to be too young for the toilet, give up the struggle, and return to toilet training at a later date. Perseverance in the face of this intense resistance has a nasty tendency to end up with self-induced, painful constipation; it's a very good problem to avoid.

The acquisition of urine control during sleep seems to be nearly independent of daytime control of urine and stool. Only a small minority of newly day-trained toddlers will be dry at night. Most girls attain nighttime control by age 3 or 4; boys tend to be a bit later. Parents who push for a dry bed too early are inventing a problem that they really do not need. Be patient; diapers are a lot cheaper than family psychotherapy.

Food. Eating patterns and preferences don't tend to change much during the third year. Calorie requirements may inch up, but the increase is usually imperceptible. The range of food choices often continues to shrink; it will get even narrower within a year or so. Most 2-year olds still eat frequently; 3 meals and 2 snacks is fairly typical. Unfortunately, snack foods often tend to be junk foods. Cookies, candy, soft drinks, and juices are handy and uniformly welcome; avoiding these inadequate but popular snacks takes some planning. Fresh or dried fruit, peanut butter on crackers, cheese, raw vegetables like carrots and celery—are all nourishing and valuable snacks. (Sometime during this year, most kids have become skillful enough eaters that they can safely be given nuts and popcorn, two excellent categories of snack food. However, some children retain an excessively casual approach to what they put into their mouths, and are better off waiting until about age 3.) If you offer healthy snacks to your children's friends, they may respond with horrified disbelief, and you will be well on your way to a reputation as the neighborhood health food nut. Your own children are also likely to balk after discovering that snacks are sweeter and more seductive at nursery school or at a friend's house. Thus, the nutritionally wise and well-informed parent is up against the persuasive power of the American advertising industry. Many dollars are spent to sell Pop Tarts and Twinkies to your children; nobody is mounting a clever campaign to push carrot sticks. Good luck.

Sleep

Parents of 2-year olds are nearly unanimous in wanting their children to continue midday naps. Happily, a majority of 2-year olds remain in substantial agreement and enjoy a regular period of real daytime sleep. Unhappily, there is a dissenting minority. Some of these children really do not need to nap. They function quite well until just before bedtime, when they are likely to become so tired that their behavior deteriorates. In this situation earlier bedtimes help, and parents eventually give up the struggle over the unwanted naps. On the other hand, some of the Anti-Nap Brigade should never have enlisted; they truly need some midday rest and become absolutely impossible without it. If a stern and unyielding insistence on naps fails to restore a livable pattern, consider offering a compromise of quiet play time in the child's room or on his bed. No TV, no music, no playmates, no adult interaction—just quiet play. If he is sufficiently tired, a nap often supervenes. If not, at least he has had an opportunity to recharge his batteries.

By the age of 2 going to sleep at night has usually been a comfortable routine for a long time. It may have become a rather complex ritual of bath and stories, depending on the family's priorities and personnel. A two-parent household with a small number of kids and neither parent working an evening shift may be able to spare a substantial amount of adult time in getting small children to bed. However, that does not describe every American family. As the third year progresses even the most idyllic, Norman Rockwell-type household may find itself coping with major bedtime battles when the resident Terrible Two decides that an early bedtime is no longer acceptable. What is to be done? The first question to answer may be "Is the kid correct?" Perhaps he needs less naptime or a later bedtime at night. There is no table of Hours Needed for Sleep to which you can refer; every child is different. Some still nap for 2 hours and sleep for 12 hours at night; others get by with 9 or 10 hours a day total sleep. What is important is watching the child. If his evening behavior suggests that he really is able to stay up an additional hour and he awakens refreshed at his usual time in the morning, then the later bedtime makes sense. If his resistance to naps does not match his actual need to rest, his evening fretfulness and morning stupor will give you the information you need to enforce the hours of sleep that he clearly requires. My own prejudice concerning this matter is that getting the kids to bed on time is even more important than it may seem to the exhausted and grumpy mother and father. The parents whose children keep adult hours never have time in the evenings for themselves, and this can be bad for mental and marital health.

Dreams, Nightmares, and Night Terrors are common at this age. As children become more verbally proficient, their descriptions of their dreams become more complex. It is often easy to relate dream content quite explicitly to the events of the preceding day. There does not seem to be much complicated symbolism involved when the child cries out in her sleep "Give me my dolly!" When a child awakens from a nightmare she is likely to be crying and upset, but she will clearly be awake, and she may tell you something about the frightening dream she has just had. In contrast, the children who experience night terrors suddenly become partially but not fully awake; they sit up screaming, inconsolable, confused, and thoroughly out of contact. These terrifying events subside slowly; it can sometimes take half an hour before the child finally calms down and returns to sleep. He will have no memory of the event the next morning. Relatively few children have night terrors; they are more frequent in boys, and they tend to run in families. Night terrors are not dream related, but may be triggered by upsetting events or excessive tiredness. They may recur sporadically for months or even years, but eventually disappear. When a child is having a night terror, the parent's first impulse is to hold and comfort him. Sometimes this seems to be helpful, but often the child only screams and struggles harder. If this happens there is really nothing you can do but leave him alone until the episode wears itself out. Very rarely, night terrors occur so often that a sedative or tranquilizer is needed for a few weeks to break the cycle.

Chapter 14

Age 3 to 4 Years

Behavior and Development

By the time the child reaches her third birthday, it is pretty clear who she is and who she will be; this is not to say that personality is set in concrete, but close to it. Of course, the first hints have been evident much earlier. Once past the newborn period, when the effects of labor and delivery can muddle the picture, temperamental differences begin to surface. Patterns of persistence with tasks, motor skills and tempo, interest in things or interest in people, general sunniness of disposition or lack of it—all are well expressed by the middle of the first year. The developmental processes that result in stranger anxiety late in the first year, clinginess in the second year, and negativity in the third year can hide the underlying personality to a degree. However, by the fourth year all of this is over with, and what you see is pretty much what you get.

My understanding from watching this unfolding is that an awful lot of personality is innate. I think the observations made by psychoanalysts about infant and child development somewhat misled us into overestimating the influence of the parents. If kids are as firmly put together in psychological terms as they appear to me to be, their ordinary experiences with Mom and Dad may have less effect in molding personality than psychoanalysts have imagined. The reports of neurotic turn-of-the-century Viennese about their childhoods may not be an accurate basis for understanding everybody else. I'm not saying that parents are unimportant or without influence, nor that a truly batty household is free of adverse consequences for its inmates, but simply that the kids come into the world with an impressively well-structured set of personality characteristics already in place. As an amateur gardener I tend to think in horticultural terms, and it seems to me that child raising is like planting tulips: If you provide a healthy place for the bulb to grow, and feed and water it just right, you will get a stronger, taller tulip. But no matter what kind of a gardener you are, when you plant a red tulip bulb, what comes up is a red tulip. Kids are not infinitely malleable, and parents are not somehow always responsible for the child's problems nor, for that matter, the child's triumphs. These innate characteristics become most evident when there are other children in the family for comparison; the differences between siblings are far greater than can be accounted for on the basis of differences in parenting. Mothers are often

EVERYDAY PEDIATRICS FOR PARENTS

intensely aware of this: "I could tell how different he was from his brother when he was still in my womb." One aspect of these differences is that the fit between a child and her parents can vary from just right, when the parents and the child are rather similar people, to just awful, when the parents and the child are different down to the bone. It can take a long time and some hard lessons before the parents make their peace with the reality of a given child, and decide that she cannot be dealt with as if she were a carbon copy of Mom or Dad. I learned a good deal about this from my son Mike. One day when trying to help him deal with a problem I said "If I were you, this is what I would do." He looked up at me very quietly and seriously and said "But I'm *not* you."

Well, anyway, 3-year olds: They are a nice bunch, by and large. They tend to be reasonable, their verbal skills are good, and disagreements can often be handled with words alone. Generally speaking, these children have graduated from the automatic negativism and assertiveness of the preceding year. More often than not, people will say about their 3-year old "He's so much fun."

Food

The 3-year old at the family dinner is the world's best argument for governesses and meals taken in the nursery. There is a powerful American myth that the family dinner is a sacrosanct and peaceful time for all to gather in amity and good spirits. Nothing could be further from the truth. In reality, dinner time is usually the hardest time of day for everyone concerned. Small children are exhausted and usually manic. They were ready for their last meal of the day around 5 PM, long before it was prepared. If they had an adequate snack at that time, they won't be hungry when dinner is ready. If they did not have something to eat earlier, some kids act as though they were having a touch of low blood sugar grumpiness and may be too miserable to even attend the meal. Few, if any, normal 3-year olds can sit still long enough to be welcome participants at an adult-type dinner, no matter how well-timed. They want to eat and run.

Furthermore, the average American 3-year old has pretty well abandoned vegetables, has not yet learned to like salads, is beginning to distrust sauces, and sees little excuse for anything much more complicated than bread, cereals, pasta, and apple juice. Like the 2-year old, he prefers to eat the largest portion of his daily diet at breakfast, and spread the rest out over lunch and snacks. Dinner is probably his smallest meal. Unfortunately, this does not fit well with the adult American pattern of dinner as the largest meal. When a mother says "She won't eat a thing" she usually means "She won't eat dinner." The remaining difficulties with the myth of the Happy Family Dinner reside in the adult realities of end-of-the-day exhaustion. If you have had a long day on the job, you are not likely to be the relaxed, interested, wise, and loving people you and your children wish you were. Perhaps everyone would benefit from a revolution of falling expectations.

So, feed the kids early, allow them to leave the dinner table quickly, and grab a little adult time if you can. There will be plenty of opportunities for intense family interaction around the dinner table when they are older.

Toilet Training. There is not a great deal to add to the previous discussions regarding this subject. For most 3-year olds, progress in bowel and bladder control is coming along nicely. A sizable proportion of children are dry and clean, day and night. However, wet beds are still the rule for many. The kids most likely to stay wet well into middle childhood are boys who are heavy, deep sleepers, and whose families have a considerable history of delayed bladder control. If your child's lack of urine control is beginning to get to you, now is the time to read Chapter 23 on bed wetting. However, it probably is not the time to do anything about it. If struggles concerning bowel movements have led to withholding stool, have a look at Chapter 22 on Constipation.

Nursery Schools

Sometime around age 3, the subject of nursery school arises. Of course, many if not most American kids have already been in some sort of day care by this age, but more formal preschool is often contemplated as the child toddles into his fourth year. The usual reasons adduced include the availability of more complex and challenging play equipment, formal academic instruction in letters and numbers, perhaps more art and music opportunities, and a bigger social scene. "He'll be bored if he stays at day care another year." There are also the intangibles; I will never forget the mother who smugly informed me that her daughter was attending a nursery school which specialized in ego development. I recall blushing with embarrassment as I realized that my own 4-year old had stayed at home with her mother and her little sister and obviously had not been given the priceless opportunity to develop her ego. It took me several seconds to recognize this as utter nonsense.

What can a nursery school reasonably be expected to do? Look at them as transitional places, where children are introduced to the more structured, school-like settings in which they will be incarcerated until adult life. They will learn to be socialized into component parts of an adult-administered youth culture, dealing with a variety of more or less interchangeable grownups, some of whom may even be well trained and have the children's best interests in mind. Some of them, however, will be trained very poorly if at all, and some of the adults, trained or not, will be bored time-servers, long past caring about their charges. In the best and happiest nursery schools, the children will learn a great deal about life with peers and grownups, they will stretch their minds and bodies and voices with new experiences, and they will walk another block along the long road toward independence from their parents. In any nursery school, good or bad, the children are also given innumerable opportunities to cope. Problems arise, toys are fought over, first friendships are formed, children are teased, lunches are lost. Learning to cope is probably even more important than learning how to swing from the monkey bars. In nursery school, kids can get practice in both areas.

Nursery schools vary in funding (private, church, public, parent-owned co-ops), pedagogical theory, academic emphasis, racial and class integration or segregation, physical amenities, and size. For many families, the high cost of privately owned, profit-making nursery schools will be prohibitive, and the choices will necessarily be limited to schools subsidized by public schools, religious institutions, or the volunteer labor of parents. Each of these possibilities has its own attraction. Public nursery schools are typically free or very inexpensive. Depending on the community, public nursery schools are also likely to offer the most diverse group of children. This may be of little significance for families residing in one-class, one-color towns. However, for cities with a richer economic and ethnic mix, publicly funded nursery schools can serve children of many backgrounds as the entry point into the wide world of diversity. There is no point pretending that mixtures of this nature are all sweetness and light. The cost of bringing together the children of differing races, ethnic groups, and social and economic classes is inevitably friction and problems of misunderstanding. The world of inner-city kids is harsh; this shows in their speech, their style of personal interaction, and their general demeanor. Blending children from inner cities and the out-lying suburbs has advantages for everyone—liveliness, excitment, learning about the real world, and unexpected friendships. Many of these advantages can also be found in parent-owned co-ops. The great thing about the co-ops is the opportunity for the participating parent to observe and interact with other children. And seeing your own child in the nursery school context provides a nice perspective which may otherwise be difficult to attain.

Many nursery schools come with a particular pedagogical theory attached, of which the most commonly seen are Montessori schools. The schools founded by Dr. Maria Montessori for the education of retarded children and, later, for children dwelling in the slums of Rome, became the laboratories where she developed a complex set of educational ideas. She stressed individual student effort, few if any group activities except in cleaning the schoolroom and serving food, the use of teaching materials in strictly prescribed ways, and limited exposure to music and art. When Montessori schools were established in the United States, these rules clashed with the more group-oriented, freer style of progressive education that had been developed in this country under the leadership of John Dewey. Strict Montessori protocol also fit rather poorly with the personal style of expressive behavior typical of late twentieth century American children. I recall the frozen smile on the face of the European-trained teacher at our first local Montessori school when one of her pupils proudly showed her the castle he had constructed with the Montessori volume blocks. She knelt down next to his masterpiece and dismantled it, block by block, as she explained to the dismayed child that the blocks were to be used to learn about size and shape, not as elements in his personal fantasy play. Later that same day, a group of girls exhibited the battleship they had built from a jigsaw puzzle meant to teach the geography of the fifty states. The American-trained Montessori teacher knew that she was being teased, and retreated as gracefully as she could manage. These two interchanges exemplified the problems of incorporating a pedagogical theory rooted in a quite foreign style of child rearing. The result was that most American Montessori education became a hybrid, bearing some relationship to its Italian ancestry, but not a great deal. Some orthodox Montessori schools still exist, and there are even two rival national Montessori education associations, co-existing in mutual disapproval. Despite the fervid claims of superiority sometimes advanced, I don't know any reason to prefer a school labeled "Montessori" to any other.

A fairly new phenomenon are the nursery schools with academic pretensions. These are often called learning centers, child development centers, or academies. I think their existence expresses a basic anxiety about the educational process. The notion that reading and writing should be force fed to toddlers, without regard to their levels of intellectual development, suggests that the proprietors and their customers are equally ignorant about the processes of learning and equally unsure that they can trust kids to learn at an appropriate age. When a child is forced to attempt material which is too advanced for him to comprehend, the inevitable failure is bound to be injurious to his self esteem and unnecessarily worrying to the his parents.

Practical considerations such as affordability and school hours that fit your family's needs will make some nursery schools more desirable than others. The adequacy of the physical plant, the presence of indoor and outdoor play space, and the quality and condition of toys and books will all factor into your decision. But most important is the professional staff. How many teachers are there? What is the ratio of students to teachers? How well trained are the teachers?— these are crucial questions. There are also some intangible qualities about each institution; some places are upbeat, vigorous, and happy, others are not. The more information you can gather about nursery schools, the better. Your friends may have useful information, and so may your pediatrician, local kindergarten teachers, and anyone else with personal or professional contacts with little kids. Ask and visit.

Safety. The appearance of a degree of reasonableness at this age can be misleading in a number of ways. We can see that 3-year olds actually have some sort of primitive understanding about limits and rules, and it seems that they should be able to understand the idea that certain objects or activities are hazardous. Well, it may seem so, but don't bank on it. Make the assumption that all the household dangers you dealt with at an earlier age are still dangerous. The street is still fatally seductive, unknown liquids in bottles still invite ingestion, hot water can still scald, knives can still cut. In short, 3-year olds require a very short leash when in the presence of the usual perils of modern life.

Siblings

If your 3-year old is your first child, it is not unlikely that you may already have presented her with a new sibling. From many points of view, 3 years or thereabouts is an ideal period for child spacing. The older child has had a good crack at being an infant and is likely to be ready for a more mature role in the family. She has probably graduated from the negativism of 2½ which has led any number of new parents to conclude that single child families make a lot of sense. (I suspect that many pregnancies are started when the first child is around 2, before she has raised limit testing to a fine art.) Another factor is that the veil of forgetfulness has obscured accurate parental memories of how hard it was to get up at 3 AM for a feeding. In any case, the urge to procreate has often overcome questions of "Can we actually afford another child?"

The majority of 3-year olds will respond with considerable distaste, not to say horror, to the advent of the little newcomer. Few events in childhood are more predictable than the abrupt reversion to infantile behavior of the displaced elder child. This may take the form of regression in toilet behavior, a return to the bottle, requests to nurse at the breast, or baby talk. Some children become angry, some seem depressed, very few are delighted. The entry of a third child into a family is quite a different matter. The oldest often perceives the new baby as a potential ally in the family competition. Already having lost his old position as only child, he may accurately foresee that one more child will not make any great difference in the power structure; he'll still be the oldest kid. The second child has naturally never experienced only-childness, so he might be expected to suffer a proportionally less severe diminution in parental attention when child #3 arrives. Unfortunately, he may find himself eclipsed coming and going. The oldest is able to command parental time with his stories about nursery school and his many well-honed and charming talents. The new one is little and cute and fussed over by every adult in sight. Consequently, the status of a middle child, especially during the first several months after the birth of a new baby, can be awfully shaky. This entire state of affairs is an excellent example of the workings of **Grossman's Law of Family Ecology: *When anything changes, everything changes.*** This particular law is neither prescriptive nor proscriptive. Its point is simply to direct attention to a process. Any major perturbation in a family will affect everything and everybody. All the usual and customary relationships will shift. You may not need to do anything about these changes, but it does help to expect them, to be aware of them, and be ready to make adjustments if indicated. In the case of the child newly appointed to the status "middle child," this probably means making the deliberate effort to find time for him, so he will have reason to believe that he still has an honored place in the family constellation. The particular symptoms of rage or regression chosen by each of your older children will gradually subside, no matter what you do. These are not permanent changes; the big kids will once again act their age. For more details on parental tactics, see the discussion concerning siblings near the end of Chapter 5.

Chapter 15

Age 4 to 5

Behavior and Development

The best way to think about age 4 is as a re-run of age 2½, but with words. More often than not, the 4-year old will have a period of intensive and annoying limit testing, most often directed against Mother but sometimes generalized against the entire adult world. This takes fairly complicated verbal forms; there is lots of name calling, especially bathroom words. Because the kids have such complete command of language, a common parental error is to suppose that the peace will be restored and rules will be respected by verbal appeals to reason. It doesn't work. The issue is not "Does she understand the rules?" but "Who is in charge?" Once again, as at age 2½, it makes sense to look at the balance of power within the family and decide whether it is time to hand over a bit more authority to the new generation. Maybe it is appropriate to let her choose her clothes for the day, or to decide not to share a favorite toy. The formal relinquishment of power in some small areas may be what is needed to satisfy the growing ego. "You're getting to be a big girl now, and you can be in charge of that." Choose these concessions carefully and sparingly. If you retreat too precipitously in the face of your 4-year old's offensive, she will continue pushing. She is still looking for clear limits and she will get frantic if she does not find them.

A few more comments about the 4-year old's love for bathroom words may be in order. This is beginning of the age of poop-head, b.m., pee-pee face, and similar terms of nonendearment. I don't fully understand the powerful attraction of the vocabulary of elimination, but it is evident from about this age on. Grownup conversation suggests that it never quite disappears. Older children and adults have learned the rules concerning this area of language, when and how it can be incorporated into speech, and what responses can be expected. The 4-year old tries on these words for size and thoroughly enjoys the discovery that he can freak out the adult world at will with a little well-placed profanity. Power of this magnitude is not lightly relinquished.

How you respond to this phenomenon depends on your own sense of the proprieties. Some people don't much mind their children's rather dirty mouths; in this case other adults, either grandparents or other relatives or teachers, may take up the task of setting limits on the children's choices of words. At the other extreme are parents who react with vigorous disapproval; there are still people who wash out their children's mouths with soap. My own view is that dirty words are not really a moral issue and it is not required that we react with punishment. It is often worthwhile to explain to a child what the words literally signify; especially when a child starts using sexual terms of which he is unlikely to know the meaning. It is also important to explain that the use of dirty words is likely to call down upon his head a considerable degree of opprobrium, at least in some settings. Although he may consider a set of synonyms for male genitalia hilarious, and his parents may simply consider the list unnecessary and redundant, the Sunday school teacher may take a darker view. Most of the time, this rather cool approach defuses the dirty word situation, and kids eventually learn to swear as circumspectly as their parents. I suspect that the whole issue can be minimized by using precise anatomical and physiological terms with our kids from the very earliest age. Most of the pertinent sexual and excretory terms are self evident. Nipple, breast, penis, testis or testicle, vagina, vulva, anus—these are all good English and socially acceptable. Female genitourinary anatomy is complicated by its relative invisibility. There is nothing wrong with teaching your girls that their urine is stored in the bladder and comes out through the urethra, but I suspect most parents settle for less precision. In any event, a matter-of-fact attitude combined with a matter-of-fact vocabulary is a good start.

Oedipus, Electra, and Other Aspects of Sexual Development

Freud was right; kids really are sexual beings. Even the most obtuse observer will note the unmistakable evidence of children's sexual interest at about this age. Four-year olds are not very subtle about this: The little girl decides to crawl into her daddy's side of the bed; the little boy rushes into the bathroom to watch his mother take her shower. Plans are often discussed: "Daddy, when I grow up, I'll marry you." Plans are suggested: "I think Daddy should get a little house all his own." Contingencies are considered. Eldest of three young boys to his mother: "If Daddy dies, you will still have Adam and Pete and me, but if you die, Daddy is just out of luck."

It seems reasonable to help children give up their interest in a sexually satisfying future with their parents. The family which has been casually and happily naked together needs to limit the visual stimulation of shared baths and beds. Doors need to be closed to decrease the auditory or visual evidence of parental love-making. And the child needs to hear that, no, she will not take Mom's place when she grows up; she will marry someone else.

Of course, not all early childhood sexuality is heterosexual. Even at this tender age, signs of what will eventually become a homosexual orientation may be seen. The clearest view into the inner life of the 4-year old child is through play. When the play patterns of little children do not conform to the sex role expectations of our culture there are at least three possible explanations. First, some of the little boys who prefer playing dress-up in their mothers' clothes will be thoroughly heterosexual in adult life, as will some of the tomboys who are interested only in boyish pursuits. These kids do not seem to be worried about sex; they are expressing the complexity of who they are, and they are playing with a variety of adult roles. Second, a few of these children appear to be acting out gender role concerns because of specific psychological problems, either their own or within their families. This group of kids are likely to show other signs of psychological strain. The sex role confusion is only a part of a larger picture of emotional distress. It is likely to require the services of a child psychotherapist to judge the significance of the behavior. Third, there is also a substantial number of little kids who begin to express what will eventually become mature, adult gay or lesbian sexuality. These children may become aware at a remarkably early age that they are truly, deeply different from their peers. Some of my gay and lesbian friends tell me that they knew from earliest childhood that their feelings about boys and girls set them apart from the other children they knew. For others, it can take years or decades for the meaning and identity of the difference to become clear, since the pressure from peers and parents alike is to conform to the ways of the majority. It can be confusing and frightening for children to contemplate the possibility that they are different in some unacceptable way.

Until recently, not much attention had been given to long-term studies of the development of adult sexual patterns. There was a lot of theorizing and an even greater amount of moralizing, but not much scientific attention. Now that homosexuality has become a topic that can be talked about and studied, it is becoming obvious that sexual orientation is largely built-in. There is an increasing body of information from family and twin studies showing that genetic factors play an important role. The inference I draw is that parents are probably well advised to let their children express themselves fully and honestly in their sex role play. Our kids are going to have the adult sexual orientation that fits them, and there is no virtue in trying to coerce them into any other. This topic is touched on again in Chapter 18 on adolescence.

Besides lusting after one or another of their parents, some children of this age are beginning sexual exploration of each other as well. They may already have learned a good deal about their own genitals; both girls and boys discover a variety of forms of masturbation. Even the most liberated, modern parents may be taken aback by infant sexuality. "I don't really mind that he plays with himself, but I wish he would keep his hands out of his pants when his grandparents are around." One effective approach to suggest is that genital play is a private matter; it's okay, but not in public. This is a concept that children of this age seem to readily understand.

How much interest in sex is normal? When does sex play among little children become obsessive rather than exploratory? What frequency of masturbation is acceptable? All these questions imply that there is some meaningful standard of what is healthy and expected rather than excessive and a subject of concern. Unfortunately, there are no such guidelines about sex. Perhaps the best way to arrive at a judgment is to look at the child's whole range of activity. If every moment of inactivity and every challenging social situation is met with masturbation, if every peer meeting turns into another round of the "Doctor Game," and if every question about life turns into a quiz about sexual functioning, a savvy parent will begin to suspect that something is awry. But take your time in reaching any conclusions; an intense flurry of sex talk or sex play may come and go quite quickly.

Sex play among young children is a great way for them to learn about each other's anatomy, and, unlike similar activity at later ages, it is free from the risks of sexually transmitted disease or pregnancy. The parent who discovers a giggly game of "Doctor" being played by a happy group of 4, 5, and 6-year olds would be well advised to back quietly away and let the game, and the attendant learning, proceed. Of course, there will be situations where this may not be possible; other parents might object, or a particular child might be thought to be too easily upset. If the children are aware that their game has been witnessed, there is the dilemma of appearing to sanction the children's sex play, something many adults would find quite uncomfortable. Sex play initiated by older children that may frighten a smaller child is another matter, and one good reason why adult supervision of children of diverse ages is a necessity. Parenthetically, this is an important consideration in choosing a babysitter. Most adolescent boys are too much at the mercy of their sexual impulses to be left as the sole guardians of younger kids.

EVERYDAY PEDIATRICS FOR PARENTS

Sexual Abuse

This leads me to the subject of the sexual molestation of children which has become the focus of a nearly hysterical amount of attention. This is partly the result of the "recovered memory" movement which claims to be uncovering untold millions of cases of forgotten incest and rape. Those who subscribe to this theory believe that memories of sexual abuse in childhood and adolescence are commonly pushed completely out of conscious awareness. The repressed memories remain in the minds of the victims but find their expression in bodily symptoms or emotional turmoil. A variety of therapies are said to enable the repressed memories to be retrieved and the symptoms alleviated. I think the practitioners of recovered memory therapies need a more thorough grounding in the evaluation of the information provided by their patients. Memory is faulty, and emotionally upset people can often be persuaded to produce whatever memories the therapist is interested in. A little more skepticism on the part of these therapists about their own theories and their patients' memories would be in order. Yes, sexual misconduct of adults with children exists; yes, it is without doubt damaging to children; yes, it is important for parents to be aware that our children can be at risk. But no one is served by the current climate of suspicion and the apparent willingness of some police and child welfare workers to take precipitate and disastrous action on the basis of next to no information.

What kinds of behavior and what sorts of bodily symptoms *should* lead a parent to suspect the possibility of sexual abuse? An increased intensity of interest in sexual subjects, an unusual focus on masturbation, undue concern with the genitals—all these symptoms might suggest sexual abuse. However, I believe that sexual abuse triggers much more nonspecific sorts of emotional distress. Symptoms as diverse as suicide attempts, school failure, depression, and anxiety may occur. Physical signs of sexual abuse may include bruising or bleeding involving the genitals and the anus. Sometimes the child's own report is enough evidence to require investigation. I think that the family should turn first to the child's doctor. He will know when and how to involve the local child protective services or the police if that is necessary.

I am also concerned about the child safety courses being offered in nursery schools and the early elementary grades. These seem to be based on the notion that small children should be taught that adults are generally dangerous and that children should take the responsibility for their own defense. This is not a burden appropriately placed on the shoulders of the very young. The world remains a hazardous place, as it has always been. Just because one set of hazards has become a popular subject for the media to exploit does not give us license to pursue quick and dubious solutions to complex and ancient problems of human interaction.

We all go through life guided by our own particular combination of trust and wariness. These habits of mind are influenced by our own perceptions of the personal worlds in which we have lived. The survivor of incest will have a different outlook and agenda than the product of a more benign family environment. Are there any reasonable ways to teach children how to protect themselves from sexual molestation? I believe the best common denominators for keeping kids safe are as follows: First, teach children to respect themselves and their bodies. A child who has been taught that a part of his body is dirty and bad may be too ashamed to tell his parents about forced sexual contact. A child who has spent his first years being coerced by harshly controlling parents may be less able to protect himself from sexual coercion as well. Second, teach children that no subject is off limits for discussion. It is difficult for some of us to hear our kids talk about the problems they encounter in their lives. We may not want to face the fact that they experience fear and pain and embarrassment. And it may be easier to minimize or deny the problems they tell us about because they discomfit us, or frighten us, or make us aware of the limitations of our power. Enough lessons of this sort teach a child that the grown-ups need to be protected from unpleasant reality. I think that if our kids like themselves and trust us, we have probably done about as much as we can do to help them navigate amid the sexual predators who really do exist.

Questions of Life and Death and Everything Else

Question time begins a lot earlier than the fifth year. One-year olds like to have objects identified and named. Two-year olds are always asking "What is it?" Even 3-year olds can come up with complex questions about existence. But by the age of 4, questions from child to parent are a constant. Perhaps I overestimate the importance of this part of child rearing, but it seems to me that the information-seeking and information-giving interchange is of real consequence. The child whose questions are met with clear answers designed for his vocabulary and present level of understanding receives not only the information he seeks, but also the underlying message that getting the right answers about the world is possible, important, and satisfying. You are teaching another lesson when you take the child along on the search for an answer. Going to a reference book, or calling on someone else's expert information to resolve a complicated question is the kind of problem solving behavior that shows by example some of the ways to learn about the world. In contrast, the child who is put off with an uninterested shrug or an annoyed "Don't bother me now!" learns not to seek knowledge. The underlying messages are also apparent; "Neither you nor your question are important enough for me to bother with." I don't wish to seem unsympathetic or without understanding of the realities of life for overburdened parents; there will be times when you just will not have the time and patience to deal with yet another question. However, there is no virtue in pretending that the child is unaware of being shunted off to one side, with whatever conclusions he may draw.

Quite a few kids this age ask questions of stunning complexity. I recall a child who asked me how the breast makes milk; try to explain the necessary physiology and biochemistry at the 4-year old level! More commonly, the hard questions involve human motivation: "Why did Jimmy hit me?"; human feelings: "Why is Mommy crying?"; and human fate: "Where do we go when we die?" About the best guide to action in these situations is to use the simplest language, the most concrete and understandable terms, and the most honesty you can muster. Not infrequently, the best answer will be "I don't know," and that's all right, too.

School

By now, many if not most American kids will have started some kind of school. For the child who has already had a year or two of day care, moving on to nursery school is typically quite easy. It is usually perceived as simply another familiar group setting. For the child who has been mostly at home, entrance into the world of nursery school can be quite intimidating: all those noisy kids, all those unknown adults, so much confusion, and no Mom or Dad. The preponderance of day care veterans seems to have made it difficult for some nursery school teachers to remember how threatening nursery school can be for the neophytes. The expectations of the adults have changed, and the newcomer is expected to fit right in. This is unfortunate and unrealistic; the process of separation may be prolonged. It may take many weeks or even months until the home-reared 4-year old can be left without tears and a struggle. He may quite enjoy the place after his mother has torn herself out of his grasp, but he may cry again when she comes to pick him up at the end of the session. All this is uncomfortable but normal; most 4-year olds adapt nicely to the school and its routine. If the adaptation doesn't seem to be developing after the first month or two, it may be best to abandon the attempt. Some children do better with a different interim place between home and kindergarten; a small play group or a peaceful family day care setting might be an easier transition.

For a minority of children, no matter how much experience they have had in no matter how supportive a day care setting, starting a new school is hard because of the child's intensely experienced shyness. There are simply some children who are socially uncomfortable, ill at ease in strange situations, and slow to make even a single friend. They may eventually learn how to move with a little more ease in school and other social situations with their peers, but these children will most likely grow up to be shy and introverted adults. The start of every school year is a misery for shy children, and the start of every summer camp will be anticipated with dread. These are children who would probably love home schooling, a tiny private school, or personal tutoring by a governess. However, none of these options is likely to be available, and for better or worse the shy kids get thrown into the maelstrom of mass education. They may not enjoy it, but they usually survive.

The entire problem of separation is a nice example of that recurrent theme of child rearing, how hard should a child be pushed, and when should a child's own rhythm of development be allowed to determine the timing of events? It may sometimes be worthwhile to frame the question of school and separation in these terms. When a child continues to resist preschool for longer than anyone expected, and for much longer than is convenient, the easy and usual adult response is to try to fix blame: "Is something wrong with the child?" "Why can't he shape up and be like the other kids?" "They enjoy the preschool; why can't he?" The second choice is to blame the parents: "Why can't the mother just leave her child promptly?" "Doesn't she see the kid is just manipulating her?" The third choice is to blame the school: "It's too big—noisy—impersonal—dirty—chaotic." "No wonder my child does not want to stay." Well, all these are valid questions and possibilities. But the other possibility is that this nice, normal child of excellent parents is not yet ready to enter into the world of the well-run and beautifully equipped preschool. Next semester, perhaps, but not now. Although this analysis may seem simplistic, it may also be accurate. If so, the parents have an uncomfortable choice: push him over this hurdle prematurely, because it is the family's only option, or wait and try again later. The decision will depend on family circumstances and on the particular temperaments of the parents, and it will not be the last time decisions of this nature will arise in the course of the child's career.

Play

Although some gender differences in play can be seen even by the end of the first year, much of the play of very young American children has a generally unisex character. By age 4 this is changing as little boys become absorbed in superhero play, begin to run in packs, are increasingly drawn to wheel toys, and manifest a generally increasing appetite for noisy, large muscle, running, and jumping activity. Little girl play is not vastly different, but their play is more likely to involve smaller groups, imaginative play with dolls and toy animals, less noise, and somewhat less vigorous activity. Increasingly, one also sees the development of individual social styles among children. Some are already clearly the leaders; they are usually assertive and vigorous kids who are full of ideas for play. These attributes may be associated with a degree of bossiness. Franklin D. Roosevelt's mother used to warn him that he would never have any friends if he didn't learn to assume a gentler manner. She was probably mistaken; children like this are usually the chosen children, the popular kids who always have an entourage on the playground. In addition to the leaders, there are of necessity the followers. If a parent happens to be a leader herself and her child is clearly in the follower category, she may be tempted to see this as a form of social failure or an expression of individual pathology. Neither of these explanations is necessarily accurate. There is room in the world for all kinds; as Milton said, they also serve who only stand and wait. A few children are so thoroughly oriented towards the adult world that they seem to have neither the skills nor the interest to make friends with their peers. Other children are socially isolated because of their shyness; they would very much like to have friends but the task seems overwhelming. There are also rare children who have what I think of as social dyslexia: They cannot "read" social cues, and they have the greatest difficulty finding their way in social situations with either adults or children.

Activity: Normal and Not–So–Normal. It is at about this age that the question of possible hyperactivity may be raised, nearly always concerning a boy. These boys do not want to sit still during show and tell at nursery school. They flit from one activity to another, resist being engaged in quiet learning pursuits, chafe at the restraints of indoor play, and often cut a wide swath of noise and confusion wherever they pass. Some children suspected of being hyperactive turn out just fine. They may never be particularly well-suited to quiet, indoor existence and may require either considerable taming or eventual transfer to a more active outdoor life. There is another category of very active boys who are socially out of step with the school environment because of their vastly different past experience. These are likely to be poor, inner-city kids whose play style tends to be rougher and more active than that of middle class children. There are even racial differences; compared to white children, from the time of early infancy, Asian children tend to be more passive and quiet, and black children generally develop motor skills earlier and use their bodies more actively.

In addition to all these quite normal variations on the theme of activity, there are also some children whose increased level of activity is truly and unhappily pathological. These are the children who, early in elementary school, acquire the diagnosis of attention deficit hyperactivity disorder (ADHD) as their behavior comes into greater conflict with the requirements that one settle down, attend to the work, and learn. At age 4 such a diagnosis is difficult to make with any accuracy, but the behaviors that prompt the raising of the question require evaluation. There are a great many reasons for kids to act wild, and some of them deserve specific attention and treatment. This topic is explored in Chapter 16 - Middle-Aged Children and Chapter 50 - Schools, Learning, and Learning Problems.

Chapter 16

Ages 5 to 9 Years: Middle-Aged Children

Growth and Development

Middle-aged children change so quickly in so many areas that generalizations regarding development tend to be diffuse or misleading, but I'll offer a few anyway. By and large, this is the age of strengthening ties of friendship to peers, increasing importance of the peer culture, immersion in school, and slowly increasing distance from the family. Boys tend to run in packs at this age. The masculine focus on competitive sports begins to emerge and the boys who are not interested in or not adept at sports may begin to be marginalized. They are not antisocial, on the contrary they may be

EVERYDAY PEDIATRICS FOR PARENTS

very attached to friends and shared activities, but they prefer less physically demanding pursuits. Yet another group of boys fail to connect with athletics because they have a more general problem of connecting with *anything* their peers are doing. Some of these boys are shy or fearful, some are truly loners. I mention these patterns because they entail significant social disabilities in participating in the masculine culture which begins at this tender age and becomes even more important in later years. Some parents insist that their reluctant athletes overcome hindrances of physique or psyche and join in. If an appropriate match between a particular child and a particular sport can be found a measure of success is possible, but often the child manages to follow his own impulses and opts out of sports whenever he has a choice.

Whereas physical prowess is the great definer of status for boys, skill in relationships tends to be the main focus for middle-aged girls. Girls are beginning to structure complex and often exclusionary friendship groups. The search for a best friend can make for highly charged relationships, and the likelihood that any group of three little girls will remain stable is nil. Someone is always finding herself odd girl out. Next week, it will be someone else.

During this period, some children move rapidly into a social world away from family. Sleepovers with friends, team sports, various clubs, hanging out with other kids as much as possible—all these define certain very independent children. Others are still tightly bound to the family at home; peer culture has not yet become the center of existence.

School

School is a big enough subject to require its own chapter, which it gets later in the book, but a couple of comments seem to fit here. The first has to do with the question of time of school entrance. The standard American pattern of kindergarten at age 5 or thereabouts began when there was no such thing as nursery school; kids stayed at home. Kindergarten was designed to be just what the German word means—"a garden for children," where they could enter gently and gradually into the adult-organized world of real schooling. Now, however, the children arrive with wildly divergent group and school experiences, ranging from several years of group day care or academically pushy nursery schools to survival on inner-city streets. In some school districts, the preponderance of academically experienced children has led to the introduction of what was once first grade learning material into the kindergarten classroom. This has had the unexpected effect of turning a substantial group of 5-year olds into instant school failures. An awful lot of kids, especially boys, are not at all ready to deal with reading and writing at this age. Savvy parents may decide to keep their boys out of kindergarten until age 6, or let them repeat it after a year of struggle. Although the older boys are more likely to settle down to learning, they are now a year older than their classmates. This is a small but quite significant difference, and it gives the older boys a permanent advantage in the one area that counts in the little boy culture—sports. Conversely, the boy who was successful as a 5-year old in kindergarten is presented with a permanent and unearned disability; simply because he is younger, he is highly unlikely to catch up to the older boys' prowess on the playground, especially if he happens to be small or slow in physical maturation. And eight or nine years later, he will still be prepubertal at a time when his older classmates are sprouting in all directions. This is a social incapacity of some magnitude and should be taken into consideration when you are faced with early versus late school entrance for your little boys.

Since girls are much more likely to be able to do academic work at age 5, the issue will come up less often with them. When it does, keep in mind the various disadvantages of being out of step in the girls' peer culture. The sources of status among girls are popularity (with other girls at this age, with both girls and boys during later childhood and adolescence) and academic success. If you are older, you may get leader status by virtue of your better developed social skills; but when adolescence arrives, you leave your sister schoolmates behind as you develop new interests and new body parts. Being the oldest girl in your class can be a lonely business in junior high.

In the preceding chapter I mentioned the problems of hyperactivity and learning disabilities, which sometimes, but not always, appear in the same child. The wide range of school readiness exhibited by 5 and 6-year olds leads to some interesting problems in figuring out whether a given child's patterns of activity, attention span, and learning style are normal or not. Ideally, I would like to have a precise and sensitive test to point to the kids who are dyslexic or hyperactive or both. Well, there is no such thing. It takes the combined efforts of teachers, parents, and pediatricians to pick out these problems, and none of these groups is particularly well trained for the task. For example, teachers may be misled by class, ethnic, or gender sterotypes. Working-class boys may look hyperactive by middle class standards. The teacher may equally be misled by a quiet, well-behaved and bright girl who sits without complaint in class, never drawing attention to herself or to the fact that her dyslexia is causing a child

EVERYDAY PEDIATRICS FOR PARENTS

with an I.Q. of 150 to do average work. School teachers are nearly all over-worked and overwhelmed by the large numbers of students that are now typical of American classrooms. It is difficult, but possible, to get to know a class of 15 or 20 kids, teach them, and eventually arrive at sound judgments concerning their strengths and weaknesses. But American teachers are faced with classes of 25 to 35 children, a nearly unmanageable mass for even the most energetic, experienced, and dedicated teacher. Despite these difficulties, teachers still serve as a valuable early-warning system. Parents will often be the first to suspect a learning problem. When a parent in my practice raises this question, I see my task as gaining a broad and balanced view of the whole child. Is the child normally active or truly hyperactive? Is his letter reversal pattern within the normal range for his age? Are there other family members who have reading disabilities or problems with impulsivity and attention? Is there a family, medical, or financial problem of which his school performance is just a symptom? Does he have an exhausted teacher who just cannot bear one more noisy little boy? In short, does this situation deserve a careful, potentially upsetting, and certainly expensive investigation right now, or would watchful waiting make more sense for a few months or so? Our current knowledge concerning these issues offer no clear guidelines. When these questions are raised, close and continuing consultations between parents, teachers, and pediatricians are needed. It is usually possible by the second grade to decide which children should have a full-scale evaluation. Psychoeducational studies of this type can be done by specially trained psychologists or by pediatricians who specialize in developmental problems. I should mention that a variety of folks without training in children's behavior and development claim to be able to offer diagnostic services of this type. This is an area in which the buyer had better be aware; it is difficult enough for the professionals, let alone the amateurs. Purveyors of vitamin cures, therapeutic spectacles, "vision training," special kinds of physical therapy, and other fanciful approaches—all should be avoided. For more about learning disabilities see Chapter 52.

The Overscheduled Child, the Sputnik Syndrome, and Baby Burn–Out

When I started practice in our suburban, university town in 1959, I was amazed to discover a previously undescribed form of child labor, the overscheduled child. These were kids who left early for school to take an elective class (music or art or a foreign language, usually), stayed late for another elective, then went to 1) dance class, 2) art class, 3) pottery class, 4) religious school, 5) Chinese language and civilization class, 6) baseball, 7) swimming, and on and on and on. At first I reacted greedily: I wanted all of that richness for my own 4-year old. Then I began to notice that these kids were, by and large, a mess. For years, they had "worked" 8 or 10 or 12-hour days at becoming skilled and wise, and by the time they hit high school they were ready to light up and drop out. That "Sputnik" generation, raised to catch up with the Russians and be sophisticated, worldly, and talented was badly served by the anxiety of their parents and teachers.

Today, in our suburban, university town, the opportunities for an enriched extracurricular education, remain as seductive as ever. Now, of course, we are supposed to catch up with the Japanese. The main difference I see is that sports are being pushed harder, and more of the special classes are given privately rather than in the public schools. Many kids are still scheduled to within an inch of their lives. In middle-class neighborhoods where both parents work and the kids are in after-school programs, ordinary, unorganized play on the block is a thing of the past.

The eagerness to push children onto the treadmill of a "full" adult life is fascinating. Parents who complain bitterly that they never have time for themselves or their kids are often the ones who carefully arrange their kids' lives so that the kids have no time for themselves or their parents. Slice it anyway you wish, there are only twenty-four hours in a day. Childhood is the time when human beings have our first and probably best chance to find out who we are. It is the time to explore relationships with all sorts of other people, our peers, our siblings, our grandparents, and the families next door. It is the time when playing is what we are supposed to do, rather than what we can slip in when we manage to steal time away from work. Middle childhood is the all-too-brief moment of grace before daydreaming is seen as laziness, before enthusiasm is seen as ambition, and before innocence is seen as ignorance. Why must we rush it?

Lying and Stealing

Lying and stealing may seem like rather harsh words to describe the behavior of young children, but since lying and stealing is what a great many children do at this age, we may as well label it clearly.

Lying surely qualifies as one of humankind's most common activities at nearly any age. In early childhood the boundaries between reality, fantasy, wishes, and prevarication are blurred. Little children have the complicated task of delineating the differences between what they want, what they would like to

EVERYDAY PEDIATRICS FOR PARENTS

have happen, and what actually occurs. When the 3-year old blames her teddy bear for knocking over the milk, she may understand that she is trying to manipulate her parents, but she may be quite unclear that her statement is an untruth. I think we complicate the job of understanding the difference between truth and fiction by raising our children with stories about talking animals, and with television and movies that simulate real life but are, in fact, only images and fantasies. It is amazing that kids sort this out as soon as they do.

In addition to becoming clear about what is real and what is not, our children must learn that it is wrong to lie for purposes of self-aggrandizement or to avoid adult displeasure. They have already been taught by adult example that untruths are perfectly all right in the service of a good bedtime story or an entertaining television program. If lies and fantasy are good enough for the grownups, they ought be good enough for the kids. Well, this is a complex problem and it takes awhile for it to be solved by some middle-aged children. Some of them never do quite get the point and reach adulthood fit only for careers in advertising or politics.

Stealing can be thought of as a kind of acted-out lying. "I see it, I want it, so it must be mine and I'll take it." I have the impression that stealing is somewhat more likely to be a male occupation in childhood as it is in later life. When adults talk about their childhood and adolescent misdemeanors, women are often rather shocked to hear the amount of petty theft men will admit having accomplished. Regarding both stealing and lying, adults have two complementary roles in teaching our children the expectations of society. Without question, we teach best by example. Children who hear their parents telling little white lies, let alone large black ones, can hardly fail to learn that truth is worth very little at home. We also attempt to teach by precept ("It's bad to tell lies") and by punishment ("Go to your room"). You can imagine how hollowly either of these lessons falls upon the ears of an attentive child who has heard her parents telling convenient social untruths day in and day out.

So, what should you do when you hear your kids shading the truth, telling small tales, and when we find purloined toys or illicitly acquired candy under their beds? First of all, recognize these activities as normal behaviors during the years when children are becoming clearer about the necessary distinctions between truth and fantasy, and between mine and yours. There is no need to take the high moral ground with preschoolers; one need be neither excessively preachy nor punitive with the very young. It is sufficient to:

1.   Point out the facts as they appear to a more or less objective adult;

2. agree that the version of the facts initially offered by the child is convenient and would have been nice had it happened to be true;

3. point out that the rules in your family are that you tell the truth even when it is uncomfortable and embarrassing.

(If the last point happens not to be the case in your family, your task is certainly more difficult.) Keep in mind that the moral education of your children does not need to be accomplished in one fell swoop. You can rest assured that you will be presented with many opportunities to help your offspring sort out right from wrong, and reality from fantasy.

Eventually you may decide that something more is required than clarification. When lying and stealing continue it certainly seems worthwhile to make clear to the child that this is hazardous, unacceptable, and expensive behavior. The family that fails to punish chronic misbehavior is tacitly accepting and rewarding it. We don't know very much about the roots of antisocial patterns in adult life, but it is quite clear that some families teach dishonesty in various forms by both precept and practice.

Safety

During the first few years of your child's life safety concerns have a certain simplicity. "This knife is sharp, so I'll keep it safely out of reach of my toddler." "This hot water heater is set at too high a temperature, so I'll turn it down to 120° F." But as your child gets older a process of allowing some exposure to hazards actually becomes necessary. "This knife is sharp, but I want to teach my child how to use it." "There is dangerous traffic on my street, but I want my child to learn to cope with urban life." Actually, I suspect that most parents deal with questions of acceptable risk in a nearly completely unconscious fashion, setting safety limits pretty much on the basis of gut feelings. If we are anxious people, it is difficult to be anything other than anxious with our kids. "Watch out! You'll hurt yourself!" is a cry from the heart. If you are not particularly anxious, you may have more choices. I recall talking with a friend near our community swimming pool one day. Looking over her shoulder I saw her son playing a game of running full tilt towards the pool and launching himself into the air as far as possible from the water's edge. I said to her "Diane, do you know what William is doing?" and she replied "Elmer, do I really want to know?" Her calm assurance that William had the sense to take care of himself was more than I could have managed, but it worked for her and for her child.

EVERYDAY PEDIATRICS FOR PARENTS

During these years, a number of new dangers need to be considered. These include access to hazardous tools, firearms kept within the house, bicycles, skates, and skateboards. Community standards will have a powerful influence on how most families deal with the dangers implicit in these devices. If every child on the street wears a safety helmet when he rides his bike, it is easy to insist that your newly fledged cyclist wear his as well. But what if helmets are proscribed by the neighborhood peer group as sissified? The tension between the folkways of the children, the expectations of the adult community, and the particular standards of behavior of a given family can be a major and persistent issue from middle childhood on. The applicable teaching is **Grossman's Law of Nonconformity:** *He who marches to a different drummer can expect to have his feet stepped upon.*

Food

For a very long time after we left Eden, the human diet was relatively simple. Our ancestral hunter-gatherer tribes grazed their limited ecosystems. A modest assortment of animals to be hunted or fished, seasonal fruits, tubers, seeds, and nuts, perhaps some wild grain, and that was about all. With the development of agriculture, most static populations came to depend on grains for the largest part of their diet. The contrast with the bounty overflowing our supermarkets today is striking. Nearly equally as impressive is the simplicity of the diets chosen by our middle-aged children. More often than not, it resembles the limited diet available in primitive agricultural communities: grains, tubers, seeds, and nuts. Grains are dominant: wheat in the forms of bread, cereals, and pasta; corn as cereal, popcorn, chips, and burritos. Tubers are represented by potatoes. Peanut butter is the preferred form of seeds and nuts. The big differences are the importance of milk and milk products and the heavy intake of sweets of all kinds. All of which makes the point that the diet chosen by your first-grader may not be so bad after all. If eggs and meat are available to provide extra iron, and some fruit is added to provide fiber and vitamin C, a reasonably decent diet is possible, even for 6-year olds.

Most kids this age like very simple food, very simply prepared, and that's okay. Leave the gravy off the meatloaf; he'll prefer ketchup, anyway. Don't expect her to try the roasted garlic or sautéed eggplant, at least not until the late teens. I have yet to see a case of growth failure due to a vegetable deficiency. It is common for kids to have strong views about the presentation of their food. They may want their sandwiches cut diagonally, and they may complain vigorously if the peas touch the mashed potato.

The best single thing you can do to improve the diet of small children is to limit the amount of junk food you bring into the house. They cannot fill up on cookies if there are no cookies to fill up on. If there are no juices or Cokes in the fridge, they will drink water or milk. If there are no Pop Tarts or Sugar Bombs for breakfast they will eat toast or corn flakes. In the absence of frozen yogurt from the freezer, they may decide to eat an orange. And even if they don't, they will probably survive.

I have to confess that I find this advice easier to give than to live by. Having been raised in a household where clean plates were expected and where refusal to eat a vegetable meant banishment from the table, I vowed to take a gentler approach when I had a family of my own. And I tried, I really did. But when I saw my children push their vegetables aside, rejected without so much as a taste, I could hear myself sounding very much like my own father: "At least take a bite!" The conservative tastes of our youngest children really got to me, and we instituted a "50 New Foods" family competition. When one of the kids had tried 50 previously rejected foods, he had the privilege of orchestrating an entire day of family activity. (They always chose the same thing: a visit to the bagel bakery, followed by a day at the zoo, and a spaghetti dinner in the Italian section of San Francisco.) By the time our fourth child had grown up and left home I had pretty well calmed down about this issue. Those readers (both of you) who are somewhat more rational about food may find this either amusing or pitiful, depending on how judgmental you happen to be. The problem is identical to the one discussed earlier in the chapters on infancy; many of us define ourselves as parents too powerfully as those who feed. Until a self-help group (Feeders Anonymous, I suppose) forms, we will have to struggle along as best we can, suppressing as much as possible the impulse to force feed our children with unwanted kale and cauliflower.

The Middle-Aged Child and the Family Dinner. In a preceding chapter I mentioned the myth of the Happy Family Dinner Hour, and how generally unsatisfying family dinners with small children were likely to be. The company of middle-aged children changes this somewhat. They are likely to have acquired fairly civilized table manners and can understand and even take part in conversation. Of course, they are unlikely to be able to sit still through a really long meal, and there are limits to how much complex dialogue they can be expected to tolerate. Within these limits, I think children's participation at family meals is increasingly important. Mealtimes can provide children with some of their best opportunities to hear the significant adults in their lives talk about the significant issues of life. These are the times when family values are *really* learned—by watching and listening and participating. If disorganization or the television is allowed to postpone or intrude upon these times, everyone loses. In American life today, time has become a precious and increasingly rare commodity. Longer work hours combined with commuting means less time for children to learn what only their parents can teach. We learn to be fathers or mothers by watching what our fathers or mothers do, and seeing how they do it. Our expectations of adult life and the roles and rules of the adult world are taught at home. Cooking, home repairs, making a bed, doing the laundry, changing the baby, coping with an angry neighbor, premenstrual tension, an inadequate paycheck, or an inadequate spouse—the skills of family life are learned in the family. We teach our kids what we think adults should spend their time doing by being the adults they watch as we spend our time. They may (or may not) hear what we say, but they *learn* what they see us do. If we are not present in their lives as models, the vacuum will be filled very promptly by society's other teachers—the movies, television, and the culture of the child's peers.

Chores and Allowances. Family life has changed enormously in the last century. A hundred years ago, most Americans still lived in rural areas. A child growing up on a family farm was immersed in the adult world in a way that could not fail to teach the lessons of adult life. Work and responsibility were the pillars of existence. Children were important as sources of family labor from an early age, and their roles were obvious and significant. A hundred years ago, a child in an urban family was also incorporated into the routine of household tasks; there was so much to be done in the era before labor-saving machines that every pair of hands was needed and used. But the role of many American children today is quite different. Nowadays, parents are home less, so there is less opportunity for the sharing of household chores. Furthermore, those chores are fewer and more easily managed. Or it may be simpler to make the bed and do the laundry yourself than it is to teach the kids and oversee their labors. Thus many children grow up nearly oblivious to the daily requirements of a functioning household because they have not been expected to contribute to it. I think it is essential to incorporate our children in every possible way into the real tasks of family living. They need to learn the skills of everyday life, they need to experience the discipline of family expectations, and they need to feel that they have a real part to play in the smooth operation of the family unit. This kind of contibution has still another advantage: It makes an allowance a meaningful reward for work accomplished, rather than an expected and automatic perquisite. It is a most useful lesson that regular effort is needed to obtain a regular income. (For even more comments regarding this issue see Chapter 19.)

Chapter 17

Preteens

Behavior and Development

Medical practice, parenting, and bird watching have in common the development of skill in pattern recognition. The bird watcher looks for the telltale combination of markings or flight pattern or song. In much the same fashion, physicians and parents become sensitized to groupings of signs and symptoms. Your preteen kids will provide you with the opportunity to note some striking patterns in human development. As they grope their way from childhood towards adolescence, some children fall into clearly recognizable types, as easily discernible as wrens are from blue jays.

The Organized Girl is a fine example. These children often begin to show themselves in early childhood by the way they line up their dolls on the shelf. They are generally choosing their own clothes every morning by the time they are about 3-years old. In school they quickly learn the rules and are teachers' helpers instantly. By the time puberty is starting, they have taken on significant household responsibility, and may calmly evaluate their mothers' methods of cooking, cleaning, and child raising, with the implicit judgment that they can and will do it better. (Not surprisingly, some mothers do not take kindly to this.) Among their friends, these girls are the leaders—they edit the school newspaper, sit on the student council, and organize the fund-raising events. All this talent may be wrapped up in a charming personality package; then again, it may not.

The Teenie Bopper is different. These children look at adult patterns of life with something between disinterest and loathing. They are early converts to the styles of the real adolescents. They are listening to hip-hop or punk or heavy metal before they are out of grade school; they demand the popularly correct brands of all consumer goods; they know which idols of popular culture are still worth idolizing and which are on the way out. The female Teenie Bopper is in a hurry for her first training bra, and for boy/girl parties. The male of the same age may find himself somewhat out of his depth with this aspect of Teenie Bopperism, although the rest of the teen scene looks awfully good to him. His parents may wonder why so many little girls keep calling him up; he may wonder a bit about it himself.

The Reluctant Scholar has often surfaced by this age. School may never have been much to his liking from the start; by the end of grammar school, he (usually he rather than she) has begun to dig in his heels. He lies to his parents about homework: "She didn't assign any tonight" and to his teacher as well: "I lost my notebook". These children are neither stupid nor emotionally disturbed. But their interests are simply incompatable with academic life. They need a nonacademic environment as soon as one can be arranged. It is a profound mistake to believe that every child and adolescent is best served by the same curriculum. By the start of junior high school, this becomes painfully obvious.

The Boy Who Does Not Like Sports comprises a small, sad category. Whether the disability is muscular, hormonal, or temperamental, he has little interest and less skill in the playground activities that enthrall his sweatier peers. This may have already become a sore subject at home if his father equates masculinity with Monday night football. Finding a substitute activity can be a big help. This might be an unusual but socially acceptable sport that requires greater skill and less brawn, such as archery, golf, or sailing. Nonphysical pursuits for competition and success include chess, photography, fossil-hunting, and other kinds of collecting.

In general, the preteen age group is notable for a quantum leap in independence from the family. An annoying symptom is the style of speech that parents of an older generation termed "sassy" and modern parents call "smartass." This is in no way a recent phenomenon; there is historical evidence that the erosion of respect for one's elders has been noted and regretted for thousands of years. However, it does seem to be particularly virulent in an age when most of the rules of verbal interaction between the old and the young (and everyone else, for that matter) have been abandoned. Parents are appropriately taken aback by the snotty know-it-alls who abruptly appear at the dinner table. My own view is that the newly sensed independence that underlies disrespectful speech can be quietly appreciated, but adults should take the opportunity to restate family expectations about the proprieties. During the tug of war that will develop during the next few years, parents must be as clear as possible about where they remain in charge and where the kids can take over. Guidelines about manners within the household are a good reminder during this transition.

The Sexual Development of Girls

Few of the developmental milestones of childhood vary as much as the timing of sexual development and the associated growth spurt that ushers in adolescence. In general, the sexual development of girls precedes that of boys by at least a year. Girls often start budding out with breasts as early as age 8, although the average time is after age 10; some perfectly normal girls have no breast development until after age 13. The first evidence of breast change is the formation of a firm, and often temporarily tender, button-like disc of breast tissue under one nipple. When this happens at an early age it is often the cause of needless alarm. The development of the other breast may start at about the same time or may be delayed for months. Pubic hair often begins to appear at this time, and the girl's height growth accelerates. The rapid increase in height and weight necessitates a larger intake of food. Most girls' appetites increase noticeably, although not usually to the degree seen in pubertal boys. Unhappily, many preteen girls are already hooked by the current American fashion of excessive slimness, and eating disorders begin to appear. (See Chapter 21 on Eating Problems.) Within about a year, her rate of growth is at its fastest, and within about 2½ years after the first breast changes, her first menstruation (menarche) will probably occur. The average age at first menstruation has been dropping in the developed world and is now 12½ to 13 years in the United States. This pattern of earlier sexual development is apparently due to better nutrition, fewer serious infections during childhood, and possibly other environmental factors such as increased exposure to artificial light. The rate of change has finally decreased in recent years. Once menstruation has begun, growth has already slowed down; after adding another 2 or 3 inches during the next couple of years, most girls will have attained their adult height.

Menstruation, when it does finally arrive, may become a regular, reliable monthly event, though it can be erratic for the first few months. The early cycles of menstruation are usually not accompanied by the production of eggs and are typically free of any menstrual cramps or other physical discomfort (dysmenorrhea). Emotional discomfort is another matter. The rapid increase in sex hormone levels and their fluctuation around the time of menses have profound effects on your daughter's mood. As time goes on, she will probably learn to live with premenstrual tension and unexpected mood swings, but in the early years of her developing sexual maturity, many girls act as if they have fallen under the influence of the Wicked Witch of the West. The first emotional displays are likely to be spread without prejudice over everyone within range.

Later, as they start to feel their ovarian oats, girls may begin to find life with Mother increasingly problematic. She may sense that life with two women under one roof in a family is not always a satisfactory arrangement. These early struggles can be expected to accentuate as adolescence comes along.

The insane sexual prudery of previous eras meant that many girls experienced their first menstrual bleeding wholly without preparation or information. There is no longer any excuse for this kind of predictable and unnecessary trauma. Don't count on schools to do the job; many girls need this information long before Health, Sex Education, or Social Living classes are offered. Parents need to teach their girls explicitly about what to expect and what to do. Girls nearly always start by using small menstrual pads rather than tampons. As she becomes more familiar and less uncomfortable with the process of dealing with her own genitals and her bloody menstrual flow, she may quickly decide that tampons are easier and neater, and less trouble under a swimsuit. The vast majority of girls have little or no hymeneal tissue at this age, so the use of small tampons is easy to master.

As one might expect, different girls respond to this developmental excitement in different ways. Some have been anticipating these changes with delight and impatience. They simply cannot wait to be launched into adolescent and adult life. But there are plenty of girls for whom budding breasts and pubic fuzz are embarrassing and unwelcome. Parents may also be divided in their views; some will celebrate the signs of growth and some will be sad to see that childhood is ending, with the storms of adolescence just over the horizon.

Responses to sexual development often depend on timing. The first girl in her class to grow breasts and shoot up in height is breaking trail for all the other girls to follow later—and she will probably hate it. It is weird and lonely to stand inches higher than everyone else except the teacher, to discover that ones interests are no longer the same as the others, and to face the future without the comfort of peers who are doing and going through the same things. By contrast, the last girl in her class to grow breasts and shoot up in height has had a terribly long time to wish something would start to happen. Nearly every other girl is interested in boys (and may have boys interested in return), is immersed in discussions of brassieres, and experimenting with makeup: she isn't, and its pretty lonely for her, too. If one of your daughters find themselves at either of these extremes, she will appreciate your sympathetic understanding, and she may need to hear that her experiences, although painful, are perfectly normal. Everyone has her own personal timetable, and you just have to live with it.

Sexual Development in Boys

The first sexual change is an increase in the size of the testes, somewhere between the ages of 9½ and 14½, with the average around age 12; a bit later the penis starts to enlarge and pubic hair begins to grow. Erections become more frequent, and sexually explicit dreams, sometimes accompanied by orgasm (nocturnal emissions, or "wet dreams"), may begin. Shortly after the first increase in the size of the testes, the period of rapid growth begins. This is nearly always accompanied by a startling and expensive increase in appetite. Height and weight grow faster and faster for about 2 years and then gradually begin to decelerate. Adult height may be reached anywhere from the midteens to the early 20s.

The early stages of sexual development seem to be less emotionally upsetting for boys than they often are for girls. Both the pituitary hormones (gonadotropins) and testosterone, the predominant sex hormone of males, increase gradually starting at around age 9 or 10, and reach adult levels in midadolescence. However, the day to day levels are reasonably constant; boys never have to cope with the monthly cyclic fluctuations that unsettle so many girls. This is not to say that these hormonal changes are without effect on behavior. The testosterone-rich blood of the pubertal boy is without doubt the cause of much parental hand-wringing and many visits to various juvenile authorities. My point it is that male hormones underlie behaviors that inconvenience people other than the owners of the hormones themselves. More about this later, in the chapter on adolescence.

The early developing boy finds himself in a different situation than his early developing sister. Increased height and heft means increased strength and a higher place on the preadolescent male pecking order. He is more likely to sense admiration from his smaller classmates, rather than feeling isolated from them. The late developing boy probably has the worst of all worlds. While his peers get bigger and bigger, changing their voices and their opinions about the opposite sex, he seems hardly to be growing at all. He often wonders whether permanent childhood is his forever, and it is not a pleasant prospect. This is a culture that values and rewards height, especially in males. It is no surprise that large numbers of perfectly normal, but late developing, boys are taken to their doctors with the request "Please give him something to make him start growing." Hormone treatments to jump-start pubertal development have been available for years. In the short run, they work; growth starts. In the long run, there is the risk that eventual height may actually be *less* than it would have been if pubertal development had been allowed to start on its own. My personal prejudice

EVERYDAY PEDIATRICS FOR PARENTS

is to deal with the emotional problems of the boy as best you can and hold out for the spontaneous appearance of the growth spurt.

Sex Education

It is often about this time that parents begin to look for guidance concerning sex education. What books to provide, who should talk to whom, perhaps we can ask the pediatrician to do this during the next check-up visit? Unfortunately, if you've waited this long, you are probably too late. It seems to me that the most important parts of sex education are about the way people relate to one another, the way the human body is viewed, and about the power relationships of the sexes. Is human interaction marked by consideration and respect, or do people exploit and dominate each other? Does the family's balance of power teach that both sexes are to be respected as important, or that one sex exists to serve the other? Is the child taught that the genitals are dirty or shameful, that masturbation is evil, or that the body is a wonder and a joy? All of these lessons are the foundation of adult sexual functioning. Teaching the 12-year old about breasts and menstruation and erections and all the rest is fine, but rather after the fact.

Still, someone has to teach the anatomy and physiology of sex. The first step is a visit to your local library to find out what books are available; the reference librarian can help. Then you may want to go to the book store; it is a good idea to have this material easily available over a long period of time, so it's worth owning the books. There are also inexpensive booklets published by the American Academy of Pediatrics and the American Medical Association; these are available from your doctor. The local Planned Parenthood office is another excellent source. In many school districts, sex education is thoughtfully and fully incorporated into the curriculum of primary and secondary schools. Oddly enough, the kids who need the most information in this area are likely to be the ones who attend private schools where sex education is frequently ignored. Parochial schools are wonderfully inconsistent; some focus wholly on Thou Shalt Not, some really teach.

When you embark on this enterprise, it will pay to have read the material before giving it to the kids; most adults need a quick review of the facts to be able to answer a question with any accuracy. Don't be surprised if your children react to your sexual pedagogy with embarrassed avoidance; you may have to persevere over a period of time. Eventually, sex can become a real subject for discussion, instead of the Great Secret, second only to the family finances as something never to be talked about. I will never forget my daughter, age 15, sitting down on the rug between her mother and me one Sunday afternoon, and asking whether we thought it appropriate for her to start having sex with her boyfriend. I thought it was wise of her to consider our opinions, and I thought it was wonderful that she trusted us enough to talk about the subject. (In case you are wondering, I responded that readiness for sex meant being ready for all its consequences, emotional and physical. Some of those consequences could be wonderful and fulfilling, but some could be deeply hurtful, and it was necessary to make a careful judgment. Years later, she told me that she had already decided that she was not ready, but she wanted to hear what her mother and I would say.)

Pushing Kids: Music Education as a Paradigm

All these issues—sassiness, independence, sex—are linked by the question of how much parents should stay in charge of their children. In many instances, this devolves into a struggle between the parent who wants the child to do something, and the child, who doesn't. Whether it is using the toilet at age 3 or working harder in school at age 13, parents must decide if, when, and how to push. A classic example is the teaching of music. I had not been long in practice before noting the common sequence of failure in extracurricular music education. The mother of a bright little 7-year old reports happily that he has started to take piano lessons; the teacher is said to be impressed by his enthusiasm and talent. At about age 8, I ask how the music is going and learn that the lessons are proceeding but under duress; he really resists practicing and the teacher wants the parents to insist on half an hour a day "so that he can make progress." At about age 9, I ask about the piano and the mother grimaces "We gave it up; I told him we were not going to pay good money for lessons when he refused to practice." In short, if one defines music as a drudgery imposed by the teacher and enforced by the parents, one can pretty well predict that a self-respecting child will decide there is nothing in it for him. The problem here lies in the music teacher's assumption that continual practice is the only road to proficiency. It is as if the teacher of pottery insisted that the weekly lessons in the studio were useless unless the child took a bag of wet clay home to work on every day. In fact, if the teacher can relax about practice when the child wants to do other things, a weekly music lesson can work very well indeed. Progress will be slow, no doubt; this is not the way to make Horowitzes, *but music will not be abandoned.* If the teacher can accept this without feeling insulted, and the parents can understand that the choice is between no musical education and a leisurely one, this laissez-faire approach can keep children learning and loving music. It may also serve as a model when other issues arise between adult goals and a child's sense of what is right for him. Sometimes we have to listen to the child.

The End of Innocence? There are certainly many children whose preteen years appear to be a seamless continuation of childhood. Their increased independence remains channeled safely within adult-approved, peer group activities and they continue to play contented childhood roles within the family. For other preteens, the world has already burst in upon them, and childhood has developed some dark-edged meanings. Parental conflict or separation, family struggles with finances or drugs or the law, the hazards of life on mean streets—all these frightening realities are part of the lives of too many youngsters. But for a happily large group of American children, these years constitute a period of immense personal growth, of a wider and wiser view of the world, of increased readiness to ride the roller coaster of adolescence that awaits them. These are lucky kids, not always easy to live with, but exciting to be around. Make sure everyone's seat belt is buckled, and have a good time.

Chapter 18

Adolescents

Teenagers and Their Doctors

When I see an infant or a child in the course of my practice, there is always another responsible adult present. More often than not, it is the child's mother, and much if not most of the medical encounter is actually between myself and Mom. Although I am a doctor for children, my doctoring is very largely accomplished through the efforts of the parent or the parent's substitute. As the child matures, her part in the visit expands. She can tell me her symptoms and ask me questions, and her mother, who is usually still present, plays a less central role. But what happens when the child patient has become the adolescent patient? What is the parent's role when the teenager can speak for herself? The answers depends on the needs and the styles of everyone involved. The pediatric visit is a great place for adolescents to practice their increasing autonomy and for parents to practice the fine art of letting go. It is also provides an opportunity for the doctor to practice the fine art of tightrope walking. It seems to me that my role as pediatrician has to expand when I am dealing with kids of this age. I want the teenager to think of me as her own doctor and at the same time I want her parents to continue to see me as a useful resource in helping them deal with whatever problems may arise. This all needs to be made explicit; therefore, sometime early in her teens I try to find an occasion to explain the ground rules within which I want us to operate. These include a promise to the adolescent of privacy. I expect her to come for visits whenever possible without her parents, and she has my word that what she tells me is privileged information, not to be shared without her permission. The sole exception to this rule is if I consider that privacy will result in serious danger to anyone. I also try to continue discussion visits with the parents alone, so that I can obtain an adult view of the teenager's life. (This ideal situation is only sometimes realized, and in the current climate of managed and therefore restricted care, it may not be easy to get your insurance carrier to pay for your talk visits with your child's pediatrician. This seems to me yet another reason to remove insurance companies from the provision of medical care.) A certain proportion of kids this age consider me to be an agent of the oppressive adult power structure and under no circumstances worth talking to. Furthermore, a proportion of parents seem uncomfortable with this proposed adolescent medical independence. I've had some college juniors appear for their annual check-ups still chaperoned by hovering mothers. When this happens I always ask myself who is having the most trouble: the parent who can't trust the teenager or the teenager who can't assert her own need to assume responsibility for herself?

Graduation from the Pediatrician. Pediatricians were first defined as baby doctors back at the turn of the century. Then our role expanded to include older children and young adolescents, and now we find ourselves taking care of young adults as well. Is this a good idea? It seems to me that most kids do well to stay with a pediatrician through adolescence. We are focused on the problems of growth and development and the diseases of youth. We attempt to understand the issues of education and independence that concern people in their late teens and early twenties. My possibly biased conclusion is that until the young person is out of the family home and launched into the adult world, he probably does best in a familiar pediatric setting. Of course, some teenagers become uncomfortable in an office full of babies. I know that some of our burly, bearded young men are embarrassed when the nurse mistakes them for fathers rather than patients. But most of them stay with us until independence and employment. I tell them that they are welcome until they get a master's degree or get married, but I've been known to make temporary exceptions to both conditions. The truth of the matter is that they are such interesting people I hate to see them go.

Growth and Development

Adolescents cannot and should not be characterized according to fashionable stereotypes. This is worth mentioning because so many parents of preteens live in dread of the Terrible Teens looming ahead. More often than not, this automatic anxiety is unnecessary. I recall the comment of a physician friend who had six teenage children; he said it was awfully noisy but wonderfully exciting. Within the limits of this generally accurate description, there are a few recognizable patterns.

Girls often signal the approach of puberty by a distinct increase in volatility of mood. Easy tears and easy rages may upset the family and puzzle the girl herself. What is happening is hormones, and it will take her a while to learn to live with them. As adolescence progresses, she is likely to be more and more in conflict with her mother. The process of becoming a woman in her mother's house implies a certain amount of rivalry between them as the girl separates and defines herself in a new way. This is often an exceedingly painful process for her mother who finds her daughter increasingly distant and hostile. It is a kind of rerun of 2-year old negativism with strange sexual overtones added. The number of ways in which the teenager chooses to explore her separateness and her independence seems to be limited only by her imagination. Green hair and a nose ring state her difference from her parents and proclaim her identification with the adolescent world of her friends. Her refusal to pick up the mess in her room and her reluctance to pursue her studies express her desire for freedom from the trammels of filial obedience. None of these behaviors is likely to go down very well with her parents, which, after all, is the whole point. The adolescent girl may be close to her father during the early teens. But the relationship between father and daughter can become quite tense as she begins to have sexual feelings for her peers, starts to date, wants more freedom to come and go as she pleases, and borrows the family car. It can be difficult for Dad to accept the reality that his little girl is not so little any more, that, in fact, she is a sexual being with her own agenda.

By the late teens, a substantial number of girls have made their peace with Mom. It turns out that there is room for two women under one roof, after all, and both mother and daughter accept that they are different and separate people. They may even become friends as they discover some feminine commonality. Not infrequently, Dad may remain odd man out for a while. This may be largely a sexual matter; it can take a long time for a girl's Elektra feelings for her father to wane, and his discomfort with the realities of his daughter's sex life can also last a while.

Personality changes in adolescent boys can be summed up in one word: testosterone. This does not always mean trouble, but it does imply a brisk rearranging of family processes and power. As he approaches his midteens, the adolescent male is becoming fairly restless. He wants a longer leash or no leash at all. He continues to shift his interests and allegiances away from home. School may appear utterly irrelevant to his world. As he becomes aware of his growing strength, his behavior may become decidedly less compliant and more challenging. This is a perplexing time for parents. When should controls be loosened? Is it worthwhile even trying to maintain the old rules? The period of male rebellion seems to be quite prolonged for many of our young men. While a substantial number of young women apparently work out their new relationships with parents by the end of the teens, my impression is that this process is extended into the twenties for many men. Perhaps it is related to the often prolonged schooling that delays financial and vocational independence. In any event, the young lions challenge the old lions again and again.

In an occasional family, none of this happens at all. The growing young man remains contentedly ensconced at home, challenges no one, continues to be involved with school, and is perceived by his parents to be an ideal teenager. I worry about these kids; why are they not moving towards independence? Is it too frightening? Is the family constellation so fragile that the boy believes that his growth would shatter it? Whatever the reason, failure to assert some independence at this age is a symptom to be studied rather than a situation for the parents to enjoy.

At this point in the chapter I would love to be able to outline a successful program for parents to follow when faced with adolescent rebellion, but, unhappily, I don't have a useful Grossman's Law at hand. About all I can suggest is the following:

1. Examine your own goals as a parent. Do you want your child to grow up? If so, this means giving over control of her life to her, not all at once, but it has to be done.
2. During the process of emancipation, it helps to keep clear about what is allowed and what is forbidden. Teenagers are continually pushing the limits

not only to test your authority and their freedom but to assure themselves that you still care enough about them to have rules you will enforce.

3. You will often be reminded of the 2-year old stage. As was the case then, it is absolutely necessary to pick your battles with care. Some fights are not worth the bother.

An unusual but important variation on the theme of adolescent acting out occurs in families where the parents are inappropriately pleased by their children's rebellious behavior. These parents seem to identify so closely with their kids that they perceive even dangerous and antisocial behavior as desirable evidences of strength and courage, rather than hazardous experiments with adult roles. Some of these parents have never really settled down to ordinary standards of mature behavior themselves. Their use of alcohol and other drugs and their patterns of sexual and social behavior may even retain a flavor of adolescence. And on the contrary, some parents regret having led such straight and narrow lives themselves, and use their children's behavior as a substitute for the wildness they wished they had experienced. In any case, teenagers whose families fail to provide guidance by example and precept are at distinctly greater risk of a variety of developmental, sexual, medical, and legal mishaps.

Sex

In a book like this, a chapter on adolescents without some discussion of their sex lives would be surprising. The only problem is knowing what to say to parents that has any likelihood of being at all useful.

In the unlikely event that they could actually talk about it, parents and their children might be able to agree on one topic: **Masturbation is good.** That statement may strike some readers as unusually direct and unequivocal in a book which I have tried to fill with pros and cons, shaded judgments, and fairly restrained editorializing. But masturbation is a valuable exception. At a time of life when the sexual impulse is amazingly powerful, especially among males, and when the task of finding a willing partner in sexual enterprise may be daunting, masturbation provides an excellent answer. It requires little effort, never results in unwanted pregnancy, and poses no risk of sexually transmitted disease. The vast majority of adolescent boys will have already discovered masturbation. If they have had accurate sex education they should know that it is harmless and healthy. There is no normal frequency to which they should attain or beyond which they should not venture. As usual, girls are different; recent studies suggest that fewer than half of American teenage girls masturbate.

Whether this is a function of their sexual parts being less convenient for self-stimulation, a less vigorous sex drive, or possibly early lessons that touching oneself is bad, for whatever reasons masturbation is not a uniform part of their lives. Very few teenagers will be interested in discussing any of this with their parents. This is not to imply that you should not try to talk about masturbation with them if it seems indicated; however, you should not expect much in the way of dialogue.

As I've noted in earlier chapters, sexual behavior (other than masturbation) is just another form of human interaction, and the way your kids act sexually depends, to a considerable extent, on how you have taught them to act in general. If they have learned that people are supposed to respect each other and themselves, there is a fighting chance that their sexual lives will be influenced by that golden rule. At least, that is the theory. In real life, how they act will also be determined by their inborn temperaments, the mores of their friends, the effects of a variety of psychoactive drugs, especially beer, and the availability of unchaperoned private places. We all hope that a healthy respect for the invasive power of viruses, bacteria, and spermatozoa will also enter into their sexual equations. But what role do parents have when kids reach this age? You have already taught your lessons about human relations, you have already developed the family guidelines about what subjects can be discussed between generations, and you have made clear how much freedom you want them to have in regulating their lives. In short, it's pretty late in the day to make any changes. This is a subtle and complex business. I wish that children could live in families where everyone is respected, where even emotionally charged subjects can be discussed without shame or fear, and where an important lesson taught is the desirability of growing up to strong and independent adulthood. This could set the stage for relationships with teenagers that allow continued, honest communication about the pleasures and dangers of sex; in all honesty I have to say that it also may not. The particular chemistry of a given family may mean that one child can talk frankly and usefully with his parents, and another may hide every part of his sexual life. Whether they appear to be listening or not, I think it is worthwhile to remind our kids that condoms prevent death and disease, and that condoms, diaphragms, or the pill will prevent pregnancy. The tendency of young people to feel immortal and invulnerable is well known, and these days is more dangerous than ever.

Homosexual Adolescents

Any discussion of homosexuality in childhood and adolescence must be prefaced with a disclaimer: Not much is known about the development of sexual preference. As societal prejudice wanes, it is finally possible for gay and lesbian adults to report on their personal sexual odysseys, and a variety of stories have emerged. However, we have no really large studies of a representative group of homosexual adults, and because so many gays and lesbians still live hidden lives, we don't even know what a representative group would look like. Children who experience homosexual feelings during childhood soon learn that expressing these feelings leads to predictable and unpleasant consequences. This is particularly true for boys who will promptly find themselves called names, ostracized, and often physically attacked by their peers. The reactions of their families is not likely to be much more comfortable. All this makes it exceedingly difficult to study homosexuality as it unfolds in the first decades of life.

As gay men reconstruct their memories of childhood and adolescence, they often describe a sense of being different from early or midchildhood on. Some, but by no means all, of these kids will be labeled as sissies. Some of them will have had a prolonged and powerful interest in dressing up in girls' clothes or engaging in girls' play. Others will have discovered that they simply failed to share the usual interests of most boys their age. For some, clearly sexual attraction to other boys is present by the beginning of the teens, if not before. However, none of this definitely predicts homosexual development. Many teenage boys are engaged in a struggle to define their sexuality, and many heterosexual boys worry about whether they are actually gay. Homosexual experimentation during this period when sexual preference is being defined is quite common among boys and young men who eventually settle into dedicated and comfortable heterosexuality.

The development of a lesbian sexual identity is equally hard to delineate. Unlike the category "sissy boy," with its clearly pejorative overtones, the category "tomboy" is unlikely to get a girl into much trouble. It is an approved youthful style which the girl is expected to "grow out of." And it appears that most tomboys do just that, changing with time into heterosexual young women. Some don't, and they probably make up a significant group of lesbians. But the early history of a great many lesbians seems no different than that of their heterosexual sisters. During adolescence the development of sexual feelings among women may be thoroughly confused by the category of the "crush," an intense and ostensibly platonic love of one girl for another girl, an older teenager, or a grown woman. This is part of the personal history of so many heterosexual adult women that it seems to signify little if anything about eventual sexual preference. Obviously, we are going to have to wait for a generation of adult homosexuals to give us a broader and more accurate picture of the growth of the homosexual identity.

What we do know is that the teenager who discovers that he or she is gay is nearly sure to find this deeply troubling. Few of these kids will know adults who are successful and open exemplars of gay or lesbian existence; role models are few and far between. For most, being gay or lesbian will be perceived as shameful, dangerous, and isolating. No one needs social support more than they do, but it is a rare high school indeed that will have a club for the gays and lesbians. If the church youth group is the center of their social life, it is even less likely to be a place of acceptance and understanding. Stepping into the world of adolescent dating and sexual exploration is daunting enough for most heterosexual kids. Think how it feels to the kids who know that a completely different sexual world is out there somewhere, hidden, hazardous, and totally unknown. One effect of all this is the high incidence of suicide and suicide attempts among homosexual teenagers. Between one quarter and one half of young homosexuals attempt suicide on at least one occasion.

A large proportion of adolescent homosexuals can benefit from skillful psychotherapy. Until the very recent past, emotional problems associated with sexual orientation were often dealt with by the therapists' vigorous efforts to erase the "undesirable" sexual preferences. This is still the preferred method for some religious counselors who define homosexuality as sin. It has taken a long time for the psychotherapeutic community to decide that the troubled gay or lesbian needs help with the troubles, not with sexual preference. Finding a therapist who is experienced and knowledgeable about all this can still be difficult. Gay and lesbian organizations or publications may be good sources of information.

The Hypochondria of Change

One way to deal with adolescent change is to worry about it, so some kids fasten all of their anxieties on their bodies. They note with alarm every intestinal gurgle, are convinced that every mole is a cancer, and avoid no-calorie soft drinks because of the chemicals. His pediatrician will recognize this syndrome when your teenager appears for a brief illness visit and pulls out a list of eighteen complaints.

A frequent item on lists of this sort is chronic fatigue. Medically sophisticated families will have kids who are sure they suffer from the recently described chronic fatigue syndrome, and perhaps a few of them do. A tiny proportion will have signs or symptoms suggestive of hypothyroidism; I have found one such patient in the last thirty years. But the vast majority will fall into one of three groups: the excessively busy, who need more sleep and fewer activities, the anxious, and the depressed. The teenager who is tired because she is too busy has probably been dragged kicking and screaming to her doctor. Indeed, she *is* tired much of the time, but she has too full a schedule to worry about it. As far as she is concerned, her tiredness is basically her mother's problem, and if Mom would just quit worrying about it, everything would be fine. She will greet with derision or rolling of eyes any suggestion that cutting out some elective activities would make it possible to get more sleep. Parents should keep in mind that the adolescent hyperactivity of which you now disapprove is simply an exaggerated form of the wonderful vigor of earlier childhood which you had once thought marvelous.

The adolescents who are anxious or depressed are another matter. In my experience, these kids put up an impressive resistance to the idea that their troubles may be of a psychological nature. They usually deny any sort of difficulty in their social or family relationships. Even when school has become a sink of failure and despair, they will report that they are actually doing fine. The predictable response to my suggestion that psychotherapy might be useful is to tell me that maybe their parents could use it, but not them, thank you. Fortunately, adolescents are often sufficiently self-absorbed that they are fascinated with simple techniques of self study. I sometimes suggest that a diary would be useful to clarify issues and feelings. For the teen with a literary bent, I may suggest that he write letters to himself about the problems in his life. Another technique I offer is to draw pictures about problems. The concept of subpersonalities, which are representations of the varying, and sometimes warring, needs and tendencies within, can be used. I will ask the teenager to draw a cartoon of each of his subpersonalities, in order to become cognizant of the inner complexity and, eventually, to accept the reality of competing parts of himself. For those who eventually accept the need for therapy, teen groups are often useful. Discovering that other adolescents have similar concerns, and learning to talk about their problems in the presence of peers can be truly liberating.

Food

Anorexia and bulimia are now epidemic among adolescent American girls. This painful social and psychological problem is discussed in Chapter 21 on Eating Problems.

The usual problems of normal teen diets are deficiencies of calcium, iron, and vitamin C. Calcium deficiency occurs because a substantial proportion of American kids grow up drinking soda pop and juices instead of milk. Fortunately, some of them automatically begin drinking milk when their growth spurts start, a nice example of the innate wisdom of the body. However, some bodies are apparently pretty dumb, and a lesson in nutritional principles is in order. For practical purposes, calcium is available from milk and milk products and not much else. It is possible to devise a diet with enough soybean curd, nuts, oatmeal, and greens to provide a modest amount of calcium, but not nearly enough for optimal bone growth. Calcium supplements are often the best answer for the teenagers who won't drink milk or eat cheese or yogurt. Generic calcium carbonate or calcium phosphate are inexpensive, but the tablets are rather large and usually unpleasantly chalky, and they tend to be constipating. Antacids like Tums or Rolaids are calcium carbonate; they come in various flavors, which is a considerable help. Calcium citrate is less likely to be constipating; unfortunately, the pills are even larger. Calcium fortified orange juice is another alternative. The soy milks sold in dairy cases are not rich sources of calcium and should be avoided. One gram of calcium is supplied by 2 grams of dibasic calcium phosphate, 2.5 grams of calcium carbonate, or 5 grams of calcium citrate. Adolescent girls need about 1.2 grams of calcium daily; adolescent boys need about 1.5 grams.

A major problem for the menstruating girl is the loss of iron with every period. Many of these kids take a minimal caloric intake in order to control their weight. If they also happen to be inactive rather than athletic, their caloric needs are quite modest, and it becomes difficult to get enough iron from a typical diet. Iron deficiency anemia results. During childhood, enriched grain products (breakfast cereals, bread, pasta) are major sources of dietary iron. If the adolescent skips breakfast (most do) and avoids bread, she will have to get by on the iron in meat, eggs (currently out of fashion), nuts, and dark leafy greens (never in fashion). The best answer is supplemental iron taken as a ferrous sulfate tablet once or twice a week or as part of a daily multivitamin and mineral tablet.

Vitamin C is certainly not hard to get in the American diet but a substantial number of teens manage to avoid it. The sources are oranges, orange juice, tomatoes, potatoes, dark leafy greens, summer fruits (especially berries and mel-ons), or, failing all of these, vitamin C tablets; 50 to 60 mg a day is enough.

Aside from calcium, iron, and vitamin C, there really are no serious defi-ciencies in the average American teenager's diet. Despite this fact, an industry has arisen peddling a variety of protein supplements and amino acids to adolescent boys eager to bulk up their muscles and improve their athletic performance. The sole reason for this hucksterism is commercial greed. Proteins and their con-stituent amino acids are easily obtained from such ordinary foods as cereals, grains, legumes, meat, milk, cheese, nuts, and eggs. A large teenage boy needs about 60 to 80 grams of protein a day. When you consider that a modest slice of pizza plus a glass of milk supplies 25 or 30 grams, it is clear that expensive supplements are unnecessary. Unfortunately, this elementary nutritional infor-mation is not understood by athletic coaches and trainers who often advise the consumption of various patent powders and pills; they should know better.

Drugs

The subject of drugs is similar to the subject of sex in that parents often want more guidance than pediatricians have to offer. However, some organizing con-cepts may be worth noting. The most important of these is **Grossman's Law of Drug Use: *Everyone does drugs.*** Well, okay, maybe not quite everyone, but awfully near. When we think about drug use we mislead ourselves if we consider only the so-called illicit drugs. What is illicit and illegal depends on where you live and when. What is more to the point is the reality that our species discovered long ago that a wide variety of substances made people feel happier, more relaxed, and generally more content with existence. These won-derful chemicals, given to us in easily available form by bountiful Mother Nature, are found in chocolate, tea, coffee, hemp, poppies, coca bushes, fer-mented beverages, tobacco, and several species of mushrooms, to name a few. The use or consumption of each one of these materials has disadvantages, some minor, such as excess weight gain from chocolate, and some major, such as uninhibited violence and homicidal automobile driving from alcohol. Despite these flaws, drugs have been in use since the dawn of history and probably before. We are drug-using animals and I see no reason to expect us to change.

So, how does this bear on the question of the use of drugs by our teenage children? First, they are raised in a society that offers chemical answers to life's questions. Advertisements tell them to take a pill for everything that hurts, that beer lubricates social occasions, that liquor is sexy or prestigous or both, and that cigarettes are the badge of the grownup. Second, they are raised in families that use drugs. They watch their parents' enthusiastic use of coffee, tobacco, and alcohol, as well as innumerable medicinal drugs. After a decade or so of this indoctrination, the majority of young people will decide that if it is good enough for Dad and Mom, it is good enough for them. They may decide to try the drug of choice of their social group, which may not be the chosen drug of their parents' generation, and may even be under a legal cloud, but these are not seriously inhibiting factors. On the contrary, they make drug use even more desirable as a statement of independence. I am not recommending that teenagers or anyone else use drugs; the decision to do so can lead to incarceration and death. What I am saying is that people *do* use drugs and probably always will. If we want to diminish the damage done by drugs, both personal and social efforts will be required. At the family level, we may want to consider how we use drugs ourselves. Does every little headache really require a trip to the medicine cupboard? We teach drug use there just as surely as do the ads for Budweiser. Can we introduce our favorite drugs in a gentle fashion as part of life, rather than as an indicator of adult stature? The child who has always been given a sip of wine when the parents drink it at dinner is being taught that alcohol is part of life, not an exotic and exciting route to sex and freedom. At the societal level we can circumscribe drug use by limiting tobacco smoking in public places and by enforcing drunk driving laws. I think we should strictly limit the way dangerous drugs are advertised; the less money spent promoting alcohol and tobacco, the fewer children will get hooked. And I think we should legalize the drugs that we currently define as illegal. The Prohibition experiment of the 1920s should have convinced us that outlawing a drug simply increases the profits from its distribution. Crack cocaine is not a good thing to use, but if it can be obtained legally for moderate cost at the corner drug store, no one can make any money from selling it on the street, and we could be all but done with a major problem of crime and public health. Finally, we need to keep in mind that the conditions of one's life have a bearing on the decision to use drugs. For a young person trapped in poverty, with no prospect of a decent job and a successful family life, the hours spent high on drugs may be the only tolerable part of existence. Until we structure a society that makes the possibility of decent lives in decent communities a reality for everyone, drugs will be abused and more lives ruined and lost.

EVERYDAY PEDIATRICS FOR PARENTS

Chapter 19

Families—Changing Roles, Changing Expectations

As an inexperienced and not terribly worldly young doctor, I had somehow retained my childhood view that grownups and their institutions were cast in concrete. It took only a short time for the vigorous, dynamic reality of family growth and change to impress itself on me. Families truly are living organisms. In the usual, heterosexual, two-parent family model, the analogy of the fertilized egg is pretty close. Two people contribute a generous portion of their genetic and other material, coming together to form a new being, an amalgam of them both. And then, in obedience to inner and outer forces, the new family, like the new fetus, grows and changes and becomes a mature but still malleable entity. Well, one need not push this tiny insight too far, but it does serve to focus one's attention on the dynamic quality of human families.

Children. Nothing shapes the developing family more powerfully than the children—their number, age, sex, spacing, and individual characteristics. The American family has gotten considerably smaller over the last decades under the influence of the interacting factors of better birth control, concern for overpopulation, and the increasing costs of rearing a child. Despite the attractive myth of the Happy Family of Ten, there is a great deal to be said for the alternative myth that Less is More. Big families mean much less parental investment in each of the children. Older kids, of necessity, take on child rearing duties, although they are unlikely to have the maturity and judgment to carry them out as well as a parent. If we want our children to learn our values and our world view, we had better be available to do the teaching, and not leave it to teenaged siblings, let alone babysitters or nannies.

Regarding the gender of children, the question of whether parents want girls or boys is so complex that I hesitate to get into it. Obviously there are powerful cultural norms at work, and each culture has individual patterns rooted in economics, rules of inheritance, power relationships, and religious beliefs. Some of this is consciously understood, but some of it is so much a part of one's upbringing that you may be acting and feeling without real understanding of the sources of your preferences. The effects of all this in American life often eventuates in a desire for at least one boy. When a couple has had two or three girls and "keeps trying for a boy" the results may include a group of girls who feel undervalued by their parents and a boy who is overindulged to within an inch of his life.

It need hardly be said that the daily mechanics of family life require as much effort as it does to work at a job outside the home. When family life and work life are completely intertwined as in family farming, each family member must take an active role. Thus, children are incorporated into the economic life of the family very early. But when family and work are separated, the situation in the home may be somewhat less coercive, and the assignment of tasks to the children becomes less automatic. It is easy for children to grow up with the notion that the functioning of the household is wholly the duty and responsibility of the parents. I think that many urban kids have no idea of how much effort it takes to get bread on the table and clean clothes in the dresser drawer. It seems to me that it is a mistake to raise children as parasites on the parents. Assigning family responsibilities appropriate to the abilities of the children means respecting their need to be useful and valued, and it teaches them something about the interdependence of family existence. The way this is accomplished will depend on the age and level of understanding of the children as well as the particular needs and style of the family. By the age of 2 or 3, many children love to take part in family chores; it is true that they generally make more work than not, but the lessons of shared labor and cooperation are taught. Older kids often complain about assigned jobs and feel put upon by even minor infringements on their chosen activities. A useful tactic is to call a family meeting and compile a list of the ways in which each family member contributes to the whole. It is impressive and chastening for the resistant 10-year old to see the list grow as one enumerates the hours every week that parents earn the money, do the cooking, make the beds, and do the errands that keep the family afloat. When his short list of duties is written and assigned he may find it easier to understand the balance of effort and his small but necessary place within it.

Another complicated topic which should be touched upon is the effect that each child has on every single person in the family. The strengths, weaknesses, and peculiarities of every family member set up a kind of force field that

EVERYDAY PEDIATRICS FOR PARENTS

impinges on everyone else. Sometimes this is wonderfully positive. For example, an older brother who is loved and idolized by a younger sister can help her to respect and appreciate herself. Sometimes individual differences can have results that are quite mixed. In one family I know, the presence of a moderately retarded child was the focus of marital struggle, but helped the other children to become mature and wise in their understanding of individual differences. The experience of living with their sister eventually directed their interests into careers of helping others. Unhappily, some personality patterns are nearly completely destructive in their impact. A child with serious behavior problems can drain a family of energy and joy, and leave the other children marginalized and emotionally battered. The presence in a family of a child with a fatal or chronic illness can have a similar effect. Oddly enough, the presence in a family of a child with unusual gifts can also pose some problems. There was a nice, average boy in my practice whose older sisters were academic superstars. I'll never forget seeing him walking to high school carrying a briefcase and trying to look scholarly, which he wasn't. As far as he could see, there was no road to success or adult approbation other than by intellectual brilliance, and the gods had not vouchsafed him that.

Parents. Once upon a time, boys and girls grew up together in homogeneous neighborhoods, went hand in hand to the one-room schoolhouse, and eventually got married, living happily ever after. I suppose there is a full 5 or maybe even 10% of truth underlying that fairy story. Our communities *were* once smaller and more stable, our neighbors looked a lot like us, and spoke the same language we spoke. There are real advantages for the people who enter into marriages based on shared life experiences, beliefs, and folkways. One knows pretty much what to expect; less excitement perhaps, but lots more stability. Of course, that fairy tale was never an accurate picture of American life. We have always been a nation of immigrants and movers about. Now, however, social bounds are increasingly elastic. We marry partners from other faiths, other races, other lands, and other socioeconomic classes. These are the factors that determine the unspoken expectations concerning human life and personal interactions that have been built into our psyches throughout childhood. When there are enough differences in the backgrounds of the newly married couple, friction, hurt feelings, and misunderstandings are absolutely inevitable.

An additional issue is the rapid change in male and female roles within the family. Mothers are working full time outside of the home, and fathers increasingly are expected to share in the tasks of running the household. Part of this new definition of the male role is the implicit and sometimes explicit demand that parents should be interchangeable parts. In this new and surprising view, being a mother and being a father have both been subsumed in a new role—being a parent. My judgment concerning this notion is mixed. I have no doubt that women can do as good a job cutting the lawn as men, and that men can vacuum and wash the dishes as well as women. The equity of sharing household chores among the adult members of a family is self evident. However, the idea that the intimate relationships involved in caring for children are equally satisfying, comfortable, and effectively accomplished by the two sexes is another matter. Raising their offspring has been the primary responsibility of females in the vast majority of animal species and the overwhelming preponderance of human cultures. The mother who carries the child in her womb and feeds it at her breast has biological ties to her child which the father simply does not have. Watch new parents as they contemplate their newly born baby. The mother is often overwhelmed with joy and love. The father is probably pleased to see his new child but he is also frequently ill at ease and anxious, wondering whether he will be able to cope with his new responsibilities. Neither his genes nor his culture have taught him much about nurturance. Now, however, his culture is telling him something new: "Get in there, and be a real parent! Act like a mother!" If his previously formed expectations of adult male life are sufficiently discordant with that new message, there will be some problems. If his wife expects him to take the same pleasure and lavish the same energy on infant care that seems second nature to her, she is likely to be disappointed. Making fathers into unisex model parents does not appear to me to be a wholly reasonable undertaking. This particular social experiment is going to need some shaking out.

Does it seem like a miracle if any marriages survive? We don't make it easy in the United States today. Marital and sexual roles are in a state of confusion, economic pressures on the family are unceasing, and divorce is now socially sanctioned and easy to obtain. It is worth considering the measures that a couple can take to minimize the risks to their union. Plato told us that the life which is unexamined is not worth living. I think the same is true concerning the unexamined marriage. The examination of a marriage begins with a close look at yourself. This can be difficult for the person raised to repress any consciousness of unpleasant emotional states. If I am angry and don't know it, there is not much that I can do about it, but a safe bet is that the angry feeling will find expression in some fashion. It may trigger a headache, a bout of drunkenness, or an episode of depressed withdrawal, but one way or another, it will make itself felt. On the other hand, if I am aware that I am angry, some choices await me.

A good start is talking about it. Obviously, the best person to have in such a discussion is the person at whom one is angry. If this turns out to be your spouse, you may feel this is too dangerous and difficult. In that case one is in grave need of a wise listener—a friend, a relative, or a counselor. Becoming aware of your feelings and talking about them is a skill that requires practice. Expressing a negative feeling and discovering that no one is destroyed in the process can help to free up the next nasty emotion that is bubbling around inside your psyche. Once out, there is at least a chance that it can be dealt with; left inside, it is simply poison. Learning to share your feelings openly will not be easy. On the contrary, it can take expert tutoring from a therapist before some people are ever able to let loose. This kind of learning may best be accomplished with both marriage partners working with the same person, ideally a psychotherapist trained in the techniques of family therapy. In the best of all possible marriages, no such third person would ever be needed because the couple would have structured their relationship from the start to include time for talking about their lives together, as well as emotional space to allow the spontaneous expression of whatever feelings happened to be around. Until we reach the time when all marriages attain that high standard, there will be adequate employment for skillful psychotherapists.

Divorce. One of the least happy aspects of my pediatric practice has been watching families come apart. Sometimes the disintegration of a marriage is prolonged and public. More often, in my experience, the problems have been successfully hidden, at least from me, and I learn about the impending or completed separation in a burst of parental tears at a well check-up or an illness visit. Ours is a psychiatrically aware community and many of these couples have already worked with therapists in unsuccessful attempts to solve their problems. Despite that, I think parents may benefit from psychotherapy during the period of separation and divorce. Apart from all the practical problems to be dealt with, the heavy weight of anger, sadness, and turmoil make clarity difficult. A skilled therapist can help parents sort out the best solutions, even if the marriage cannot be salvaged. Many of these problems will involve the children, and if they are old enough a family therapy approach that includes them may be ideal. At any age, children will be confused, frightened, and angry about divorce. They generally welcome the neutral, sympathetic help of a therapist.

Older children are often deeply ashamed of their parents' divorce. They may have no one to talk to outside of the family; within the family, feelings may run so high that safe discussion seems impossible.

The response of children to separation is often surprising to the parents. You may be so involved with your own miseries that there may be little emotional energy to spare for the kids. You may want to believe that their quality of life will not change. But it will. Their feelings of fear and anger and abandonment are quite real, and often quite realistic. "Who will take care of me?" is a common and perfectly reasonable concern. Many children will blame themselves for the divorce. At a simple, common sense, nonpsychiatric level, it is terribly important for parents to tell their children that the divorce is not their fault; it is the responsibility of the parents themselves.

In the rancorous atmosphere that surrounds many divorces, parents may find it hard to keep in mind that the children are not divorcing anybody. On the contrary, they need to hold on as hard as they can to *both* parents. This is made much more difficult when one parent pours out scorn and fury about the other in the child's hearing. Poisoning a filial relationship may be tempting but is certainly not useful. Using a child as an intermediary to take messages from one to the other can also put the child in an impossibly painful situation.

One of the most contentious aspects of divorce is child-sharing and custody, an area of rapidly changing practices. In the past, the children typically stayed with the mother; the father was limited to brief weekend and vacation contact. A mother had to be grossly incompetent to lose custody. All this has changed. Mothers as well as fathers work outside the home, and they are aware of the problems of single parenting. Fathers increasingly want a real role in the upbringing of the children. The old pattern marginalized his importance. The weekend Daddy played no real part in the everyday issues of raising his children. His role was so limited, it was virtually impossible to develop and sustain a normal pattern. As paternal ties frayed, many men all but disappeared from the lives of their own children.

Joint custody is the solution which has became popular. The idea is simple and attractive. Each parent provides a real home for the children, and the children shuttle back and forth on some kind of agreed rotation. (A much less common approach, sometimes termed **nesting,** is for the children to stay in the family home and the parents to come and go from their individual abodes; this is rarely attempted and even less commonly succeeds.) Joint custody clearly helps keep fathers involved; if you are spending several days every week with your children, it is harder to drop out. It maintains a reality-based kind of parenting; each parent must oversee homework and household chores. It protects mothers from the pressures of working all day and single parenting all evening. It also forces the parents to maintain a nonmarital but co-parental relationship or partnership which in the early years of a divorce can be excruciating. Most ex-spouses learn to tolerate each other after a few years, although this may initially be hard to imagine.

From the children's point of view, two houses sometimes mean no home. The unsatisfactory nature of the arrangement can be appreciated if one contemplates from a parent's point of view the nesting strategy described above. There is also the matter of the distance between the houses; two neighborhoods or two different cities means disruption of friendships. Where do the kids attend school, and who has to take them there? For the infant and toddler, being away from either parent for several days can be exceedingly stressful. The mother is likely to be the primary care giver in the early years, and separation from her is particularly difficult Clearly, even the most flexible arrangements can fail to meet everyone's needs, but on balance, some sort of shared custody makes the most sense, most of the time.

Stepparenting. What commonly follows after divorce is the acquisition of a new marital partner, and thereby the creation of a stepparent. The usual first stage of this process is dating, which can be remarkably difficult for the adults and children alike. The appearance of Dad's or Mom 's new date is awful confirmation that the separation is real and the destruction of the former family is complete. It may also interrupt Oedipal feelings; many a child has crept (or been invited) into the erstwhile marital bed when one partner has left it. When a more or less strange adult stays overnight in that bed for the first time, a certain amount of ill will can be expected.

If the new relationship becomes permanent, the stepparent is faced with the complex task of developing a truly parental role in the family. This means becoming a rule maker and rule enforcer, taking over a fair share of the tasks of parenting, joining in the play and recreations of the family, and making ties with the extended family. In short, acting like a mother or a father, rather than some sort of adult boarder. Sometimes real parental and filial love blossom, which makes the role easier to fill; sometimes it doesn't. Becoming a stepparent requires an extraordinary degree of maturity and commitment. You are marrying a great deal more than a spouse. From the point of view of a mother or father, the new marriage requires a leap of faith that this new person will be a good parent for his or her kids. Watching the process develop can be a prolonged ordeal, and it does not always go smoothly.

"Blended Families" is the currently fashionable term for families formed when the new marital partners both bring children from a previous marriage into the new union. What a dreadful misnomer. It conjures up such conflicting and misleading images: either a gloriously happy group of perfectly mixed and matched children (one little boy of hers, one little girl of his, etc.) or a pulverized mess of partial survivors of a trip through a family food processor. Call them what you will, preformed families of this sort are a fact of life in America today. With the wisdom of Solomon and the patience of Job, a great deal can be done with the raw materials of two families trying to survive under new management. There are numerous cases on record where this has been accomplished without the intervention of pastoral counselors, family therapists, or the sheriff's office. However, for most such families considerable time and effort will be needed for the kids to decide that stepdad is really okay, that the new stepsiblings are not total idiots, and that their own lives are not permanently blighted. The time it takes for the new stepparents to reach similar conclusions is not likely to be much shorter. Balancing all the claims for love, attention, and money among his, hers, and possibly even theirs, figuring out what is fair and what isn't, and settling on a new set of family rules that makes sense to everyone involved are among the challenges that keep boredom at bay.

Writing this chapter reminds me forcibly of my own experience of divorce, remarriage, and stepparenting. There were surely many times during the first years of our multifamily odyssey when the safe arrival of our family ships in port seemed in question. Love between stepparents and stepchildren takes time, and the intensity of your ties to your own flesh and blood never weaken. There is always room for guilt, anger, and jealousy. Happily, there is also room for healing, peace, and joy.

How to Be a Stepchild. If I had a chance to meet with the children in a newly forming stepfamily, these are some of the words of advice I would want to give them. **1) Stay out of the crossfire** if you can. If you are already a child of divorce, you have had some practice with this. You may have learned to tell a parent you do not want to hear how awful your other parent was. When your parent and stepparent argue, suppress the natural tendency to kick someone in the shins; adults do not like being kicked. **2) Recognize that this new adult has replaced the absent parent in your home, but not**

in your heart. You do not have to reject the father who is no longer present in order to accept and even love the stepfather who is here now. Nor need you hate the stepfather in order to remain true to your dad. With luck, you can find what is strong and valuable to you in each relationship; do not expect this to happen fast. **3) Don't let anyone convince you that you have to love your stepsiblings;** you may, in time, and they may love you. Initially, however, life may feel like you are in a litter where the piglets outnumber the teats. **4) Get all the help you can.** Trying to deal with these painful and scary changes is not child's play. The other people in your life will be sympathetic and they may be able to offer either good advice or a shoulder to cry on. Grandparents, aunts and uncles, your own doctor, teachers, youth group leaders, family psychotherapists—there are a lot of folks out there who will want to be useful. Give them a chance.

I know that I am asking the child to hang in for a long haul, because the formation of a well-functioning stepfamily is always slow and rewards are not quickly forthcoming. However, that is the reality for everyone involved in a divorce. The remarkable fact is that a substantial number of these new family structures work very well; given enough time, lots of effort, and some really good luck.

The Many Models of Family Life

For Americans at the very end of the twentieth century the **nuclear family**––two parents plus some children—remains the standard and expected model. Most of us were reared in such groups, although the frequency of divorce means that our expectations of nuclear family permanence may have become shaky. But even if our own experience fails to confirm its reality, the nuclear family is thrust upon us as the good, the proper, the American way to live. The family portrayed on television, like the radio family of an earlier era, consists of Mom, Pop, and the kids. When an exception to that ubiquitous image comes along, it becomes an object of critical comment.

The strengths of this family structure depend on the strength of the surrounding supports. In good economic times, when one wage earner can support a family in reasonable comfort, a single pair of parents can handle most of the children's needs and still take pretty good care of the household and one another as well. It may be politically incorrect to say so, but the old, familiar middle-class model—father works at a job and mother runs the house and the kids—was often quite comfortable despite the limits it placed on both parents, especially on the mother. Stay-at-home moms meant that stay-at-home babies could get the intensive attention that small, growing beings require. Mom was also likely to be home when the older children returned from school; she could supervise snacks, play, homework, and household chores. Family dinners were more common, too. The children in families like this had a fighting chance of seeing and spending time with both parents who had the energy to focus on them, help them, guide them, and teach them. Family cohesion, never easily achieved, could be sought with some possibility of success. And community functions, from the Red Cross to the PTA, could benefit from the volunteer efforts of the women who did not have the additional pressures of full-time employment away from home. The surrounding supports needed by nuclear families also include neighborhoods where children can find playmates, schools that are at the least educationally adequate and physically safe, communities that provide libraries, recreational and sports facilities, peer groups, religious organizations, and opportunities to explore art and music and nature. For a considerable number of white, middle-class families during the last half century, situations of this sort have actually existed.

Unhappily, this Norman Rockwell picture of the happy, secure 1950s family will fail to convince anyone who remembers the era. The disadvantages of nuclear family life, even in the best circumstances, are real. Perhaps foremost among them is the isolation. The post-World War II flight to suburbia, and the concomitant explosion of detached, single family dwellings, effectively defined middle-class life. Trapped in their perfect homes, often living far away from their relatives, lacking an easily accessible web of friends and a caring community, families like these often failed to function to anyone's satisfaction. Women found their abilities ill-used, their contact with others limited, and their personal development stunted. Then their husbands came home tired and tense after a long, tedious commute which could add as much as two to three hours to the workday. The myth of the happy nuclear family turned out to have little congruence with day to day experience, although it continues to dominate our national images of how family life is supposed to be.

The current variation on this theme is the **nuclear family with two parents employed outside of the home;** this has become the dominant pattern in a society where one income fails to provide enough money for the lives we choose to lead. The ecology of the two worker family is vastly different. For a woman, a theoretically stimulating life outside her home has at least the potential for a new fullness of experience and personal growth. For a man,

EVERYDAY PEDIATRICS FOR PARENTS

the fact that another income is available takes away some of the financial pressure. However, the changes in his wife's existence may carry all sorts of possible meanings for him, some liberating, some threatening. Through her work, she may become more independent, more worldly, with greater self-assurance, and a broader view. She will also become even busier, and she may need her husband to shoulder more household and family responsibilities. At the very least, the dynamics of power within the family will change. Meeting the needs of the children becomes an exercise in family acrobatics. Schedules must be coordinated, child care found, extracurricular activities choreographed, household help hired, and older children may need to take on quasi-parental duties. Family pressures ratchet upwards, especially in times of illness, school vacations, and any other interference with the precariously balanced patterns of everyday life. For two working parents to find the time, energy, and patience to meet the needs of their children, a certain amount of superhuman ability may be needed. Supermom and Superdad have hard rows to hoe.

The next most rapidly growing pattern is the **single parent family.** Single parenthood is seldom a deliberate life style choice; it is usually the result of an unplanned, unwedded pregnancy, or the effect of the death of a spouse or of a divorce. However, some people do become single parents quite deliberately. This has always struck me as a little like volunteering for a chain gang: long hours, low pay, demanding bosses, and not much free time. A choice like that is a powerful testimony to the need to be a parent. Single parenthood is most often single motherhood rather than single fatherhood. The situation of the single mother is surely the most eloquent testimony to my argument that human life is meant to be lived in the setting of a supportive family. The sheer amount of time and energy it takes to care for a human infant makes the task of single mothering a form of cruel and unusual punishment. When do these women find time to wash their hair or go to the toilet or eat breakfast sitting down? Of course, with luck, there will be friends to help, neighbors to pitch in, and reliable babysitters available, but the chronic strain of the daily single mothering of an infant or small child can hardly be exaggerated. It inevitably leads to someone being shortchanged; that someone is always the mother and often the infant as well. The psychologist Urie Bronfenbrenner once wrote that every child needed somebody who was absolutely crazy about him. It is awfully hard to stay crazy about the baby to whom you are in permanent and solitary thrall.

The task of the single father may, in some ways, be even worse. He will have all the duties of single parenthood but few of the skills. By upbringing, and perhaps by nature, American men know next to nothing about the ordinary care of infants. These are mothering skills and they are best learned by watching and assisting mothers. Not many little boys are encouraged to practice taking rectal temperatures or feeding the baby her first spoonfuls of rice cereal. And in my experience, not many little boys would stick around for the lessons even if they were offered.

From the child's point of view, having a single parent means growing up in a household where there are no models for married life. It usually means lacking a father to whom one can relate, and that means losing many opportunities to learn something about the male sex. Whether you are male or female, it helps to have a grownup man around the house to give you some notion of what they are like.

The current American experiment in single parenting should be viewed as just that: an experiment in raising children without the kinds of family structure that young humans have had for the last few million years. Maybe babysitters and day care centers will prove to be effective at teaching children to be loving, working, interactive members of society and leaders of families. Maybe not.

Extended, multigenerational families have been the standard way to live for most of human history, and that structure remains the dominant pattern in many parts of the world. Extended families have become the exception in America today. They are most common in socioeconomically marginal situations, like the matriarchal African American families where a woman and her children and grandchildren live together, or immigrant families where three generations plus aunts and uncles and cousins share a dwelling. The advantages of multigenerational living are manifold. It is cheaper, there are likely to be extra hands to help with the chores and with child rearing, and it is a kind of protected environment, especially valuable for newcomers to this country with limited language skills and unfamiliarity with local customs. It is also a fertile field for conflict. The multigenerational family in traditional societies defines power in a fashion that shows everyone his place. It might not be a very nice place, but at least everyone knows the rules. In the traditional Japanese family, the power of the husband's mother may make life bleak for the young wife. When these patterns are transplanted into American soil there are no longer social sanctions to keep them alive, and new arrangements of intrafamily authority arise. If a Japanese couple have moved to the United States and the husband's parents come here to join them, the older generation will discover a very different set of family expectations. The mother-in-law may find that her

EVERYDAY PEDIATRICS FOR PARENTS

daughter-in-law has enjoyed some of the freedom of her new American friends, and she may be unwilling to resume her subsidiary and subservient role. The power has shifted and the old relationships no longer work. We are a nation which gives little or no automatic privilege to our elders. Grandparents may voice their opinions, but their children and their grandchildren will probably listen critically if they listen at all. We prize modernity and we denigrate old country ways; that does not leave much room for the wisdom of the older members of the tribe.

Communal families have a long history in America. Always based on an organizing idea, either religious, philosophical, or political, groups have come together to live and often to work as an extended family. The mostly religious colonies of the nineteenth century and the mostly political communes of the last few decades have had a generally similar history: They flourish, stumble, splinter, and fade away.

Our experience here in Berkeley has included two rather divergent groups. The sociopolitically motivated communes that thrived in the 1960s and 1970s were based on a heady blend of radical political ideas, relaxed sexual mores, and a good deal of marijuana. The political ideas led to schisms, the sexual practices played hell with family structure, and the marijuana made clarity of thought increasing unlikely. The religion-based groups made demands of their adherents to live ascetic and sometimes contemplative lives in the midst of an antiascetic and uncontemplative majority culture. Both types of commune, religious and political, promised to provide a ready-made community and a defined identity for their members. People joined these groups with enthusiasm but generally drifted out or were thrown out as the contradictions between theory and reality became intolerable. Some of the children who lived in these communes seemed to thrive; the environment was supportive and generally happy, and there was always someone around to play with. Some children became prematurely independent. It was as if they learned that multiple parent figures were not really parents at all, and they had better figure out how to take care of themselves. And some of them seemed to become resigned to the continual coming and going. The child learned that the adult to whom he became attached last month had packed up her sleeping bag and her guitar and moved on, and he thereby learned not to care too much for anyone. You may have noticed that I have described our communes in the past tense; this is not wholly accurate since a few, mostly religion-based, living groups still struggle on. I think the communes were attempts to invent brave new worlds somehow resembling the ancient tribal structures of the past. Unlike those earlier groups, the communes of the 1960s and 1970s had no roots in contemporary life and they withered. The experience of these recent attempts at the creation of new communities does not lead me to be optimistic about this form of family life for the future.

Gay and lesbian families are a small but increasing factor in American life. In places like the San Francisco Bay Area where I live, it is gradually becoming safer to live openly in a homosexual relationship, and lesbian households with children are now commonplace. In contrast, such families are literally unlawful in some parts of the country. A recent court case in which a child has been taken away from its mother simply because she is a lesbian living with her lesbian partner illustrates the still tenuous social and legal status of homosexuals today. It is interesting to speculate on the relative rarity of gay men or gay male couples living with children. One of the most common scenarios in gay life is that of the man who lives more or less uncomfortably in a heterosexual marriage, becomes a father, and then at some time avows or discovers his true homosexual identity. Predictably, this leads to divorce and the setting up of two households. It seems to me that his role as a father often becomes even more attenuated than that of divorced heterosexual men. This may be the result of adverse pressures from heterosexual society, or simply an expression of the homosexual condition, as varied as that appears to be. It has been only within the last few decades that the community of gay men have had the opportunity to develop social structures that can help provide a foundation for gay family life. As gay religious groups, political clubs, and other organizations arise, support for gay fatherhood is increasing. But so far, gay men or gay male couples living with children are still relatively few in number.

In our pediatric practice we have a fair number of lesbian women who had been married and are now raising the children of that union, either alone or with a lesbian partner. We also have lesbian families where one or both partners chose to become pregnant by artificial insemination and raise their children together as two moms. The obvious issue in families such as these is what role will men play in the lives of these children. How will they learn anything about the usual relations of married heterosexual couples? How will they learn how men act within a family setting? How do the boys of lesbian couples learn what it is to be an adult man? Of course, quite similar questions arise when one considers the situation in the households of single, heterosexual women. For some lesbian mothers, the answer to these questions is the less exposure to your ordinary, run-of-the-mill male, the better. Others anticipate that their children are more likely to be straight than gay, and they recognize the necessity of learning as much as one can about both sexes while growing up. So they arrange as much contact as possible with heterosexual families, men friends, and male teachers or mentors in the lives of their children. A nearly parallel situation exists in gay male households and in the families of heterosexual men who are single parents. How this will work out is anybody's guess. I hope some graduate students somewhere are embarking on longitudinal studies to provide some answers.

"The ideal human family structure." Wouldn't it be great to have a category like this? Reading over my comments on all the ways human beings live and rear our young, I am struck by the number of difficulties I ascribe to each. Isn't there a right way to do this? Perhaps so, but its nature eludes me. My conclusion is that we humans are driven to procreate, and each of us had better give some thought to the pitfalls inherent in every one of the alternative ways in which we attempt to manage the process and its products. At some point in the distant future we may even know enough to devise social and governmental supports for the best family programs, but for the present it is hard to make a convincing case that anyone knows just what those patterns might be.

Chapter 20

Food and Nutrition

I s a book written by a doctor the right place to look for accurate information concerning nutrition? I have to admit that physicians have justly earned the reputation of nutritional nincompoops. The problem was that, until quite recently, most medical schools provided little or no instruction in the field. I presume this was largely because nutrition is mostly concerned with health, a difficult concept to define or study, and medical education is mostly concerned with disease, which is easier to define and more likely to be funded. When I entered practice a number of mothers assumed my ignorance and attempted to educate me about their True Beliefs Concerning Nutrition. I was given a variety of publications clarifying the mysteries of food and drink. The claims made were often exciting, sometimes upsetting, but rarely well supported. Sorting the wheat from the nutritional chaff was not always easy. I found this quasi-scientific nutritional literature extremely frustrating because it promised so much but provided so little evidence to compel belief. Well, things have not improved.

Over the years the roles, advantages, and risks of vitamins, sugar, fats of all varieties, additives, preservatives, pesticides, yeast, carbohydrates simple and complex, fiber, excess protein, calcium, zinc, trace minerals, fluoride, and heaven only knows what else have all been explicated by an amazingly diverse group of cranks, zealots, conservatives, liberals, Greens, and an occasional real scientist. Who should we believe? The claims of the obvious crazies are the least of the problem. The most serious offenders in the nutritional nonsense sweepstakes have often been physicians. Previously reputable doctors have written whole books alleging the most egregious nonsense about food additives, pesticide residues, yeast, fluoride, and cows' milk, as well as flooding both the popular and the professional press with undigested and premature pronouncements about the dangers of numerous other foods and food constituents. The spectacle of doctors rushing into print with overheated warnings about the new Disease Risk of the Month has become a professional embarrassment. Scientific skepticism is appropriate for scientists but may not serve all of our requirements. The food we provide is essential for our children's growth, it is a sign of our caring, it is a symbol of our family life. And according to all sorts of people who claim authority in such matters, it is a sure way to shorten our children's lives by giving them cancer or coronaries. It is difficult indeed not to be impressed and frightened by the "experts." The magic amulet to wave in the face of these purveyors of doom is **Grossman's Law of Medical Skepticism: *50% of what we know is not true, but we don't know which 50%.*** Translation: The first reports of a new nutritional hazard are best ignored. If there is any truth in it, someone else will restudy the subject and begin to build a case that may be worth listening to.

Avoiding Allergy. Is it possible to decrease your children's risk of developing allergies? After seventy years of investigation the results are still unclear. I think a fair summary is as follows.

• If women with a personal history of major allergic disease could avoid the most allergenic foods throughout pregnancy, the incidence of allergic disease in their children might diminish. Unhappily, the category "most allergenic foods" contains such basic items as milk, milk products like cheese and yogurt, egg white, wheat, corn, fish, oranges, peanuts, and soybeans. Omitting all of these foods from the diet during pregnancy would be practially impossible and nutritionally disastrous, so the issue remains of academic interest only.

• Early introduction of allergenic foods during the first year of life increases the incidence of infant eczema and possibly other infant allergic disease, especially asthma and allergic rhinitis. It is not clear that protecting children from these allergens in infancy changes their *later* risk of allergic disease. There is much more to say about allergies and it can be found in Chapter 40.

Growth and Nutritional Needs. In the short run children's appetites are inconsistent and unpredictable. A given child will eat vastly differing amounts from day to day for no discernible reason, and the differences between kids is amazing. Some observers believe that appetite increases just before frequent, small growth spurts and decreases thereafter, but this is not yet well documented. If it turns out to be true, parents might be able to tolerate with less anxiety the periods of diminished appetite.

In the long run, children's appetites reflect the rate at which the child is growing. Babies grow fast, especially during the first four to six months, and they usual triple their birth weight by the end of the first year. The rate of growth of toddlers and young children is much slower, and it stays slow until late childhood. Appetites during early childhood tend to be modest. Most young children really eat only one or two good meals a day; they would generally rather snack. At the end of the first decade or early in the second decade, the growth rate accelerates. The growth spurt of the adolescent girl starts around age 10 to 12 and is accompanied by a noticeable increase in food intake. Boys start their growth spurts at 12 to 14; their adolescent appetite will be much more impressive and decidedly more expensive to fuel. During periods of slower growth and smaller appetites, most children not only eat less, they also narrow their range of preferred foods. Starches are the mainstay of children's diets during these periods especially. There is only a rough correlation between appetite and activity level, but generally children do eat more when they are most active. Eating is also a socially driven activity. You can get satiated chickens to eat more if you introduce some hungry chickens into their pen. It is the same with kids; they tend to eat more when they are with their friends.

Avoiding Nutritional Imbalance. Is it impious to discuss junk foods, juices, and milk in the same paragraph? Probably, but an old point is to be made again—nothing in excess. Fruit juices, the symbol of good health and proper parenting, are crummy foods. Except for the vitamin C in orange juice and grapefruit juice and the vitamins C and A in tomato juice, they provide sugar and water and that is about all. Aside from their vitamins, they are the nutritional equivalents of ginger ale. They limit appetite, displace more useful foods, and rot teeth, especially when consumed slowly and frequently from bottles. Anything more than a few ounces a day of citrus or tomato juice should be thought of as a sweet treat. I think that fruit juices and fruit drinks should be marketed with a PG–17 rating on the label; parental discretion is advised. Milk is better, but it has its problems. Because it is low in iron, an excess of milk in the early years will predictably lead to iron deficiency anemia. You see, nothing is sacred after all.

Junk foods? Well, some of them actually have redeeming qualities. There is vitamin C in french fries (13 mg in a regular order at McDonald's) and there is a significant amount of calcium (581 mg) and protein (39 gm) in a 10 oz. serving of pizza. True, junk foods are generally very poor sources of minerals, vitamins, and fiber, and they tend to be major sources of salt, saturated fats, and sugar. Sweet junk foods like candy, colas, cookies, and pastries are loaded with what the nutritionists call "empty calories," by which they mean sweets and fats which have little nutritional value other than as energy sources. One really must consider each item on its merits, in so far as it has any. Perhaps the most important lesson is that every morsel that passes a child's lips does not have to be maximally nourishing. Kids thrive on varied diets. The applicable rule is **Grossman's Law of Junk Foods: *Junk foods are like television; we are not going to keep our kids away from either, but we need to limit the ingestion of both.***

If you are interested in the details, buy a copy of Bowes and Church's *Food Values of Portions Commonly Used.* 16th edition. (Philadelphia; J.B. Lippincott Co., 1994); it is the standard source book of nutrition information. Browsing through it is unexpectedly revealing. Since scientific study of nutritional requirements continues to refine our knowledge of the subject, various official groups prepare recommendations from time to time. One of the most comprehensive of these is the Recommended Dietary Allowances report of the National Research Council, 10th edition, 1989, part of which is reproduced on pages 190–91. The recommendations of other groups differ in rather minor ways.

Vitamins

Are there good reasons for adding supplemental vitamins to the diets of healthy American children? This question is actually more complicated than it may appear because it is necessary to draw a clear distinction between 1) the amounts of vitamins necessary to promote normal growth and avoid deficiency diseases, and 2) the amounts allegedly needed to decrease the risks of degenerative conditions such as cancer and cardiovascular disease in later life. We know the amounts of vitamins needed for optimal growth in childhood, and a decent American diet can provide these vitamins without recourse to vitamin supplements. (The addition of vitamin D to cows' milk and B-complex vitamins to white flour products are exceptions to this rule. These vitamin fortified foods have made an important contribution to the public health, and are among the reasons why additional vitamin supplements are so rarely required.)

Do supplemental vitamins decrease the incidence of disease at older ages? Population studies suggest that diets high in fruits and vegetables are associated with lower risks of several kinds of cancer and possibly heart disease. This has led to the hypothesis that the so-called antioxidant vitamins A, C, and E found in fruits and vegetables may be the protective substances that make such a diet healthier. But fruits and vegetables are a lot more complicated than their vitamin content. They contain many substances that may have a role in disease development or control. Furthermore, fruits and vegetables may replace other foods which may have adverse effects on health. The complexity of this whole subject has not prevented the popularization of wondrous claims for the efficacy of various vitamins as disease preventatives. Actual evidence for these claims has been scant. The one unequivocal success story is the prevention of certain birth defects by supplemental folic acid, one of the B-complex vitamins. (Folic acid is present in vegetables, especially leafy greens, and in nuts, whole grains, and liver. The FDA has now required folic acid supplements to be added to flour, which seems like an excellent idea.) Other dietary supplementation trials have been less successful. A ten-year study of beta carotene, a vitamin A precursor, showed no evidence of any decrease in cancer rates. Another major study of beta carotene plus vitamin A supplementation actually indicated an increased incidence of lung cancer and a higher rate of death. A study of adult cigarette smokers in Finland given beta carotene plus vitamin E also showed an increase in cancer. Studies of vitamin E supplementation have yielded rather confusing results. Certainly, at the time this is being written, a cautious observer can only conclude that vitamin supplements have not been proven to prevent or delay these diseases. Therefore, what I have to say relates only to the much better understood area of the normal requirements of these substances.

Food and Nutrition Board, National Academy of Sciences–National Research Council
Recommended Dietary Allowances, Revised 1989

Category	Age	Weight		Height		Average Energy Allowance (kcal)		Protein	Fat–Soluble Vitamins		
	(years)	(kg)	(lb)	(cm)	(in)	Per kg	Per day	(grams)	Vitamin A (micrograms retinol equivalents)	Vitamin D (micrograms)	Vitamin E (micrograms α-Tocopheral equivalents)
Infants	0.0–0.5	6	13	60	24	108	650	13	375	7.5	3
	0.5–1.0	9	20	71	28	98	850	14	375	10	4
Children	1–3	13	29	90	35	102	1,300	16	400	10	6
	4–6	20	44	112	44	90	1,800	24	500	10	7
	7–10	28	62	132	52	70	2,000	28	700	10	7
Males	11–14	45	99	157	62	55	2,500	45	1,000	10	10
	15–18	66	145	176	69	45	3,000	59	1,000	10	10
Females	11–14	46	101	157	62	47	2,200	46	800	10	8
	15–18	55	120	163	64	40	2,200	44	800	10	8

EVERYDAY PEDIATRICS FOR PARENTS

	Water-Soluble Vitamins								Minerals	
Vitamin K (micrograms)	Vitamin C (mg)	Thiamine (mg)	Riboflavin (mg)	Niacin (mg)	Vitamin B_6 (mg)	Folate (micrograms)	Vitamin B_{12} (micrograms)		Calcium (mg)	Iron (mg)
5	30	0.3	0.4	5	0.3	25	0.3		400	6
10	35	0.4	0.5	6	0.6	35	0.5		600	10
15	40	0.7	0.8	9	1.0	50	0.7		800	10
20	45	0.9	1.1	12	1.1	75	1.0		800	10
30	45	1.0	1.2	13	1.4	100	1.4		800	10
45	50	1.3	1.5	17	1.7	150	2.0		1,200	12
65	60	1.5	1.8	20	2.0	200	2.0		1,200	12
45	50	1.1	1.3	15	1.4	150	2.0		1,200	15
55	60	1.1	1.3	15	1.5	180	2.0		1,200	15

But first, a few grumpy words about "natural" and "organic" vitamins. I must say that this is one of my pet peeves. The notion that a molecule of a vitamin knows its own father, so to speak, is one of those profitable folk beliefs which deserves early retirement. Vitamin C is vitamin C, whether it was manufactured in a factory or isolated from the juice of acerola berries. You will certainly have to pay a higher price for the latter, but there is simply no earthly way the two kinds of vitamin C can differ from one another. If you are buying vitamins, buy whatever is palatable and inexpensive. The products in supermarkets and drug stores are no different from the stuff in health food stores. It is also worth mentioning that highly advertised brand-name vitamins are absolutely indistinguishable from the plain vanilla vitamins sold as generic or store brands. Compare the labels and save your money.

Vitamin A is easily available from milk, butter or margarine, cheese, eggs, carrots and other yellow, red, and green vegetables, and many fruits. Developing a deficiency of vitamin A would be quite difficult for American children these days although this is a common problem among the poor of third world countries.

The B-complex vitamins are widely distributed in cereals, pasta and bread, nuts, peanuts, milk products, meats, and many vegetables. Your children are not going to develop the vitamin B deficiency diseases pellagra or beriberi on an American diet, and extra B vitamins will only serve to fortify their urine.

Vitamin C is a little less ubiquitous, but it is still not easy to avoid. It is abundantly present in oranges, grapefruit, pineapple, berries, melons, tomatoes, potatoes, leafy greens, and cabbage family vegetables like broccoli. The one case of vitamin C deficiency I have ever seen occurred in a family which faithfully followed a macrobiotic diet utterly deficient in practically everything.

Vitamin D is in D-fortified milk (nearly all cows' milk sold in the U.S. is fortified), fatty fish like salmon and sardines, eggs, and liver. It is also derived from the action of the ultraviolet rays of sunshine which convert a fatty substance (7-dehydrocholesterol) in our skin to vitamin D. This is a remarkably efficient process, requiring only a modest amount of sunlight to impinge on a small area of skin. A child from one of the northern states who drinks nonfortified milk directly from the family cow and who stays indoors during a long winter could manage to get vitamin D deficiency rickets. This was a common occurrence in cold climates before vitamin D fortification of milk became the rule. It is not easy to become vitamin D deficient these days, but it can be done.

Vitamin E is another easily available substance found in many foods including fats and oils, whole grains, meats, potatoes, other vegetables, and some fruits. The only known cases of deficiency occurred a few years ago in premature babies fed an improperly processed commercial baby formula.

Vitamin K is synthesized in the intestine; deficiency can occur in some diseases of intestinal absorbtion. It can also occur in infants during the first weeks of life; fortunately, this has become a rarity since vitamin K is now given routinely to newborn babies.

So, who needs extra vitamins? Children with cystic fibrosis and other mal-absorption diseases, some food-allergic kids on restricted diets, and any children whose diets are grossly limited by their own food preferences or other factors. One child in my practice confined herself to a diet of milk, white bread, peanut butter, and liverwurst for about two years. Giving her a multivitamin seemed like a pretty good idea. I suppose we should add to that list the kids whose parents are sure that extra vitamin C prevents colds. The evidence that large amounts of vitamin C actually does much of anything is not all that impressive. However, the stuff is nearly harmless, and it is cheap if purchased as bulk ascorbic acid powder, granules, or tablets. Surely the largest group "needing" extra vitamins are in families where a great deal of parental anxiety is focused on food. As much as I dislike teaching children that good health comes out of a bottle of pills, giving the kids an inexpensive, generic, children's multivitamin may take some steam out of those households. If so, it is not a bad investment.

Minerals

Iron. In earlier times, when our diet contained more whole grains and when our food was cooked in cast iron pots, Americans were less likely to become iron deficient. Nowadays, we eat less meat and fewer eggs, both excellent iron sources. We are an increasingly sedentary nation, and our children, like the rest of us, burn fewer calories at work and at play, and therefore are likely to eat less food. And like the rest of us, many children and adolescents diet to lose weight. Any significant decrease in total food intake may cut iron consumption to inadequate levels. This is a particularly common situation with teenage girls who recurrently diet, are apt to be less active than in earlier childhood, and lose blood with every menstrual period. Miss Average Teen can get pretty pale in a hurry. Comprising the other vulnerable group are babies and toddlers on fresh cows' milk which provides practically no iron and can cause intestinal blood loss. If a child is addicted to the bottle, the intake of iron-containing solids can be severely limited. However, for children in general, the iron fortification of cereals, breads and other flour-based foods, and the iron in peanut butter saves the day.

Calcium. This is one mineral that may need to be added as the dietary sources are really quite limited. Milk and milk products are certainly the richest sources; eggs and soybean curd (tofu) have fair amounts. The canned soy formulas for infants are fortified with calcium to equal the levels in human milk; however, the fresh soy milks sold in grocery dairy cases have much less calcium than real milk and are not an adequate substitute. There is some calcium in broccoli and other leafy greens (although perhaps not well absorbed), and in almonds. Calcium-fortified orange juice is another source. This is not a very long list, and kids who drink little milk and eat little cheese can end up somewhat lacking. The long-term effects of inadequate calcium during the growth years are not wholly clear. There may be some adverse impact on adult height and an increased risk of osteoporosis in later life.

Supplementation by calcium carbonate, calcium phosphate, or calcium citrate is not difficult if the child can swallow a tablet; kids get quite resistant to chewing the flavored wafers (like Tums) which all taste chalky. The calcium syrups are exceedingly expensive and disgustingly sweet. For further discussion concerning milk and calcium, see the section on lactose intolerance in Chapter 42 on Gastrointestinal Problems.

Fluoride. The effect of fluoridated water in controlling tooth decay (dental caries) is a true public health success story, and the leadership of the dental profession in fighting for fluoridation has been exemplary. Fluoridated tooth paste, rinses, and local treatments have also helped, and tooth decay has diminished even in nonfluoride areas. If your local water supply is fluoridated, your children will grow up with about one third to one half the number of cavities that they could expect in a community with fluoride deficient water. Keep in mind that fluoridated water only works if the children actually drink the stuff. Some families manage to avoid dental health by installing fancy filtration systems that remove the fluoride from their tap water. Others buy bottled waters which are not good fluoride sources. This is unfortunate and unnecessary since most American water supplies are both safe and acceptable to taste. There are also some kids who never learn to quench their thirst with anything other than a soft drink or a glass of fruit juice. The moral of this story is: Contact your water company and find out if your water supply is fluoridated. If it is, make sure to teach your children that water is good to drink, and expect fewer dental bills.

If not, obtain a prescription for fluoride from your doctor or dentist. This is a decidedly less desirable way of getting fluoride into people's teeth because it is expensive, time consuming, and hard to remember for the fifteen or so years required. There is some confusion about when fluoride administration should begin because the amount of fluoride supplementation previously advised was a bit high. Consequently, the exceptional parents who followed the prescription perfectly, never omitting a dose, found that some the their children developed fine white streaking of the teeth. These fluorosed teeth were hard as rock and wonderfully resistant to decay, but looked a little unusual. It seems to me that the best solution is to lower the dose, and this has now been done. What makes sense is starting it prenatally by giving a fluoride tablet every day to pregnant women from the middle of pregnancy when the first baby teeth begin to develop some enamel. Infants raised in areas with fluoride-deficient water should receive fluoride drops, and later, switch to chewable or swallowable tablets. Some physicians and dentists advise waiting until about 6 months of age before starting any fluoride at all. This will diminish the decay preventive effects on the baby teeth but will retain most of the effect on the adult teeth, so it is not a bad compromise. Because the adult teeth are still adding enamel until the midteens, fluoride should be continued until that time. If all this seems like a lot of trouble, a useful alternative is to organize community support for water fluoridation. It is cheaper, it reaches nearly every child, and community action is a great way to meet people.

Zinc. Very rarely, an otherwise normal child will manage to become zinc deficient because of a bizarrely limited diet. This leads to disorders of smell and taste, loss of appetite, and growth failure. The sequence is not easy to accomplish because zinc is widely distributed in quite ordinary foods, but some kids can do it. Zinc deficiency can also accompany some unusual malabsorption states but these are rare.

Trace minerals. A few years ago, an industry arose involving testing hair for mineral constituents, including a grand variety of trace elements. These hair analyses were then used as the basis for amazingly fanciful prescriptions designed to cure the deficiencies allegedly discovered. This particular form of technoquackery seems to have run its course. If anyone suggests to you that your child suffers from a lack of trace minerals, ask him for his proof and examine his professional credentials. You may find a deficiency of both.

Protein. A standard American diet supplies plenty of protein for standard American children. Remember that milk has about 1 gram of protein per ounce, a slice of bread has 2 grams, a serving of dry cereal has 2 to 4 grams. The recommended level of about 1 gram of protein per kilogram (2.2 lb) of body weight per day is easily met. A large proportion of our dietary protein is incomplete, lacking essential amino acids; this is especially true of the vegetable protein in cereals and legumes that make up a large part of the diet of children. What this means is that an incomplete protein will be partly utilized by the body as protein and the rest will be used simply as an energy source, like fats and carbohydrates. In the usual course of events, we don't ordinarily eat only one food at a meal. Fortunately, a mixed diet of incomplete proteins works very well; for example, rice protein plus bean protein is more complete and therefore more fully utilized than either alone. The same is true for wheat plus peanut; the peanut butter sandwich is truly the staff of life for the American child. Is there any advantage to pushing the protein content in our children's diets? It does probably make people taller and bulkier to have been given a high protein diet throughout childhood. Whether this is actually a good thing is another matter. Some evidence from animal experiments suggests that such a diet is associated with a shorter life span. My conclusion is that our present knowledge suggests that our kids are getting plenty of protein. There is certainly no need for the amino acid or protein supplements which are promoted as health producing or muscle building. About the nicest thing one can say about such products is that they are nasty and expensive frauds.

Carbohydrates. For years, carbohydrates were the least honored constituent of our diets. People seemed to think of starches as merely fillers, perhaps because they are low on the food chain and therefore less costly than proteins. Today, the contributions of complex carbohydrates to a balanced diet are now increasingly celebrated. Fortunately, carbohydrate-rich, starchy foods are what children mostly want to eat: cereal, bread, pasta, rice, and potatoes. Of course, they also favor sugar, a simple carbohydrate, and as every health food expert knows: Sugar kills. I regret to say that this inaccurate lesson has been learned by every literate parent in the United States. This notion reflects an interesting tendency in American life toward puritanical disapproval; if something produces pleasure it must be evil. Well, what is actually known about the health and nutritional effects of sugar turn out to be much less dramatic. It is true that sugar per se is an "empty calorie" food, carrying no vitamins or protein or minerals; thus, a large sugar intake can degrade the diet by displacing more complete foods. It is also true that a high sugar diet increases tooth decay. That is the complete list of the ill effects of sugar. Can sugar make

EVERYDAY PEDIATRICS FOR PARENTS

children hyperactive? This is piece of popular mythology for which there is no scientific support. I think the idea started because there actually are a few children with a sensitivity to chocolate or other constituents of candy and other sweets. This is a kind of allergy known as the tension-fatigue syndrome, and these kids can become unpleasant after eating a candy bar. The mistake was to put the blame on the sugar in the candy rather than whatever it was the child really reacted to. If you are convinced that sugar as such makes your child crazy, try a simple experiment: Have someone dose his orange juice with extra sugar or give him some plain, unflavored rock candy one or two days a week without telling you which days. Then try to guess when he got the extra doses of sugar.

People are often surprised to learn that white sugar, brown sugar, honey, molasses, and sugars from fruit are all essentially the same thing physiologically since they all end up in our bodies as glucose. It is true that molasses contains a little iron, and traces of B vitamins and calcium, and honey has tiny amounts of B vitamins and iron as well, but none of these substances is present in significant amounts. For practical purposes, they should be considered to be sweeteners like ordinary sugar. In short, the case against sugar has been grossly overstated, and we can all relax.

Fats and Cholesterol. Let's begin with some definitions. Fats are made of chains of carbon atoms each of which is also attached to one or more hydrogen atoms. The resultant fatty acids are combined with glycerol to form fat. If each carbon atom in the chain is attached to as many hydrogen atoms as it has room for, it is termed saturated. If one of the carbon atoms has a double bond which could accept one more hydrogen atom, the resultant fatty acid is termed monounsaturated. If more than one bond is double, the fatty acid is termed polyunsaturated. Cholesterol is quite different from these simple fats. It has a complicated structure of four linked rings of carbon atoms plus an attached chain of carbon atoms; all of these carbons have hydrogen atoms attached.

The function of fats in our bodies is complex. Certain polyunsaturated fats are needed for the development and workings of various body systems, especially the nerves, the brain, and the skin. Our bodies are unable to synthesize these essential fatty acids which must therefore be obtained from our diets. Essential fatty acids are found in breast milk, in oils derived from plants (especially canola and soy), fatty fish, whole grains, and nuts. Fats are the most concentrated energy sources of all our foods. A diet highly restricted in fat is likely to have inadequate calories to sustain normal growth in childhood. Fats are also an important source of flavor and desirable texture in foods. A truly low-fat diet tastes unbelievably dull.

The absorbtion and transport of fat within the body is also rather complicated. Most fats are split into fatty acids in the small intestine, coated with complex substances called lipoproteins, mixed with some cholesterol, and then absorbed into the blood stream. Cholesterol itself is mostly manufactured in the liver, and is also partly derived from the food we eat. There is a high concentration of cholesterol in breast milk, liver, egg yolk, and moderate amounts in butter and meats. Chemically, cholesterol is a steroid with many important functions. Not only does it serve to transport fat, but cholesterol is also the material from which the body manufactures the steroid hormones of the endocrine glands, the bile acids used in digestion, and the myelin which is an important part of the nervous system. Cholesterol in the blood stream is in various combinations each of which has a specific function and each of which has particular significance for health. LDL (low-density lipoprotein) cholesterol is used to transport fat into the body's cells. An excess of LDL-cholesterol is associated with an excess of coronary artery disease and heart attacks. In contrast, HDL (high-density lipoprotein) cholesterol removes fat from the body's cells; the more HDL-cholesterol, the less risk of coronary artery disease.

It is my opinion that the relationship of fats to human health has been characterized by an excess of medical zeal and a shortage of medical facts. Theories have been tangled up in careers and egos, and researchers have rushed prematurely into print. Humility has been in noticeably short supply. The hypothesis that heart disease is caused by diet has sometimes seemed to be preached with religious fervor, rather than scientific objectivity. As is often the case in theology, schisms have now appeared. Monounsaturated fats like olive and peanut oil have been welcomed back into the fold of healthy foods, and polyunsaturated fats have lost part of their good reputation.

So, where does this leave us in our quest for The Right Fat? I think present information makes the following summary a reasonable starting place. 1) Moderate decreases in total fat intake are harmless and probably healthy. Because fat is a major source of calories, severe decreases in fat are usually unwise for growing children. 2) Fully saturated fats are the most likely to raise LDL-cholesterol levels. A modest decrease in the use of these fats by limiting fatty meat, butter, saturated cooking fats (like Crisco and lard), and saturated oils (like palm and cottonseed) makes sense. 3) Monounsaturated olive and peanut oils are probably the most desirable dietary fats from a cardiovascular point of view. In general, these fats tend to increase HDL-cholesterol, which is desirable. 4) Substituting polyunsaturated fats for saturated fats in your diet turns out to be a two-edged sword. The problem is that polyunsaturated fats tend to decrease blood levels of LDL (that's fine) but also tend to decrease levels of HDL (that's a major mistake). It now appears that any substantial increase in polyunsaturated fats in your diet is unwise. In terms of their effects on the coronary arteries, they may be somewhat better for you than the fully saturated fats, but not all that much. 5) Apart from the whole issue of fats and cardiovascular health is the importance of the polyunsaturated essential fatty acids; these must be included in a healthy diet. 6) When polyunsaturated fats are artificially partially hydrogenated to make them solid at room temperature, an unusual type of fat is produced called a *trans* form, which is a sort of mirror image of the usual, naturally occurring *cis* form. Partial hydrogenation is the process used to produce soft margarine and hydrogenated peanut butter, the kind that does not separate. Inspection of the contents lists on packaged foods reveals that partially hydrogenated fats are very heavily used in a vast variety of prepared foods. Very small amounts of *trans* fats do occur in nature in animal fats, but our bodies don't seem well suited to handling the immense burden of *trans* fats provided by the partially hydrogenated oils. The evidence gathered about this science fiction excuse for food is that it is certainly no healthier for the heart than ordinary saturated fat and may actually be worse. *Trans* fats actually raise LDL (bad), usually lower HDL (bad), raise triglycerides (also bad), and raise a specific blood fat called lipoprotein(a) (bad for people who have an inherited abnormality in the way their bodies metabolize this substance). Some manufacturers of margarine have taken this seriously and have begun to reformulate their products to exclude *trans* fats. The Dutch have already begun to state the *trans* fat content of foods on their labels as a warning to consumers. 7) Lower LDL-cholesterol levels are associated with less coronary artery disease, so dietary measures aimed at lowering LDL may be useful. Keep in mind the fact that the liver manufactures most of the cholesterol in the body. The most important dietary factors tending to increase LDL levels are your intake of saturated fats and *trans* fats, not your intake of cholesterol itself. This is complicated, because many foods are sources of both cholesterol and saturated fats. Meats, in general, are pretty good sources of saturated fat, but only modest sources of cholesterol. In contrast, eggs have less saturated fat than most meats but lots more cholesterol. Since dietary fat intake is more of a problem than dietary cholesterol intake, it therefore seems to me to be a mistake to cut down the use of eggs in children's diets. They are great sources of iron and protein, and kids usually like them. The conclusion that eggs are healthy and useful foods for nearly everyone is gradually slipping back into mainstream nutritional teaching, but it is embarrassing for the experts to admit past errors, so the change is being made rather quietly.

What follows from all this is the wisdom of choosing a prudent, moderate fat diet. In short, switch to 2% rather than whole milk (or even switch to skim milk for older kids who eat well in general); cut visible fat off meat; choose lower fat meats like chicken and fish; use saturated fats like butter sparingly; use olive oil, peanut oil, or other monounsaturated oils; use modest amounts of polyunsaturated oils of which canola and soy are particularly valuable because of their high concentration of essential fatty acids; increase the use of whole grains, legumes, fruits and vegetables; decrease the amount of sweets, desserts, and artificially hydrogenated fats. These are mild diet changes which are likely to do no harm at all and will probably do some good.

Proposals to change the American diet in more radical ways should be approached with considerable caution. It is wise to keep in mind that large scale experiments in nature can be hazardous. Well-meaning enthusiasm for change brought the starling to North America and the rabbit to Australia; the Aswan Dam did more for schistosomiasis than it did for Egypt; DDT just about did in the pelican and the falcon.

A few more comments about cholesterol and then I'll leave the subject alone. Some researchers have suggested that cholesterol tests should be done routinely on all children. Their idea is that if high levels are found, firm dietary measures should be taken to lower them and if that failed, drug treatments should be instituted. There are, however, a few tiny objections to these ideas. 1) The cholesterol levels of children are not constant. They vary unpredictably over time. Many children with elevated levels at one age will be found to have lower levels later, without any intervention at all. If we treated all these kids, we would be wasting an immense amount of effort, time, and money. 2) High cholesterol or LDL-cholesterol levels are not actually very good predictors of eventual coronary artery disease. Large numbers of people with high cholesterol live out a full life span without any heart trouble at all. Treating these folks is a waste of time. Other risk factors like cigarette smoking, high blood pressure, and obesity are more important. 3) Dietary interventions have only the most modest effects. We would have to use drugs the safety of which has never been demonstrated in children, and the side effects of which are known to be unpleasant for many

EVERYDAY PEDIATRICS FOR PARENTS

adults. Furthermore, the commonly used cholesterol-lowering agents are known to increase the incidence of cancers in laboratory rats and mice. Do we really know that putting millions of children on chronic drug treatment for the rest of their lives is a good thing? Such an assumption requires an impressive leap of faith which I don't intend to make. 4) A staggering expenditure of money would be needed to pay for the required blood tests every few years and to purchase the drugs. Who is going to foot the bills? And lastly, 5) do we really want to raise generations of pill-popping, hypochondriacal children, some of whom would be convinced that they could die at any minute, and others of whom would seize on the entire process as a perfect opportunity to fight their parents? What an appalling prospect.

Fiber. Fiber is the stuff in foods that used to be called roughage. It includes the materials naturally found in plants that are largely indigestible within the human gastrointestinal tract. The completely indigestible fraction called **insoluble fiber** includes cellulose and lignin, derived from the outer layers of seeds, grains, fruits, and vegetables. **Soluble fiber** is made up of pectins, gums, and hemicellulose derived mostly from fruits and seeds. It dissolves in the colon where it is partially digested by the resident bacteria; the fatty acids thereby produced serve to nourish some of the cells of the large bowel. First, let's dispose of the question of soluble fiber and blood cholesterol. It has been discovered that oat bran and certain other sources of soluble fiber will decrease LDL-cholesterol by a modest but reliable amount. Unfortunately, the quantities (1 to 2 ounces a day) of oat bran that are required make this of largely academic interest. How many oat bran muffins and bowls of oatmeal will any child willingly consume, day after day, year in and year out?

Both soluble and insoluble fiber do seem to have significance for health by virtue of their gastrointestinal effects. Fiber passes into the large intestine, makes the stool bulkier and softer, and decreases intestinal transit time (the period from ingestion of food to evacuation of the residue as stool). Evidence is accumulating that a diet rich in fiber (whole grains, nuts, fruits, and vegetables) is associated with less intestinal cancer, diverticulitis, and possibly appendicitis. Any diet high in fiber is likely to be high in minerals and vitamins, and low in fats and sweets. Diets like this tend to be associated with lower risks of heart disease and obesity. A high fiber diet is also the best single treatment for constipation. Unfortunately, most American kids eat refined grain products with little fiber. They also avoid most vegetables and frequently take their quota of fruit in the form of juices which have had most or all of the fiber removed.

Converting kids to a diet higher in fiber is by no means easy. Choosing breads and cereals that include whole grains is a start. Limiting sweets, desserts, and sweet drinks (including fruit juices) so that whole fruits are chosen instead, and including more legumes, vegetables, and salads are all appropriate measures, but family eating patterns tend to be firmly fixed. Good luck.

Vegetarian Diets. In my experience, families who have adopted a vegetarian diet are generally well informed and well fed. They have all studied Frances Moore Lappe's excellent book *Diet for a Small Planet* (New York: Ballantine Books, 1991). They know about the incomplete vegetable proteins, and they understand how to improve protein quality by using mixtures of grains or legumes. Most of them use milk products, making a good vegetarian diet a lot easier, and protecting themselves from vitamin B-12 deficiency. They will get adequate iron from cereals and legumes, although this can be a problem for adolescent girls and women who lose iron with each menstruation.

In painful contrast, there is the rather common situation of the carnivorous family suddenly confronted with a newly hatched vegetarian child. This can occur even with young children but is more likely to be part of an adolescent's struggle for self-definition. The majority of these young people eventually drift back to their former dietary habits, but while it lasts vegetarianism can be a set-up for a great family struggle. The first necessity is educational; parents and child alike need to learn the basic facts of vegetarian nutrition. (Either *The New Laurel's Kitchen* by Laurel Robertson, Carol Flinders and Bruce Ruppenthal. Berkeley CA: Ten Speed Press, 1986, or Frances Lappe's book noted above is all they need.) The second issue is whether the whole family will change its diet; most families will not. This means parallel dinners, at least. Who has to do the extra work? If the teenaged vegetarian wants to change her diet, she will generally be willing to plan her meals and cook them herself. If her agenda is fighting her folks and engendering extra parental guilt, the kitchen will become quite a battleground. The ensuing conflict has the characteristics that psychiatrists refer to as "overdetermined," which is to say, there is more here than meets the eye. Even if you are not particularly controlling, you may well be concerned that your child will waste away to nothing on a diet of tofu and beet greens. Furthermore, the reasons for her decision to become a vegetarian may carry political or ethical implications. Often the child is abjuring meat because of her concern for animal rights or her views about the ecological impact of eating too high on the food chain. If so, you may well take the implication that she considers your meat eating coarse, unfeeling, or politically incorrect. This may lead

EVERYDAY PEDIATRICS FOR PARENTS

to a certain amount of friction between the two camps. If peace is to be restored, it will be necessary to bring out all the issues for family discussion. A clear statement that "I think you are all unfeeling wretches because you eat harmless quadrupeds" is probably easier to deal with than a steady diet of raised eyebrows and audible sighs when the vegetarian member of the group sees what everyone else is consuming.

Additives, Coloring Agents, Salicylates and Other Chemicals.
This whole area is full of land mines. There is considerable scope for paranoia when one thinks about terrible substances being added to one's food. Even paranoids can have enemies, as the saying goes, and there are indeed real examples of poisoning by food impurities. The real dangers are bad enough; when you add the imagined dangers, it is not surprising that food additives are a touchy subject.

An additive that has received considerable attention is monosodium glutamate (MSG), a flavor enhancer. It is widely believed to cause the "Chinese restaurant syndrome" of headache, breathing discomfort, and various other disorders of sensation. Evidence that such a reaction exists is surprisingly skimpy, but probably a few people do have adverse responses to MSG. There is a similar dearth of evidence that food colors and salicylates in food cause much trouble. The "Finegold diet," promulgated some years ago, attempted to cure hyperactivity and other behavior problems thought to be caused by these substances. The theory remains largely unsubstantiated, although there do seem to be a very few children who have behavioral changes after certain foods. More about this in the Chapter 38 on Allergy, page 370–71.

The problem which currently causes the greatest concern to parents is pesticide and other chemical residues in foods. Do these substances actually cause cancer? You may be as surprised as I was to learn that there is serious scientific dispute about the whole subject. The size of the pertinent literature is matched by the intensity of feelings involved, which is a pretty good sign that not enough is known. I have been most impressed by the studies of Bruce Ames and Lois Gold. (See their chapter on cancer in *The True State of the Planet*, R. Bailey, ed. NY: The Free Press, 1995). They have concluded that the alleged risks have been greatly overemphasized by serious methodological errors. In particular, they argue that administering vast amounts of any substance to laboratory animals proves a lot less than is sometimes claimed. They point out that similar studies indicate that chemicals occurring naturally in foods (celery, potatoes, carrots, oranges, mangoes, mushrooms, bread, coffee, and meat, to name a few near the top of their list) are more likely to cause cancers in mice and rats than the synthetic chemicals we have all learned to fear. Using the standard methods of the toxicologist, lettuce turns out to be 200 times more dangerous for lab rats than toxaphene, and 40,000 times more dangerous than lindane. Industrial and agricultural exposure to heavy concentrations of some synthetic pesticides is surely a hazard. However, this cannot be translated into an automatic assumption that tiny amounts of these substances in our foods is an equivalent problem. This is a subject which needs study more than headlines. Until that occurs, I expect that we will continue to experience fiascoes like the poisoned cranberry scare of the 1960s, the nitrite scare of the 70s, and the Alar in apples scare of a few years ago. All of these turned out to be embarrassingly overblown, but not before parental paranoia had been turned up another notch.

None of this is meant to deny that there are contaminants in our food and water that constitute significant hazards to our health. Fresh eggs in many parts of the country are infected with the salmonella bacteria, making it necessary to assure that eggs are thoroughly cooked. Our meats can be contaminated with a dangerous strain of the bacterium E. coli, and fresh seafood can carry a variety or viruses and bacteria. These are not particularly common problems, but they require that we pay some attention to the sources of our foods, and they require a higher level of government inspection at food processing plants. Contaminated water supplies will always be a threat, and continued investment in clean water processing plants will always be a necessity. This does not mean that we should all start buying bottled water; on the contrary, municipal water supplies are often the safest and best tasting waters available. It does mean that all of us should make sure that our own city's water system is well managed. The biggest water problem today is an increased lead content in some parts of the country. Where water is soft (which means low in dissolved calcium) and where old pipes may have lead fittings, lead can be increased to potentially dangerous levels. These levels increase when hot water stays in the pipes for a prolonged period. If you have soft water and lead in the plumbing, it is wise to flush out the hot water every morning for a minute or so to get rid of last night's new lead accumulation. Your local water company can tell you whether your tap water poses any problem and what you need to do about it.

Chapter 21

Eating Problems

There can hardly be a more necessary biological function than the act of feeding your children. The bond between infant and mother in particular is forged in the process of feeding. For many mothers feeding becomes and remains the defining experience of being a parent. Therefore, the amount of emotional energy that parents invest in the questions of what and how much to feed their children should come as no surprise. This is the context I try to keep in mind when I try to understand why a particular parent in my practice is so concerned about whether to give yellow or green vegetables first and other similarly earth-shaking issues.

There are other factors that increase the tension around feeding. The infant's physical growth is often perceived as validation of successful parenting; the big, plump infant proves the parents' success. No one ever coos over a baby "Oh, what a darling, scrawny runt; you're certainly doing a great job with him." As the child grows, sheer bulk loses its cachet; in fact, only large boned and heavily muscled males are supposed to be really big after about age 1. Current social norms rapidly differentiate acceptable and nonacceptable shapes. In the United States today, the range of approved body styles has become remarkably narrow, but the range of real anatomic variability in our species remains exceedingly wide. It is as if all dogs were supposed to be the size of cocker spaniels when in fact dogs continued to come in sizes that range from Great Dane to Chihuahua. The despair and concern among the owners of aberrant canines can be imagined. And so it is with the parents of aberrant children. American parents want their kids to look like the standard television family's children; moderately plump in babyhood, thereafter lean and muscular if male, lithe if female, above average in height, tanned and blond if white, not too dark if black, preferably curly haired, but not too curly. Unhappily, most of the time kids diverge from this idealized model. Parents sometimes try to change reality by urging more exercise or manipulating the diet. One of the most useful facts parents need to know is that body size and shape are hardly amenable to these corrective efforts. The plump kid is probably going to be plump, often along the lines of his plump parents; the skinny kid will not build massive muscles, no matter how much protein powder he consumes. Infinite perfectibility is a damaging and stupid myth.

The current American horror of obesity is actually a quite recent fad. It is worth recalling that overweight has not always been the object of so much disapproval. In societies of scarcity, to be fat means that one is rich and successful. The phrase "to carry weight" with one's peers implied the connection between power and bulk. Recall the pictures you have seen of Diamond Jim Brady or J.P. Morgan; they are not skinny squash players. The favorite actresses of their day could be described as pleasingly plump or even generously endowed. Shakespeare's Julius Caesar said "Let me have men about me that are fat" a viewpoint that would now get him in trouble with the cardiologists.

A reasonably balanced view of obesity needs to recognize that a modest amount of overweight in childhood is of little significance for physical health. It is also important to avoid the notion that being fat means that one is morally flabby. It seems clear that body shape is powerfully influenced by heredity. Twin studies and studies of adopted children confirm this. In the presence of adequate calories, children are going to grow pretty much as their DNA wants them to grow. Recent discoveries of fat-controlling hormones in our brains have begun to clarify the mechanisms that make some of us fat and some of us thin. Neither parents, diets, weight reduction programs, drugs, or anything else has more than a peripheral effect. This somewhat uncomfortable but inexorable fact leads directly to **Grossman's Law of Weight Control: *If you can't do anything useful, don't do anything at all.*** The reason behind this piece of advice is simple. When doctors or parents or weight reduction clinics urge, or the kids themselves chose a course of weight reduction that is going to fail, the child is injured. The sequence is nearly invariable: 1) Weight is lost. 2) Everyone feels triumphant and wonderful. 3) Weight is regained. 4) Everyone feels awful and defeated. The child is confirmed in the view that he is a moral as well as a physical slob, with no will power at all.

I think that the most useful message we can give to a plump child is that people come in all shapes and sizes, and not much can be done about it. Try to help the child accept the fact that she is a curvier shape than the fashion models and that the fault lies in society's screwy norms. Add to this a modest amount of information about the virtues of physical activity and the caloric content of foods and you will have given her the best available advice about weight. Neither you nor your child will be satisfied, but you will at least have spoken up for sanity and perhaps helped a little to protect her from the damaging social pressure to be slim.

Of course, skinny kids have social pressures too, but they seem much milder. The very slender boy will yearn for more muscle from middle childhood onwards. He may need to hear that special diets are quite useless, and weight training exercises not much better. Slenderness in girls is only rarely perceived as a problem in childhood, although these children may want to be less linear once adolescence arrives. It is no easier for a thin child to put on weight than it is for a fat child to take it off.

Anorexia and Bulimia. Back in the 1930s the Duchess of Windsor said "You can never be too rich or too thin." This nonsense qualifies her as the patron saint of the current American epidemic of anorexia nervosa and bulimia. Anorexia nervosa is characterized by severe weight loss, avoidance of food coupled with intense preoccupation with eating, excessive exercise used as a way to control weight, and a seriously distorted self-image. The anorexic girl sees herself as disgustingly fat even when she has lost weight to the point of near starvation. Bulimia is characterized by binge eating, usually in secret, plus self-induced vomiting or the use of laxatives to control weight. Bulimic girls are often able to maintain their weight at a desired level despite repeated bouts of massive overeating. They fear overweight but they do not have the same delusions of fatness that drive the anorexics.

The first medical descriptions of anorexia nervosa appeared late in the 19th century, but for many years the condition was exceedingly rare. Then an increase in the number of cases began to attract medical interest in the 1950s and 60s. Even then, anorexia remained an unusual problem. The physicians who studied anorexic youngsters during this era focused attention on specific psychologic patterns within these families. The girls (rarely boys) were usually adolescents with smart, demanding, and controlling parents. The girl's struggle to separate from her mother and to accept her own developing sexuality appeared to be central issues. Many of these patients were profoundly emotionally disturbed. Even with skillful and prolonged treatment, the eventual outcome was often dreadful. Some of these kids literally starved themselves to death, and among those who survived eating problems and emotional turmoil often persisted for decades.

These cases of classic anorexia were rarities. In our pediatric group practice, we saw one every few years. But in the last two decades, anorexia and bulimia have become absolutely commonplace. At any time in our current practices there are likely to be several anorexics and even more bulimics. A few of the anorexics are indeed severely disturbed girls with life-threatening disease, but most of them seem different. They may have similar psychological and family problems, but at a less severe level. They develop insight and understanding more easily, and they seem to recover more rapidly and more completely. It is my sense that they are basically sturdier people, less in the grip of family struggle than the classic anorexics, but perhaps more influenced by social pressures to be slim.

When a teenager becomes anorexic parents often applaud the initial weight loss, and sometimes seem to ignore the changes in eating habits. Anorexic kids typically increase their physical activity to burn calories, and this fits so nicely with the current fad for slenderness and exercise that dangerous amounts of weight may be lost before anyone notices that something is wrong. When she finally is taken to her doctor, she will strenuously resist the diagnosis of anorexia, and she will undoubtedly resist the therapy.

Bulimia is a different story. The bulimic girl overeats, often in private, and tries to control her weight by vomiting and taking laxatives. She may continue to eat normally when she is with her family and her friends, and her weight may remain well within normal limits. She is less likely to overexercise and she tends to have a somewhat less distorted view of her own body than does the anorexic. Bulimic kids can hide their disorder for years. Occasionally parents will notice the scrapes on the back of the fingers caused by self-induced vomiting, and sometimes dentists will see tooth damage from the vomited gastric contents.

Now that large numbers of anorexics and bulimics are being recognized, family studies have suggested that a genetic factor may sometimes play a role. There appears to be an increased incidence of depression and drug abuse in their families, as well as more than expected numbers of anorexics and bulimics among their mothers and sisters.

A child or teenager with anorexia or bulimia needs a skillful psychotherapist, preferably one who will work with the family as well as the patient herself. Some therapists work with groups of anorexics or bulimics, a good measure of how common these conditions have become. Recently, there is interest in the use of antidepressants, especially for bulimics. They also need a pediatrician who will monitor their physical condition and hospitalize them for their own protection if the weight loss becomes life threatening. I urge parents to cease telling the child how much and what to eat; feeding is a function that must be taken over by the girl herself. This is because increasing control of her own life is a necessary part of her recovery; the struggle over food is really a symbol for the more general issues of maturing and becoming an individual. The pressure on these families is intense and prolonged. The parents are faced with a child's suicidal rebellion, and they are frantic with worry for months. They feel fury at the child's dangerous behavior and at the same time blame themselves for the illness. They need continued support from the pediatrician and they need a good psychotherapist for themselves. In some of these really tough cases I have sometimes felt the need for a little personal psychotherapy myself.

The socially aware reader will have noted that I have not mentioned the most common feeding problem in the world today—not enough to eat. Even in the United States, 1 out of 3 children grows up in a home in poverty, and poverty means hunger. Glib advice falls silent in the face of that painful reality.

An unusual cause of undue slenderness which is beginning to be noted is the child who fails to grow normally because of his parents' fat phobia. It is certainly understandable that the barrage of admonitions to eat less fat and fewer calories in general has pushed some well-meaning parents over the edge. Because fat is the most concentrated calorie source, a truly lowfat diet in childhood can make it quite difficult for the child to grow. Moderation in all things: Kids need fat in their diets. For details, see page 197–201. in Chapter 20.

A variety of illnesses cause weight loss, but the other symptoms of disease nearly always bring the child to medical attention. However, one illness that can sneak up without much warning other than initial weight loss is childhood diabetes. So, any significant weight loss during childhood is likely to signal a real problem and must not be ignored.

Chapter 22

Constipation

The term "constipation" is used in two different but related ways. Constipation means infrequent stools, and it also means hard, painful stools. These different meanings are related because stools passed infrequently do tend to be hard, and therefore, painful. Normal stool frequency is partly a function of age. During the early weeks of life, babies have several stools every day, typically 1 or more bowel movements during or after every feeding. By a few months of age, 1 or 2 stools a day is usual. Breast fed babies may eventually have stools as infrequently as every few days, or even every other week. After infancy, the range of normal, comfortable stool frequency is roughly from 2 or 3 a day to 1 every other day. So much for definitions.

Since I was educated as a Freudian, my early understanding of constipation was psychological; there were all those anally retentive people who could presumably be analyzed into comfortable regularity. Well, perhaps there are some such aspects to the problem, but at least in my own pediatric practice, family genetics, diet, and activity patterns seem to be the major factors in determining the frequency of bowel movements.

Beginning with genetics: There really are constipated families. Whether these people have unresponsive bowels or super-efficient water recycling mechanisms I don't know, but the mother who reports constipation in her infant and comments that half the adults in her family need laxatives has my full attention. These children often have a recurrent pattern of constipation which requires careful dietary manipulation for years.

Diet is certainly the most important factor in bowel function. It is usually said that breast fed babies are never constipated, and like so much that is "usually said," this is nearly true. The once-every-feeding, loose to watery stools of the nursing infant commonly diminish in frequency during the first few months, sometimes to a single stool every few days. The record in my practice is 1 stool per 2 weeks. These infrequent stools are soft and painless when they are passed; however, some babies will be fretful for as much as a day prior to producing a generous stool. It may be worth giving them an occasional feeding of sugar water or molasses water to awaken the somnolent large intestine. A teaspoon of sugar or half a teaspoon of molasses in a 4-ounce bottle of water usually works, but larger doses may be required. Adding sugar or molasses to the formula is also useful for constipated bottle babies; molasses is more effective but messier. One half to 1 teaspoon of either can be added to as many bottles a day as required; increase the dose gradually until the baby is having stools often enough to be comfortable. Malt soup extract is a more expensive alternative; it requires a larger dose, it smells funny, and it doesn't work any better. Whichever of these carbohydrate stool modifiers you use, remember to experiment from time to time with diminishing doses. Babies typically outgrow the need for them. Very rarely, constipation may actually be due to food allergy; you may need to change from a cows' milk formula to soy or Nutramigen.

When constipation is present in infancy, your baby's doctor has to consider some quite uncommon anatomic abnormalities, including Hirschsprung's disease (in which the lower bowel lacks some necessary nervous tissue), and rectal or anal malformations. Recently, the claim has been advanced that a slight displacement of the anus is a common cause of constipation; I keep looking for this problem but so far without success. Medicine has a long history of similar ideas that this or that organ is a source of trouble because it is slightly out of place. Optimistic but useless operations were once done to hoist up sunken kidneys, sagging stomachs, and tipped uteruses. I suspect that the case of the migrating anus will prove to be as fanciful.

When solid foods are introduced in the middle of the first year, constipation problems increase; this is usually caused by an excess of baby cereal. Temporarily stop the cereal and add fruits, either cooked and pureed, or raw and mashed up. Peaches, plums, apricots, berries, mangoes, papaya, cherries, or kiwis work better than applesauce or bananas. After the constipation is corrected, resume cereal slowly.

The worst transition is to fresh milk. To avoid constipation at weaning from formula or breast, fresh cows' milk should be added a little at a time over a few weeks. In terms of stool frequency, it does not usually matter which kind of cows' milk is given. There are a few kids whose bowels seem happier with milk of a higher fat content, but this is unusual and unpredictable.

After infancy, the important dietary factor in constipation is lack of fiber. Unfortunately, the American child's diet of peanut butter on white bread, pizza, sugery cereals, sweets, soft drinks, and apple juice doesn't provide a great deal of indigestible roughage. In the healthiest of all possible worlds, everyone would eat a diet with more whole grain cereals and breads, more complex starches like dried peas and beans, more vegetables and fresh fruits, more water and less juice and soda pop, and fewer concentrated sweets. Well, it would be nice, but diet changes of that magnitude are exceedingly difficult. Any family embarking on such a change should expect vicious resistance from the defenders of the status quo. Change is probably best accomplished with tiny, baby steps. Substitute whole wheat crackers for saltines; sneak some dried fruit and oatmeal into the cookies; change from white Wonder Bread to a denser white bread, and then try some mixed grain bread. At some point the troops will notice that healthy food is infiltrating the family diet; they will rebel, and it may be necessary to retreat temporarily. This is not a struggle for the faint of heart.

Lack of water seems to be a problem for a few children; it should not be solved by offering juice, because the extra calories may replace solid foods which could have provided fiber as well. The way to deal with this issue is by prevention. We encourage the problem by offering juices or soda pop as thirst quenchers. It is possible to reach adult estate in America today without having noticed that thirst is a condition in which the body lacks water rather than apple juice or a Pepsi. If these sweet beverages are relegated to the status of occasional treats rather than members in good standing of the basic food groups, children will use water when thirsty, and the problem of dehydrated bowel movements will be avoided.

Nondietary causes of constipation include failing to provide enough time for the child to recognize the urge to eliminate and do something about it; this is no mean feat on busy schoolday mornings. The small child may also need some place to plant his feet if there is any need to strain; this is one reason potty chairs on the floor are better than the ones that perch on the regular toilet seat.

Constipation may also be caused by acute illness, with the attendant drop in appetite and activity. Bed rest for any reason is a powerful constipater. Certain drugs may also be factors; the likeliest offender is codeine which we often use to suppress cough or relieve pain.

During the period when toilet training is underway, the bowel movement may become the center of a vigorous power struggle between parents and child. Refusing to use the potty and fearing disapproval for using the diaper may set up a considerable case of constipation. Unfortunately, the current American custom of bowel training at 2 to 2½ years coincides with the period of the child's maximum independence needs. It is a good trick to convince a wily and surly kid that using the toilet is somehow in his best interests, and not just a present to his parents. Rewards help; for details see pages 122–23.

Withholding Stool. The most difficult problems arise when a child has had a painful, hard stool and fears the next bowel movement. This often starts the common pattern of withholding stool and getting more and more plugged up. Mineral oil given by mouth will usually suffice to soften and lubricate the stool; it usually takes a few days to work. Mineral oil is best given shaken with a little orange juice; start with ½ tablespoon twice a day and increase slowly until the stools are so runny that the child can't withhold them. Then slowly decrease the dose over several weeks, during which time the hope is that the child will decide that bowel movements are acceptable. An expensive alternative to mineral oil is lactulose, an unabsorbable sugar which increases stool water content; sometimes it works fairly well. Docusate sodium (Colace, etc.) is a mildly effective lubricant cathartic. Docusate's popularity is largely due to its ease of administration rather than any notable efficacy. It does not suffice in the treatment of withholding. There is also a large group of drugs called stimulant laxatives. These include phenolphthalein (Ex-Lax, Feen-A-Mint, Correctol); cascara and aloe (Nature's Remedy); and bisacodyl (Dulcolax). Bisacodyl is probably the best of these but, in general, stimulant laxatives should be avoided because they can cause severe cramps, may fail to soften the stools adequately, and may be habituating. Obviously, attention must also be paid to the antecedents of the withholding, or the cycle may just repeat itself.

Chronic Constipation. Every so often, constipation becomes a protracted and difficult problem, persisting despite diet manipulation and drug treatment, or recurring as soon as treatment is decreased or stopped. This is particularly likely to happen in the early years of childhood when toilet training is still an issue, and withholding stool becomes the child's chosen method of avoiding the whole affair. The child's theory seems to be "I just won't have bowel movements anymore, and then maybe they will get off my back." This line of reasoning is understandable but not helpful. To enable the child to move, so to speak, from this untenable position consider setting up a few sessions of brown clay play. You will need a potty chair, a few dolls or stuffed animals to represent a child and miscellaneous parents, and a supply of some soft brown clay or play dough. Inviting Mr. or Ms. Recalcitrant to join you, you say "Let's play that the doll doesn't want to use the potty." Most children in the age range of 2½ to 4 years will be interested and usually enthusiastic in playing out their own issues in this setting. Parents sometimes find that it takes a few tries before a child decides that this somewhat unexpected adult offer should be accepted; generally kids dive in from the beginning, and they completely take over the doll play. Two or 3 such sessions often lead to some inner resolution which will probably not be expressed in words, but will be obvious because the stool withholding begins to diminish. I must add that some parents are appalled by the idea of amateur play therapy of this sort. If it feels weird to you, don't do it.

Stool Soiling (Encopresis) may result from a number of causes. Sometimes complete toilet training seems not to be accomplished for years, and a little soiling of the child's underwear comes to be accepted by child and family as just the way things are. More often soiling begins when a child who has previously mastered toileting becomes constipated, withholds stool, and overflows. Not infrequently soiling is part of a problem in child-family interaction. In any case, the child over the age of 4 or 5 who allows part or all of his stool to escape into his underwear is signaling that something is amiss. As a pediatrician, I approach this symptom warily; this is a situation where treatment really has to be tailored to the situation. I am particularly skeptical of the routine aggressive use of powerful laxatives and multiple enemas. This blast-it-out and wash-it-clean approach is too likely to be perceived by the child as a punitive attack. A carefully chosen combination of proper diet and stool softeners, plus clearly defined and understood parental expectations is often the best way to begin. Sometimes counseling or psychotherapy is also needed, and, if so, a family psychotherapy approach is often the most useful. Stool soiling is frequently a game with many players, and the psychotherapist will want to have them all on the field.

Chapter 23

Bedwetting and Enuresis

If you try to teach 5-year old children to read, a very large number of them will fail to master the task, and you will be well on the way to creating a cadre of children with reading problems. If you wait until age 6 or 7 before this attempt, the proportion of failures will be much smaller, maturation of the necessary neural networks having taken place. Therefore, many fewer of these children will be defined as having reading problems. Exactly the same is true with bedwetters. If you provide your children with big enough diapers for a long enough period of time, and keep your expectations sufficiently relaxed, fewer of your children will be labeled bedwetters, either by you or by themselves. In short, lack of control of the process of urination during sleep (the medical term for which is primary nocturnal enuresis) is not a disease, it is one stage in a developmental process.

Like all biological functions, the acquisition of control over urination during sleep is subject to immense variability. There are a few children 18 or 20 months old who awaken dry in the morning and toddle off to the potty. In contrast, there are 7 or 8-year olds who sleep peacefully through the night in a bed awash with the results of multiple urinations. Heredity plays a role here; parents and children often have identical personal histories of prolonged bedwetting. Older children who wet their beds are also usually described as wonderfully deep sleepers: "You couldn't wake him up with a cannon." A quite different matter is secondary enuresis, the resumption of frequent bedwetting by the child who had already achieved and maintained night dryness for months or years. (An occasional wet bed, especially if it follows a particularly exhausting day or an exceptionally exciting or upsetting event, usually means nothing at all.) The children who resume bedwetting may have any of a variety of illnesses, including urinary tract infection, urethral or vaginal irritation, pinworms, or diabetes. Even more likely, they may be reacting to psychological stress. If your child recommences and continues bedwetting after a substantial period of night dryness, he needs a visit to his doctor for a physical examination, a urinalysis, and a urine culture. Most of the time, these studies are all negative because the problem is in his head rather than in his bladder. A close look at his school and family life will usually provide the clue to what is bothering him.

Daytime enuresis is more complicated. Once again, adult expectations are a factor. Many quite normal 3 and 4-year olds still wet themselves fairly regularly during the day, and it is usually a mistake to define them as abnormal. On the other hand, by the age of 6 or 7 years, more than an occasional daytime dribble deserves some attention. Some of these children show other signs of neurological or developmental delay. A very few will prove to have infection or some other abnormality of the urinary tract. There is even a theory that some of them have a learned dysfunction of urination, that is, they have learned to urinate in an improper fashion, but this idea strikes me as unduly fancy and quite unlikely. Most of these kids seem to me to be peeing on their parents; the wet pants are a part of a larger family struggle.

What to Do About the Wet Bed. First of all, don't expect too much; excess optimism leads to disappointment. About 50% of children will be dry at night by age 3, the girls tending to develop bladder control earlier than the boys. By age 5, about 85% are dry, and by age 8, over 90%. This process is largely automatic, although it can sometimes be speeded up a bit. Keep in mind that if either you or your spouse was a bedwetter to an advanced age, this pattern is likely to repeat itself.

Second, try to define this as a problem for the bed rather than for the child. This is a situation in which gratefulness to the inventor of the automatic washing machine can take the place of fury at the child. The availability of large diapers or "pull-ups" is another help. If this is not acceptable to the child, protect the child's bed with a large rubber-backed cotton felt pad. As the child gets older, he can take responsibility for airing his bed every morning, changing it when necessary, and helping with the family laundry. This is a nonpunitive but precise message to him that a dry bed is a valuable goal.

Eventually, family and social pressure may make more active measures advisable. Behavior modification techniques such as rewards for dry nights are sometimes remarkably effective. A prominently displayed star chart or calendar with a star for each dry night and a specific reward for a defined number of stars is the usual tactic. The child can help make the star chart, and he will probably want to paste each star in place after a dry night. Figure on some tangible reward for every 5 to 7 days of continence; don't make him wait so long that he becomes discouraged. The interesting thing about this method is that it can be abandoned once a dry bed is achieved, with only a small likelihood of relapse. Real learning seems to take place. If this fails, alarm devices are the next step. These consist of moisture detectors worn in the child's underpants with a wire connected to a buzzer near the child's ear. (The earlier models which had a moisture detecting pad placed under the bed sheet were much less reliable.) When he begins to urinate, the alarm sounds, awakening him and usually his parents. He is then supposed to go to the toilet to finish urinating. The theory is that he will awaken sooner and sooner, eventually somehow learning to respond to the preceding neural stimulus of a full bladder. Presumably he will either inhibit the impulse to void or he will awaken and trudge to the toilet instead. The theory carries little conviction, but the practice often works. Problems arise when the child manages to stay asleep despite the noise of the alarm; parents and siblings are often more easily aroused than the patient. An extra loud alarm is available with some of these gadgets; this is by no means uniformly successful, and may just make the rest of the family even angrier. Alarm devices are useless if the child is not motivated to become dry. It is also a waste of time to use them before age 5 or 6 at the earliest.

The last resort is medication. The drug imipramine decreases or stops bed-wetting at least half the time, but relapses are disappointingly common. Unfortunately, imipramine is not a completely safe drug, especially at high dosages. It can cause abnormalities in the electrical system of the heart as well as other adverse effects. At times the combination of imipramine plus an alarm device is helpful. Some families use imipramine for a few days or weeks to help a child control bedwetting during a vacation or at summer camp, expecting that relapse will occur later. A recent contender for the dollars of the parents of bed-wetters is desmopressin (DDAVP), a hormone made by the pituitary gland. It has the effect of decreasing urine output, the theory being that these kids just don't concentrate their urine at night in the usual fashion. Unhappily, relapse after the conclusion of therapy is the rule, and the cost is astronomical. Even if it worked, I would have grave doubts about the good sense of using anything as powerful as a pituitary hormone in such a cavalier fashion.

As you stand in the bedroom of your enuretic youngster, breathing in the uriniferous fumes and contemplating the soggy bed, it may help a bit to keep in mind the damp, unhappy reality that some kids take forever to sleep dry. It can be a long wait until nighttime continence is finally established in the teens, but it does eventually happen.

Chapter 24

Habits

In this chapter we will briefly consider three common habits of childhood: thumb- ,finger-, or pacifier-sucking; attachment to favorite objects like blankets and stuffed animals; and masturbation. These behaviors have in common their frequent appearance and the amount of concern they generate among parents. They also share the characteristic that their importance and meanings depend on the age of the child and their places in the child's life.

Thumb–Sucking and Pacifier–Sucking. It is quite obvious that all of us mammals have a built-in need to suck. A good thing, too. Babies need to be fed, and it is a great help to one and all that the method is already hard wired into our brains before birth. Sucking starts early; even before birth, sonograms often reveal the fetus peacefully sucking on its hand or arm. Every pediatrician has seen infants born with sucking blisters on a wrist or arm caused by this prenatal behavior. Immediately after being born, baby mammals, humans included, seek the mother's nipple. We don't usually let our new babies find their first meal all by themselves, but in fact, given the right situation, that is actually a task they can manage (as I mentioned in the discussion of the newborn in Chapter 5.) The importance and the power of the need to suck remains impressive right through infancy and well into childhood. At later ages most of us seem to substitute other kinds of oral activity, such as eating and drinking, but we clearly continue to get considerable pleasure from our lips and mouth.

Although the physiological reason for sucking is to acquire nourishment, the need to suck and the need to eat are not the same thing. Babies will begin to suck on any available object when they are hungry and waiting for a meal, and they will generally quit sucking when they are fed and satisfied. But if the meal is too fast, either from an overloaded breast spurting milk or from a bottle with too large a nipple hole, the baby may still want to suck some more despite its full stomach. Many a breast feeding mother has had her feelings hurt when her infant turns away from her nipple and puts a thumb in its mouth. For most human infants and children, nonnutritive sucking is an important and normal behavior for many months or years.

Well, we all seem to understand and accept sucking behavior in infancy, but how about older children and their thumb- or pacifier-sucking? Here is where the trouble begins because, after all, thumb-sucking seems so babyish, and we live in a culture that has a very small tolerance for babyish behavior. For a 6-month old, fine; for a 1-year old, still okay; but for a 2-year old? Isn't he ready to give that damn thing up? Our frontier mentality—grow up fast and leave home—has little use for a slow and peaceful transition from infant dependency to the tough, lonely status of adult life. Count on it, public display of thumb-sucking in early or middle childhood will be met with disapprobation from many quarters.

Aside from complete strangers treating your child as an emotional basket case, are there any problems with thumb-sucking? In infancy, the child who spends long hours with his thumb may be sending a message: "I need and want lots more adult attention." When other important human needs are unmet, the familiar and comforting thumb may be the best the child can do. At later ages, continuing or frequent use of the thumb may be harder to figure out. Some kids keep a thumb (or a pacifier) in the mouth even during perfectly satisfying play with peers or parents. Their message may be that they are happily wedded to the habit and it doesn't interfere with other, equally desirable activities; why not do both? However, a heavy dependence on the satisfactions of the thumb in middle childhood does raise some questions. By this age, most kids have fairly easily and spontaneously outgrown their earlier love affair with thumb or pacifier. They have learned other ways to cope with difficulties, and found other sources of emotional comfort. They have also noted that continued thumb-sucking is no longer socially acceptable, and, like all the rest of us, they want to be socially accepted. So, the middle-aged child who still really needs his thumb may be telling us that his world is out of kilter. If we look hard enough, we may find out how and why.

The other (and potentially expensive) problem is with the teeth. Habitual use of the thumb or pacifier can certainly push the baby teeth into unusual positions. If the child eventually gives up the habit by age 5 or 6, the adult teeth generally come in quite nicely. Continuing the habit into later ages can sometimes cause orthodontic problems.

The question of thumb versus pacifier continues to be hotly debated among parents. It sometimes takes the form "Which is more disgusting, a 5-year old with a pacifier or a 5-year old with his thumb in his mouth?" When you hear the debate framed in this fashion, you should be aware that you are in the presence of an emotional intensity that probably precludes good sense. The rational bases for comparison are few. Thumbs are handy, and they never fall out of the crib and under the bed. Pacifiers are, in theory at least, under the control of the parents. From the orthodontic point of view the differences are probably unimportant.

Parents or orthodontists may decide that this habit has to go. What then? 1) Give some sustained attention to the question "Does my kid suck his thumb because he is just an unhappy little person?" If the answer is "Yes," you and the child have more important things to do than worry about the thumb. 2) If the answer is "No," ask yourself if the antithumb crusade could be rescheduled for next year. This is a situation like bedwetting; the longer you wait, the more spontaneous cures. If she gives up the thumb next year without a struggle, everyone wins. 3) If you are bound and determined to proceed, make it worth her while. Punishment really does not work, nor does painting her thumb with bad tasting junk, and antithumb-sucking restraints are too medieval for most contemporary parents. You may want to consider an orthodontic appliance called a rake; these are metal gadgets glued behind the front top teeth. It makes thumb-sucking a bit more difficult, and some older children actually say it helps remind them not to suck. However, for most kids the best route is "behavior modification," a fancy phrase for rewards. The rewards can be symbolic, like star charts for recording days free of thumb-sucking, or more substantial, like collecting points to be traded in on a major prize.

If your child's source of soothing has been a pacifier rather than a thumb, you will be able to set some limits on where and when it can be used. This may make the process of weaning a bit smoother. The disadvantage is that taking a pacifier away is pretty much a matter of applied external power; from the child's point of view it must feel like "me against them." In contrast is the child who finally graduates from her thumb or pacifier on her own. She can feel that she has been in charge of this little piece of growing up, and that sense of autonomy and mastery is a lovely thing to have. I learned something about this process from my daughter Deena. As an infant and small child, she had been deeply and seemingly permanently attached to her pacifier. One morning she abruptly announced that since she was soon to be 4 years old and would be starting nursery school, she no longer needed a pacifier. While her mother and I looked on in amazement, she thereupon deposited it in the trash can. It was as nice an example of maturation as one could want.

Love Objects (Transitional Objects, Security Objects). Why do our nice, emotionally healthy, thoroughly beloved, darling children need these things? The filthy but favorite blankie, the tattered teddy bear, the much chewed Raggedy Ann: Sometime in early childhood most kids have one of these terribly important objects which provide them with a sense of comfort and safety. They seem to function as a material bridge to Mom. Especially when she is absent, the love object reminds the child of her warm and loving presence, and serves to tide the child over until her return. Is this okay, or do we have to worry about it? Maybe if we were better parents our kids would not need these crutches? I suppose you have to examine each family and each child one by one, but even the happiest kids in the strongest families with the most available mothers have security objects, so it is hard to get worked up about it. Of course, it is a matter of degree and timing. Just as with thumbs and pacifiers, so it is with love objects. You begin to wonder about the third grader who can't go anywhere without his blankie. But what is most important is not the fact of the security object; it is the whole child and how that child seems to be functioning in the world. If the child and the world are getting along pretty well, and the security object does not dominate life, why fret? Many a college freshman has her favorite teddy bear next to her pillow, and she will probably manage to turn out to be a successful wife, mother, astronaut, and futures trader. Here is a good place to practice trust in the mysterious process of growing up.

Masturbation. L. Emmett Holt, M.D., Professor of Diseases of Children at Columbia University School of Medicine, was one of the most eminent pediatricians of his day. His book of advice for parents was once in every up-to-date home. (I still have my mother's copy, with her name written carefully inside the front cover and the record of the monthly weights for my first year written inside the back cover.) Here is what Dr. Holt had to say about masturbation in *The Care of Infants and Children*, 12th edition, 1924.

"To what does masturbation lead? It increases the nervousness of the child, exaggerates the lack of self-control and when practiced frequently often leads

EVERYDAY PEDIATRICS FOR PARENTS

to impairment of the general health, lowered moral sense and sometimes to other sexual propensities...Masturbation is the most injurious of all the bad habits, and should be broken up just as early as possible."

The views of John B. Watson, Ph.D., the founder of Behaviorism and a major figure in American psychology for many years, are equally definite. In his *Psychological Care of Infant and Child*, 1928, he opines "The most important reason of all for breaking this habit is this: *If it is persisted in too long and practiced too often it may make heterosexual adjustment difficult or impossible.*"

I include this advice, considered to be first-rate at the time, as a reminder of the fallibility of "experts." We are all the creatures of our cultures, limited by how little we really know, and without doubt, knowing many things that are not true.

Writing in the 1940s, two decades after Dr. Holt and Dr. Watson, Dr. Benjamin Spock ushered in a new era of child raising. In *The Common Sense Book of Baby and Child Care*, he described masturbation as normal behavior of infants, children, and adolescents. The Freudian revolution had taken place, and doctors could look at the phenomenon of children's sexual interests and activities as healthy and desirable, the necessary preparation for adult sexual life. Half a century later, Dr. Spock's view continues to make sense. The facts of the matter are that babies learn to touch their genitals because it feels good. Some of them learn to stimulate themselves to a kind of infant orgasm. In early and middle childhood sexual self-stimulation continues, as well as sex play among peers. (The old psychoanalytic idea that there is a "latency period" in middle childhood without as much sexual interest and activity does not appear to be true.) And of course by the age of adolescence, masturbation is nearly universal among boys and extremely common among girls. All through adult life, masturbation remains an important form of sexual activity. Masturbation starts early, and it never goes away.

These undoubted facts and the Freudian understanding of childhood sexuality as normal have been current and increasingly accepted for many decades. However, I have the impression that infant and early childhood masturbation remains an uncomfortable issue for many parents. We can watch as our kids comfort themselves with pacifier and favorite blanket, and the picture seems sweet and peaceful. But when she places her free hand on her clitoris and begins to rock back and forth, we are not so sure. I suppose this is to be expected. We in the West are the heirs of nearly two thousand years of religious teaching that sex is bad and nasty. It is hard to ignore this pervasive antisexual attitude.

So, what is to be done about babies who masturbate? Babies masturbate for two reasons: It feels good, and it can lead to a nice, relaxed state. It seems to me that frequent and compulsive masturbation is a rarity in infancy. If a baby is spending really large amounts of time in this private behavior, perhaps her message is that she needs more public life, that is, more adult attention. Masturbation in young and middle-aged children is more common than in babies. Three and 4-year olds are full of interest in the body, and their focus on sexual anatomy can become intense. This is the age when "playing doctor" becomes popular, and the discovery and exploitation of genital pleasure is to be expected. So, how much is normal and how much is excessive? I think it was Dr. Kinsey who commented that earlier students of sexuality seemed to define "excessive" as "more than I do." This kind of measurement is not a great deal of help in any situation, and it is obviously useless regarding kids. About all you can say is that the amount and intensity of sexual interest and activity have to be judged within the context of the child's whole pattern of life. It would be peculiar and worrisome if masturbation seemed to be the center of attention in the life of a young child, but occasional masturbation as one among many happy pursuits need raise no alarm.

Alarmed or not, most parents tend to find their children's public masturbation socially undesirable. As a matter of manners rather than morality, it is necessary for children to learn the rules regarding the private nature of various body functions. Just as you would teach your kids that one does not pick one's nose or pass intestinal gas in public—same thing regarding masturbation. For their own social protection, children need to understand that masturbation in public is likely to bring disapprobation. This can be a bit tricky if you would like to teach the apparently conflicting lessons that sexual activity is indeed a good and desirable part of human life, and at the same time sex is private behavior.

About masturbation in adolescence, I can only suggest that every parent should say "Hooray!" It signifies a lively and healthy amount of necessary sexual interest and energy which might otherwise be expressed in some less safe and desirable fashion. Consider that it carries absolutely no risk of either sexually transmitted disease or pregnancy, nor will its practice lead your teenager into bad company. Masturbation: the parent's best friend.

The list of children's self-stimulating habits also includes head-banging, rocking, and hair-stroking or twisting. These less common behaviors have much in common with thumb-sucking and masturbation; they may express and relieve emotional tension, and are, generally speaking, not particularly

EVERYDAY PEDIATRICS FOR PARENTS

important. For all of these habits, the question to be asked involves balance; what part does this habit play in the child's life? The 6-year old who can never be without a pacifier, or the 3-year old who masturbates every time he is not busy doing something else, or the 10-year old who twists patches of hair off her head—these kids are probably telling us that something is out of line in their lives. They are sending nonverbal messages of discomfort, and we need to decipher the code. But for the very large majority of children, habits like these are simply part of normal behavior, and the less the adult world fusses about them, the better.

Chapter 25

Bones and Joints

Congenital Orthopedic Deformities

We all expect our newborn babies to be flawless and beautiful, and fortunately most of them are. However, a fair number of them come equipped with thighs, legs, or feet in somewhat twisted positions. The vast majority of these kids have what are termed **minor positional deformities;** feet turned in or turned out, asymmetrical legs, thighs that don't line up straight, and the like. For many years this was typically the excuse for a considerable amount of unnecessary orthopedic attention. The problem was that these minor variations were not clearly differentiated from the rare and important major abnormalities of position that did indeed need vigorous treatment. Fortunately, some brave souls decided that it would be a good idea to watch and wait instead of rushing ahead with orthopedic interventions. It was soon discovered that the normal processes of bone growth reversed the peculiarities of position in the large majority of instances. As news of this crept through the medical community, doctors began to relax a bit and substituted close and careful observation for the previously approved regimens of braces and casts. The positional deformity often righted itself, and in the event that a child did not spontaneously straighten out his foot or his leg, there was still plenty of time to treat. Of course, there remained the severe deformities like club foot (a tightly turned in foot which appears tipped on its side with a tight heel cord and often a twisted leg); these require prompt and prolonged treatment with casts or surgery or both. There is also the subtle but important problem of dislocated or unstable hips which also needs careful evaluation and treatment.

The minor positional problems are generally the result of crowded living quarters within the uterus. During the last months, your baby doesn't have a whole lot of extra room unless you have provided her with an unusually capacious womb. Not infrequently, the random movements of the unborn child result in a "position of comfort" in which one limb or another is so limited in mobility that it becomes somewhat twisted. After the baby is released to the outside world, she can move freely, and the normal processes of muscle action and bone growth begin to return the limb to normal. This healing process can often be sped up by gentle massage and stretching exercises. With rare exceptions, the days when casts, splints, and corrective shoes were *de rigueur* have passed. If your doctor refers you to an orthopedist who is devoted to active treatment of this sort, you might do well to get a second orthopedic opinion. There is often more than one way to skin a cat.

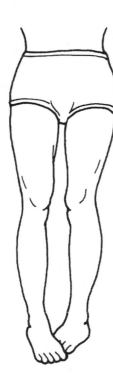

Anteversion of The Hips is one of the less common of these intrauterine position problems, is also the least likely to resolve completely. In this condition, the femurs (thigh bones) are twisted medially (*medially* is doctorese for toward the center or midline). To visualize this, imagine your baby lying flat on her back with her thighs and legs outstretched. Now imagine standing at her feet and grasping each knee in one of your hands. Rotate her right thigh clockwise with your left hand, and rotate her left thigh counterclockwise with your right hand. You have now rotated both thighs medially, and this is the state known as anteversion of the hips. The lower extremities thus rotate towards the midline; instead of pointing straight ahead, the knees point somewhat towards one another. This may become more obvious as the child grows. It can be confused with tibial torsion, described below, since both conditions turn the feet inwards. However, unlike tibial torsion, anteversion of the hips may persist. This is an essentially harmless anatomical variant which should be recognized and ignored because there is nothing useful to do about it. The hips are built this way and no one has figured out any effective intervention short of major and hazardous surgery.

Tibial Torsion is quite a different matter. Here the tibia (the main bone in the lower leg) has more than the usual mild bowing seen in most babies. The medial twist of the tibia turns the ankle and foot inward into a striking and sometimes asymmetrical pigeon-toe. In the recent past, this used to stimulate a frenzy of treatment. The minimum effort was the application of splints attached to firm, high-topped, orthopedic shoes. The shoes were rotated outward to put a twisting pressure on the tibia. This long ordeal of many months eventuated in straighter tibias, but the effects on the knees were not always good. At present, a reasonable approach is watchful waiting, or what English doctors used to call "masterful inactivity." Over a period of 3 or 4 years, twisted tibias grow into a straighter shape; it is a slow process. A remarkably severe case or one with striking asymmetry between the two sides might rarely lead one to consider splints, but avoid them if you can.

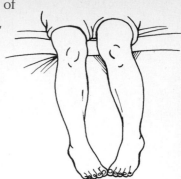

Calcaneovalgus Deformity. A common and even less important deformity is the foot bent up and back against the front of the shin, the calcaneovalgus deformity. These are quite flexible feet and ankles; when you hold the foot you can easily bend it down to a proper position. In some instances the forefoot is bent laterally (to the side) as well. All this self-corrects within months. Your baby's doctor will check the lower extremity reflexes and muscle activity to avoid confusion with some rare neuromuscular disorders; that is all the medical attention that this transient deformity requires.

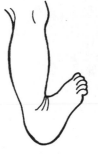

Metatarsus Varus. Deviation of the forefoot towards the midline is termed metatarsus varus or metatarsus adductus. In this common condition, the soft tissues of the inner edge of the foot are contracted but the foot can be pulled rather easily into a neutral, straight position. Left alone, metatarsus varus may improve to a degree, but complete resolution cannot be counted on. This is one positional deformity where treatment is a sound idea. Stretching exercises should begin in very early infancy. Hold the hindfoot (the back half of the foot) so firmly in one hand that it cannot move, and with the other hand bend the forefoot laterally (sideways). The hand holding the hindfoot presses against the outside edge of the baby's foot and acts as the point around which the bending motion occurs. The stretched position is held for several seconds and then relaxed. Repeat the stretching several times over a 2-minute period. The force exerted is guided by the baby's tolerance; if you pull too hard, she will fret. Try to pull the forefoot past the midline into a position where the forefoot actually points out rather than in; after the first few days of stretching this should be accomplished with ease. At least 2 or 3 sessions

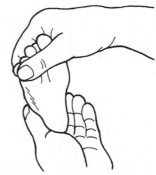

a day are needed to make reasonable progress, and many months will be required to bring the feet into a true neutral position. These feet tend to slip back into their original deformity if stretching is abandoned too early. Rarely, an outward-flared, stiff shoe or orthopedic boot can be used for follow-up control. At times, stretching does not succeed, generally because neither babies nor parents enjoy the process. If redoubled efforts remain fruitless, the baby will need corrective casting by an orthopedist.

Congenital Dislocation of The Hip is another condition in which intrauterine position and crowding play a part, although gender and heredity may be more important factors. This disorder runs in families and is much more common in girls than in boys. It is most likely to occur in first-borns, probably because the uterus tends to be a tight fit the first time around. Some cases of dislocation of the hip are truly congenital, that is, they are present at the time of birth. However, some children have a hip which is not completely dislocated, but is unstable or dislocatable. There are also children whose hips appear to be absolutely normal at birth but are discovered to be dislocated months later. This is an important orthopedic problem, and you will notice that your baby's pediatrician checks the baby's hips repeatedly during well baby visits. I have not included a sketch of hip dislocation because there is rarely much to see. Sometimes one hipbone looks more prominent than the other, or one lower extremity looks a bit short, and sometimes the bottom of one but-tock looks a bit lower than the other, but these are not uniform or reliable signs. All this variability means that the diagnosis is tricky and time consuming, and the choices of therapy are not always straightforward. This is a situation in which your pediatrician and orthopedist will need to work together.

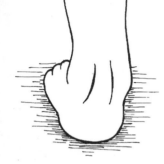

Flexible Flat Foot. After infancy, other developmental foot problems can make an appearance. One of the most common is flexible flat foot. Of course, the pudgy foot of the baby with its pad of fat obscuring the arch looks flat. As a more mature shape evolves after the first year, truly flat feet are often seen. Flat feet are best revealed when the child is standing and the feet are bearing weight. When you look at your child's feet with the child lying down, you will usually see a rather shallow longitudinal (front to back) arch. Seen from the rear with the child standing, the arch of the flat-footed child collapses, the heel slants inward (the inside of the ankle is lower than the out-side of the ankle) and the Achilles tendon (the heel cord) looks concave. The foot is said to be pronated. These kids often have generally loose ligaments, with

EVERYDAY PEDIATRICS FOR PARENTS

more than usual flexibility of all their joints. In early and middle childhood flat foot deformity is nearly always painless and with time, most improve. A few children remain flat-footed into adolescence, but only rarely does this become the source of discomfort. In these instances, firm arch supports are a real help; sometimes plastic orthotics prescribed by a podiatrist are necessary.

Bunions. A less common condition is hallux valgus (which means that the end if the big toe is angled toward the other toes) and the development of bunions. This condition seems to depend on two factors. First, there is probably an inherited tendency for the long foot bone (the first metatarsal) behind the great toe to deviate toward the midline (toward the inner side of the foot). This tends to pull the base of the great toe in the same direction. Second, there is the countervailing force of the shoe, pushing the end part of the great toe in the opposite direction. The result is an increasing prominence and angulation of the joint between the end of the first metatarsal and the base of the great toe (the first metatarsophalangeal joint). This is the deformity which is termed a bunion, and the problem is that it is painfully constrained by the inner border of the shoe. This condition is much more common in girls and women, because the design of their shoes from infancy onwards is so ridiculously unanatomical. The pointed-toed shoe should be avoided whenever possible. In order to accomplish this aim, you may have to dress your daughter in boys' shoes (which is likely to be strenuously and successfully resisted after the first few years), or you will have to declare a pair of shoes to be outgrown before your daughter's toes have grown into the pointed tip. It does help to chose fabric topped shoes rather than leather. The fabric is less firm and therefore less able to deform the underlying toes. Sneakers and athletic shoes are also somewhat more likely to be responsibly designed, but finding properly made shoes remains a frustrating exercise for girls and their parents.

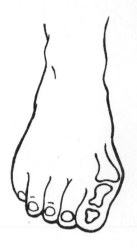

Ingrown Toenails. The shoe industry is also partially responsible for the condition misnamed "ingrown toenails." This tends to be an affliction of big adolescent males with wide forefeet. The basic problem is lack of space; even the currently popular soft footwear of the young is designed with inadequate toe room, both vertically and horizontally. At every step, the toes are constricted and formed into a sort of digital wedge pushing into the tip of the shoe. The adolescent foot grows with astounding speed, and shoes are often worn for months after the available toe space has been used. This tends to be obscured by the design of the shoe which retains some apparent space at the central tip of the

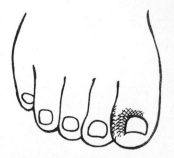

shoe where it is not useful. The effect of this wedging is to push the great toe toward the second toe which cannot move out of the way. The soft tissue of the inner aspect of the great toe is trapped between the great toenail and the second toe. It responds by becoming swollen, and it overgrows the inner edge of the great toenail. If ignored for long enough, a red, tender, pus-filled mass develops.

Treatment is slow and relapses are common because the feet keep growing and the shoes don't fit. The following approach works fairly well.

1. Get rid of the offending shoes. If possible, the teenager should wear sandals, go barefoot, or wear a shoe with the toe cut away until healing has occurred.
2. Soak the foot for 10 to 15 minutes at least twice a day in hot, soapy water.
3. After the soak, express any pus from around the nail, and push the swollen soft tissue away from the toenail with a cotton swab. Careful! This hurts.
4. If the infected area is oozing pus, apply a blob of antibiotic ointment (like polymyxin/bacitracin) and cover with a small bandage.
5. Let the great toenail grow out; when it needs trimming, cut it straight across rather than convex. (Sometimes a spicule of nail is present, buried under the swollen tissue at the edge of the nail; if so, your doctor will need to trim it off. This hurts, too.)
6. A systemic antibiotic taken by mouth may be needed for 1 or 2 weeks if the infection has been ignored for a long time and a really nasty mess has resulted.
7. In rare instances, it will be necessary for your doctor to numb the toe with a local anesthetic and remove about 1/3 of the nail from the border next to the second toe. The nail will slowly grow back to its usual shape, giving plenty of time for healing to occur.
8. The last resort when recurrences continue is to destroy a part of the nail bed so that the nail is made permanently narrower.
9. Prevention consists of warning kids with big, wide feet that cramped toes cause a lot of trouble. They need the bluntest, widest-toed shoes they can find.

Properly fitted shoes can go a long way toward preventing certain foot problems. Unfortunately, shoe salespeople have convinced many of us that fitting a shoe is an esoteric and difficult art, best left to its practitioners in shoe stores. This is nonsense. Parents may safely be guided by **Grossman's Laws of Well Shod Feet:**

1. ***Shoes are basically protective garments.*** They should keep feet comfortable, somewhat cushioned from hard surfaces, dry during wet weather,

and free from a variety of road hazards like broken glass and dog feces. With the rare exception of orthopedic shoes for true deformities, shoes do not aid in the development of normal feet. The longer babies and children can go barefoot, the better.

2. ***As Thomas Jefferson said about government, the least shoe possible is best.*** Heavy, stiff, high-topped shoes are too hot, too hard to put on, too expensive, and too hard to fit accurately. Soft sandals and moccasins are best for babies and toddlers.

3. ***Feet grow.*** The child being fitted should stand up in the new shoes. There should be at least ½ inch of space ahead of the great toe, with plenty of room vertically as well as horizontally. The streamlined, downward-slanted style that looks like it is pretending to be a running shoe is ridiculous; it doesn't even make sense for runners. A boxy toe is best. There must also be room for growth across the ball of the foot; one should be able to pinch up loose fabric or leather at the widest part of the forefoot. The ball of the foot should be at the widest part of the shoe.

4. ***Some used shoes are perfectly fine.*** Shoes are expensive; hand-me-downs are acceptable if they fit and if the previous wearer did not grossly distort the shape of the shoes.

5. ***If it is tight, get rid of it.*** Shoes should not be worn when the available toe and forefoot room has been outgrown. This often means new shoes of a larger size every month or so during the adolescent growth spurt. Given the cost of the fancy shoes teenagers wear, following this advice may require a second mortgage; I know, and I'm sorry.

Chapter 26

The Skin

In Praise of Skin

Any discussion of skin should begin with a note of appreciation and respect for this very well designed and efficient organ. Doubtless, skin is not without its problems and limitations, but consider that one basic model has to serve whether it is worn in Alaska or Zaire, and that it can usually be counted on to last for the better part of a century. During its tenure on the outside of our bodies it must remain water repellent, flexible, capable of manufacturing our requirement of vitamin D, act as a layer of insulation, resist soaps and cosmetics, heal its own wounds, and, if possible, look attractive to others. All in all, this is an impressive set of tasks, and our skins perform them in a generally admirable fashion.

There has recently arisen a revisionist theory of skin that stresses its weaknesses. In particular, the increasing incidence of skin cancers has led some observers to suggest that skin and sun should have as little contact as possible. This advice is based on the observations that excessive sun exposure, such as is experienced by people who work outdoors all the time, ages the skin and leads to the common types of skin cancer, and that repeated episodes of true sunburn seem to be linked to malignant melanoma, a highly dangerous disease. The risk for all these cancers is linked to the color of the skin; fair skin is much more easily sun damaged than darker skin. This leads to **Grossman's Law of Sun Exposure: *Everything in moderation.*** I am aware that this is not a strikingly new or original idea, and the reader may have even heard that it can apply to subjects other than sunburn. What it implies in this instance is that a modest amount of sun is actually a good idea, and that long exposure to sun despite a heavy coating of sunscreen may be unwise. The child who is covered with 30 SPF sunscreen may stay in bright sunlight for quite prolonged periods of time without burning. We know that currently available sunscreens certainly do not protect us from the full range of the sun's radiation. What we don't know is the effect of many hours of exposure to whatever rays do manage to get through the sunscreen. By actually increasing the hours our children are allowed to play outside in the sun, we may be allowing more sun injury to occur. Furthermore, skin exposed in the normal, unprotected fashion to the sun develops pigment which is protective against sunburn. Children will remain as pale as parsnips if their parents follow the currently fashionable advice to slather sunscreen over every square inch of skin, and insist on hats, long sleeves, and long pants in all weather. If they are inadvertently exposed to sun without their usual armoring, their likelihood of real sunburns will be greater. Since inadvertence is a hallmark of childhood, this seems to be a foolish practice.

The following makes sense to me: Let the kid have a little sun on her bare skin, with the aim of slowly building up a modest tan. Use a medium strength sunscreen when prolonged sun exposure is anticipated, and use the full panoply of protection when excessive sun is unavoidable. Keep in mind that skin burns most rapidly during the hours from late morning to midafternoon,

EVERYDAY PEDIATRICS FOR PARENTS

during summer when the sun is high, at the beach or on the water where reflected sunlight is an additional factor, and at high altitudes and low latitudes. Even water-resistant sunscreens wash off; reapply after prolonged water play.

Infant Skin

The skin of newborn babies is a fairly effective and reasonably healthy material, if we would only leave it alone. Unfortunately, patterns of skin care in infancy tend to be quite intrusive and vigorous, and even the best designed infant integument can get into trouble. The first mistake we make is the excessively thorough bath soon after birth. The lubricating vernix (the pasty white covering that the protects the skin of unborn babies) is scrubbed away and the baby's skin responds by becoming dry and cracked. By the second day one often sees a little bleeding, especially at the wrists and ankles. This should be a hint that we are doing something wrong, but the routines of hospital nurseries are immune to rationality. Luckily, infants heal quickly if parents restrain the impulse to bathe the newborn. Most babies do very nicely with a bath every few days, plus an occasional rinse of the diaper area. Any mild soap will suffice; there is absolutely no reason to believe that special soaps are particularly useful. It is often suggested that infants should be sponge bathed rather than be immersed in water until the navel has healed; great efforts are typically expended to keep the cord stump dry. I have seen diagrams explaining how to fold a cloth diaper to avoid touching this supposedly vulnerable area, and there are paper diapers specially tailored with a navel cutout. This notion would be hilarious if it were not so much trouble. The umbilical cord has been soaking in fluid all of fetal life. How continued intermittent moisture could be dangerous is a considerable enigma.

Washing the baby's face and hair is best done with a baby shampoo. The significant difference between these products and standard shampoos is the presence of a buffering agent which decreases the amount of eye irritation.

About the only other rules for the routine care of infant skin are to avoid overheating the baby with excessive clothing and overheated rooms, and avoid cosmetics like baby oil, powder, and lotion. They are absolutely useless, and anyway, babies smell much better without them.

Baby Acne. Within the first weeks of life, a substantial number of infants develop tiny red or white pimples and pustules, first on the scalp and forehead, then extending down the face and onto the shoulders. This is most commonly seen in babies with oily skin and often is accompanied by the greasy scale of seborrhea (see below). Left alone, baby acne subsides over a few more weeks. It tends to flare up temporarily when the baby is overheated. Gentle washing seems mildly helpful, but resist the urge to squeeze, pop, or scrape them off. In extreme cases when the baby's prematurely adolescent appearance is upsetting everyone, you can calm down both the baby's skin and the baby's grandparents by applying a small amount of ½% hydrocortisone cream two or three times a day for a few days.

Seborrhea. Sometimes baby acne segues into the more chronic problem of infant seborrhea. This disorder of scaling has several presentations. The most common is cradle cap, the yellow-brown scaly or greasy material that clings to the infant's scalp. You will notice that cradle cap is heaviest over the fontanels (soft spots) where you have probably been afraid to scrub vigorously. This is one condition for which frequent and muscular washing is often all that is needed. At the start of the bath, work up a lather on the scalp and let it sit there until the rest of the baby is clean, then scrub the scalp with a wet wash cloth. After rinsing and drying, use a baby brush and comb to remove the loosened scale. Rarely, you may need to use a medicated dandruff control shampoo or even a prescribed cortisone-type liquid. More widespread forms of seborrhea show up as scale which looks like finely crushed potato chips clinging to the eyebrows and cheeks, and reddened, moist areas in the creases of the skin. Seborrhea can become quite generalized over the trunk and it is not always possible to differentiate it from infant eczema. Unlike seborrhea, eczema is an itchy rash, and the elbow and knee creases tend to be red, often with some central pallor in the crease. I think there are some children who have both, a seborrheic eczema that is widespread and persistent; these are hard to control. In general, seborrhea is best dealt with by frequent bathing to remove the scale. Medicated soaps and cleansers with sulfur or salicylic acid can be used; cleansers containing tar are also effective but most parents object to having their infants smell like a newly paved street. Hydrocortisone creams at ½% or 1% are also effective. Secondary infection with bacteria or yeast may require treatment as well. When seborrhea affects the face and neck, irritation by saliva and food tends to make it worse. The use of a barrier cream containing silicone can be a great help. These are not widely marketed, but your friendly neighborhood pharmacist can find some for you.

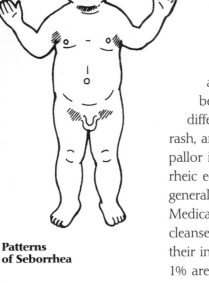

**Patterns
of Seborrhea**

EVERYDAY PEDIATRICS FOR PARENTS

Eczema. The typical appearance of eczema in early infancy is the red-cheeked baby with red elbow creases, rubbing her face back and forth to relieve the itching. The rash may spread to the trunk, arms, and legs; on the extremities eczema is most concentrated on the wrists, elbow creases, knee creases, and ankles. In later infancy, the rash on the body may appear in round patches. When eczema is severe and persistent, the most easily scratched lesions become thickened, and secondary infection with bacteria is exceedingly common.

A predominant factor in the development of infant eczema is food allergy. If your baby is breast fed, and if fresh cows' milk, orange juice, egg white, and wheat are kept out of her diet, she is a lot less likely to develop infant eczema. In later infancy, other foods are possible culprits, in particular peanut butter, corn, soy, fish, and shellfish. Another important cause of eczema in infancy and later childhood is allergy to the house dust mite, a tiny bug which inhabits bedding, stuffed animals, and upholstered furniture. (See page 361 for information on controlling house dust mites.) Other factors are increasingly important at older ages: contact irritants like wool clothes and various household chemicals, and a tendency to dry skin. The fact that the causes of eczema change with age is one reason for the disagreements between pediatricians and dermatologists about the management of eczema. Dermatologists rarely have the opportunity to see the classic food-triggered eczema of infancy. They tend to treat eczema with little regard to allergic factors and therefore miss the possibility of effecting a prompt cure by diet changes.

Some rules governing successful management of eczema are independent of the cause. In general, eczematous skin is dry, and anything making it drier will usually make it worse. Bathing removes the skin oils whose function it is to maintain moisture within the skin. Soap is the worst offender but even water alone can be damaging. Bathing should be minimized; baths should be brief and soapless if possible. If some kind of cleanser is needed, use a mild soap like Dove or a soapless lotion like Cetaphil. Immediately after a bath while the skin is damp, a cream can be used to trap some of this water within the skin. Eucerin, Cetaphil, Keri lotion, Nivea cream and many other similar products are available. For really mild cases of eczema, lubricating and moisturizing lotions or creams used twice a day may be all that is needed. The mainstay of skin medication is old faithful 1% hydrocortisone cream. It works, it has little if any systemic effect, it rarely stings, it is available without a prescription, and it is

Behind the knees

Patterns of Eczema

wonderfully inexpensive (especially if you buy it by the pound). A small application 2 or 3 times a day will control the majority of eczemas. Unlike the more powerful topical steroids, it can be used (but sparingly) on the face and in the diaper area. One percent hydrocortisone fails when used on old, thickened eczematous patches. These are hard to handle even with the strongest skin ointments your doctor can prescribe.

The dietary approach to eczema is easy if your baby has not yet started solids. Eczema due to food allergy in a wholly breast fed infant is a great rarity. In such a case, a rational approach would be a hypoallergenic diet for the mother. At a minimum, this would mean excluding milk, milk products, eggs, wheat, corn, soy, oranges, peanuts, fish, and shellfish from her diet for a 2 to 3-week trial. If her baby's eczema starts to subside, she can then reintroduce foods into her own diet, one at a time, every 3 to 5 days and watch what happens. If the baby is formula fed, switch to a casein hydrolysate like Nutramigen. If the taste and expense of Nutramigen are problems, a soy formula can be tried, but many allergic infants will not tolerate soy any better than cows' milk. During dietary trials, you may be tempted to start topical treatment with skin creams as well. If at all possible, resist the urge; it will complicate your subsequent efforts to understand what happened and why.

The older infant who develops eczema after the introduction of solids poses a harder problem. Of course, the rash may have flared up within a few days after starting a new food. If so, stop the new food and watch what happens for at least a few days. The trouble with this approach is that eczema itches, and the inevitable scratching can keep it going very nicely even if the original cause has been removed. If there is no obvious candidate for exclusion, stop all the allergenic foods mentioned above, or, if necessary, all solids of any kind. If you simply must feed some solids, the following foods are least likely to be allergens: lamb, white potato, sweet potato, spinach, carrot, pear, peach, apricot, plum, and rice (including rice crackers and baby rice cereal). A period of 2 to 3 weeks on an elimination diet that includes only these foods will usually lead to improvement. It is crucial to study labels. Foods fortified with vitamins and minerals pose no problem, but additions of flour, starches, sweeteners, and flavorings should be avoided. Elimination diets are really difficult to manage. There is always an older sibling or a grandparent giving the baby an unauthorized treat, or there is an unexpected additive to an otherwise innocent jar of baby food. Furthermore, eczema waxes and wanes without obvious cause. You may have to remove and return a food from the diet on more than one occasion to convince yourself of its effect. Families can get very tired of diet manipulation, but it does work. Chapter 38 provides more details.

Diaper Rashes. Note the plural. "Diaper rash" is a wastebasket diagnosis, and like all wastebaskets has a variety of contents. What these rashes have in common is occurrence in an area of skin subject to multiple indignities including immersion in urine and stool, abrasion from diapers, increased heat due to occlusive coverings, and nearly constant moisture. This last factor explains why the diaper area is so unlikely to be involved in infant eczema; the hydration reverses the skin dryness which is a major component of eczema.

Most diaper area rashes are transient and unimportant contact irritations set off by the neglect of sufficiently frequent diaper changing, by careless hygiene, or excessively tight diapers. The currently popular paper diapers with elastic edges often cause linear patches of skin redness around the thighs, especially if the baby is too plump or too muscular for an easy fit. Rarely, the offending contactant is something in the urine; I have seen an occasional case due to sensitivity to orange juice. Treatment consists of correcting the apparent cause, exposing the diaper area to air and a little sun, if available, and protecting the skin with a barrier ointment. All the various zinc oxide–based diaper rash ointments work quite well. If a gathered-edge diaper is the problem, the gather can be broken or a different kind of diaper used. You may need to use ½% to 1% hydrocortisone cream if the rash seems unusually inflamed, but this is not often necessary.

Ammonia burns were once fairly common causes of diaper rash. When cloth diapers and plastic or rubber diaper covers were insufficiently laundered, ammonia was sometimes produced by bacterial action on the urine. The diagnosis was straightforward: A red, often slightly scaly appearance was most marked where urine contact was greatest, plus the unmistakable stench of ammonia, especially strong in the overnight diaper. Treatment required vigorous laundering and disinfection of the diapers and diaper covers with bleach or other germicides. This problem has largely disappeared with the availability of automatic washing machines, better detergents, and paper diapers.

Any diaper rash which fails to improve with the usual measures is likely to have an infectious component. Bacterial infections are typically small, red, pustular rashes on the buttocks and around the anus. Treatment is frequent and careful washing, plus the use of topical antibiotic cream like polymxyin/bacitracin a few times a day. These heal very slowly. Yeast infection is much more common. These may accompany an illness for which the child has been given antibiotics; the antibiotics temporarily suppress the usual bacterial flora of the baby's gut, allowing an exuberant blossoming of the yeasts which normally live there in relatively small numbers. Occasionally, a mother with a vaginal yeast infection is the source of a yeast rash in her baby, and sometimes yeast rashes arise for no apparent reason at all. In small infants, there is often a coexistent thrush, a yeast infection of the mucous membranes of the mouth. Yeast rashes have a flat, red, central area often starting around the anus or the genitals, with tiny flat to raised "satellite" lesions at the edges where the rash is extending onto healthy skin. If you happen to treat the rash with a steroid cream, the appearance will be much less red, even though the yeast infection continues unabated. Treatment for yeast rashes is exposure to air and sun, frequent diaper changes, and the application several times a day of an antiyeast cream. The best are the broad-spectrum antifungals like clotrimazole and miconazole which are available without prescription; some of these are labeled for use against athlete's foot or for vaginal use, but they work just as well against yeast diaper rashes. Some other antifungals are also effective but they are available by prescription only and are usually more expensive. Nystatin (Mycostatin) was the first reasonably effective antiyeast topical medication; it is much slower to act than the newer agents and for no apparent reason is still sold only by prescription. I consider it an obsolete drug and see no rationale for its continued use. If the baby also has thrush, treat it with clotrimazole topical antifungal cream. (This drug is frequently used in tablet form for thrush infections in adults, and it is very well tolerated. Nearly all of it goes right through the gut unabsorbed. There is no FDA approved cream for use in the mouth; the creams marketed for vaginal or skin use work nicely.) It should be wiped on the inside of the cheeks and on the tongue after feedings several times a day. This is much more efficacious treatment than the commonly prescribed, expensive, foul-tasting, and wimpy nystatin liquid.

Toddler Skin

Eczema. During the early years of childhood eczema continues to be a major problem. The appearance of the rash gradually evolves into a scaly, patchy, dry eruption that may be present anywhere from scalp to feet. When eczematous areas are infected, they look redder and may be weepy; old, thickened patches may also harbor a vast bacterial flora. Contact irritation and vigorous scratching play increasingly important roles in keeping eczema active, although food, other allergies, and dry skin are still crucial as underlying factors. House dust mite and cat allergy in particular need to be considered. Tests for antibodies against specific allergens may clarify the causes. This is done with skin scratch tests after about age 3 or blood tests at any age. Cat allergy has always been difficult to manage. To say that families have a hard time deciding whether to keep the kid or the cat may somewhat overstate the case, but not by much. It has recently been argued that cat saliva is the specific allergen, generously spread by the kitty all over her fur and from there throughout the house. Frequent bathing of the cat plus exceedingly meticulous housekeeping, including walls, floors, and furniture may be helpful. Desensitization shots are a last resort. House dust mite control has never been easy either. The child's bedroom at least must be kept in Spartan simplicity to minimize living space for the mites and to facilitate cleaning. This requires that floors be without carpets, furniture without upholstery, and mattresses and pillows covered with dust-proof enclosures. Special vacuum cleaners and fancy air filtration systems are often suggested as well, but there seems little evidence that they are effective. Extending dust control to the entire house makes the process even more onerous. Few families will really work hard enough or persevere long enough to dent the population of mites. The recent commercial introduction of benzoyl benzoate powder as a household mite killer may turn out to be useful, but my bets are on the dust mites.

Keratosis Pilaris. "What are these funny little bumps on her arms, Doctor?" If the little bumps are tiny hard points surrounding a minute hair, sometimes with a little surrounding redness, and they are on the outer surfaces of the arms, perhaps the legs, and sometimes the cheeks, they bear the impressive name of keratosis pilaris. Each bump is a plug of dead skin cells in a hair follicle. This condition often accompanies dry skin in general and eczema in particular. Most of the time, keratosis pilaris persists for a few years in childhood, and typically diminishes or disappears in adolescence. Urea cream, 10 or 20%, will smooth it out temporarily but the little lumps recur.

Insect Bites and Stings. It is quite remarkable how picky insects can be in their choice of victims. Families will commonly relate that only a select few of their members are bitten by house spiders or fleas or whatever. Frequently the children are favored, and insect bites in kids are often dramatic in appearance. The red, swollen area around an ordinary bug bite can be 2 or 3 inches in diameter, and blistering is by no means rare. Redness and swelling around a bee sting can extend from the foot half way to the knee and can last for days;

sometimes there is even a little fever. None of this means anything; the bites are not infected, they itch and are tender but rarely hurt, and no significant medical intervention is needed. First aid for insect bites is usually limited to tender, loving care. Holding an ice cube to the bitten area may give everyone something harmless to do. My partners and I have had the impression that antiperspirants (which contain aluminum salts) minimize the discomfort of bee stings, but placebo-controlled studies have yet to be done. Parents are often concerned that these relatively severe local reactions may presage dangerous, life-threatening systemic reactions in the future; they do not. True allergic reactions to insect stings are not common in childhood, but they are a much more serious matter. Some of these reactions take the form of **hives,** large swellings that can appear anywhere on the skin or on mucous membranes such as the mouth and in the respiratory tract. Even rarer are instances of **anaphylactic shock,** in which there is an abrupt collapse of the circulatory system. ***These are medical emergencies requiring immediate treatment with adrenalin and sometimes other drugs.*** Any child who has had such an allergic reaction requires careful evaluation to determine the specific insect cause. Families must learn how to minimize the risks of insect stings, and arrange for the prompt treatment with adrenalin if needed. Desensitization shots are now available which decrease the risk of further reactions.

An interesting variant on insect bites is **papular urticaria,** a strange rash of small, firm bumps intermixed with ordinary insect bites. It looks as if the skin were reacting in a bite-like fashion even in areas where there were in fact no bites. Anti-itching antihistamines like hydroxyzine (Atarax, Vistaril) or diphenhydramine (Benadryl) by mouth or anti-itching creams applied locally are comforting.

Middle–aged Kids' Skin

Lice. Of all the small animals that infest the skin of children, the head louse (Pediculus capitis) is the most common, the least harmful, and the most trouble. The shock, horror, and shame of the parent confronted with a lousy child are often remarkable. Furthermore, the response of school teachers to an outbreak of head lice in the classroom suggests that bubonic plague cannot be far behind. A few facts: 1) Treatment of head lice can be limited to the head and the few objects directly in contact with the head, like pillow cases, brushes, and hats. Sterilization of the entire house or surrounding city block is not indicated. Objects thought to be infested can be washed with soap and hot water, dry cleaned, or just sealed in paper bags for 3 weeks to starve the lice to death. 2) The excellent nonprescription shampoo permethrin (Nix) really kills lice and nits wonderfully efficiently; one treatment will nearly always suffice, but a repeat treatment a week later will make everyone feel better, especially the drug manufacturer and the pharmacist. Unfortunately, there are recent reports of permethrin-resistant lice. Malathion is a fine louse killer but it is not currently marketed for this purpose. Lindane (Kwell) and pyrethrins are not as toxic to the nits; at least one and preferably two repeat treatments are a good idea. Some lice have developed resistance to lindane, so it is not always effective even if used repeatedly. 3) It is fairly difficult to get rid of lice which have taken up residence in long, thick, or curly hair; in this situation don't bother with anything less effective than permethrin. 4) If reinfestation occurs, treat your whole family, babysitters, and close friends. 5) Nits are the tiny eggs that the lice attach to the hair near the scalp. They look like miniature grains of rice, but they are hard to see without excellent illumination and a small hand magnifier. A nit present on the hair shaft more than ½ inch from the scalp is either empty because the louse has already hatched or dead because it was already treated with an insecticide. The point of all this detail about nits is that school personnel sometimes demand that kids be nit free before readmission to class. This is a lot of work and a waste of time if the nits are dead. If all else fails, a vinegar rinse 15 minutes before using a nit comb will loosen them from the hair shafts. Nit combs are usually available at pharmacies, and also are included with some antilouse shampoos.

Scabies. Sarcoptes scabiei is a tiny mite that burrows just under the top layer of the skin. As it moves about, it leaves a trail of minute eggs, bits of feces, and miscellaneous mite debris, all of which cause irritation, itching, and a rash. Mites move from one victim to the next with astounding ease; this is a highly contagious infestation. During recent decades, a worldwide epidemic of scabies has changed this from an infestation of the poor and homeless to a common problem in every social class and at every age. If your child has scabies, you will most likely find yourself looking at a hard-to-describe, finely bumpy, rather sparse, and highly itchy rash which you have already treated over several days with hydrocortisone which didn't help. The diagnosis is not easy; your child's doctor may initially be as puzzled as you are. Treatment needs to be carried out quite precisely. 1) *Every* person who has been in physical contact with the child should be treated. 2) Hot launder sheets, pillow cases, and clothes. Dry clean anything not washable. 3) The best treatment is the prescription topical cream permethrin 5% (Elimite); this is *not* the nonprescription permethrin 1% lotion (Nix) used for lice. The skin should be clean, cool, and dry; don't apply the medicine immediately after a hot bath. The permethrin cream should cover the body from soles to scalp. Wash it off the next morning. 4) Neither the rash nor the itching will improve for days; the scabies mites will be dead but their bodies and their metabolic products will remain in the skin. No new spots will appear. Repeated application of permethrin is not needed but oral anti-itching medicines (hydroxyzine or diphenhydramine) may be used. 5) Recurrences of scabies usually means continued exposure to an untreated case.

Impetigo is an infection of the skin caused by the common bacteria streptococci and staphylococci. It usually appears as a reddened, raised, scabby, or crusted patch, commonly around the nose or mouth, or at the site of a scrape or small cut. Children's skin generally does a good job of resisting bacterial infection. If your child develops impetigo, there are often extra factors which have allowed the germs to break through the ordinary barriers. A chronic bacterial nasal discharge will suffice. Hot, muggy weather also increases the incidence and virulence of impetigo. Casual hygiene and multiple abrasions characteristic of small boys in summertime explains a good many cases. Family or classroom outbreaks are the exception; impetigo is not all that contagious. The precise roles played by strep and staph germs have exercised investigators for years. It is clear that impetigo accompanied by blistering (bullous impetigo) is a staphylococcal infection. It needs to be treated aggressively with antistaph antibiotics. The other, ordinary forms of impetigo may be strep, staph, or both. Mupirocin (Bactroban), a prescription-only cream, generally does a nice job against either or both of these germs. If the disease is widespread or unusually virulent, an antibiotic by mouth will be needed.

Hot Tub Folliculitis. Now here is a disease of affluence! This is a rash of rather small bumps on the child's trunk; it is caused by a pseudomonas bacterial infection spread in hot water. Topical polymxyin/bacitracin ointment is curative. Proper maintenance of the hot tub will prevent recurrences.

Molluscum Contagiosum. This viral infection is spread in water as well as by close personal contact. The lesions start as tiny, less than 1/16-inch in diameter, firm, raised bumps, and mature into 1/8 inch firm, pearly to pink papules. Most of the bumps have a dimpled center, but you may need a magnifying lens to see this clearly. The natural history of molluscum is interesting. The rash may remain confined to a few spots, or it may spread with hundreds of papules. At

EVERYDAY PEDIATRICS FOR PARENTS

some point, redness may develop around a few of the papules; this is a skin reaction which may precede the spontaneous disappearance of the entire eruption. Sometimes the lesions disappear quite rapidly without any preceding inflammatory response. If you can be sufficiently patient, molluscum usually disappears in the fullness of time. If treatment is indicated, your child's doctor can pop the little bumps out of the skin one at a time with a sharp instrument, or they can be destroyed by applying a blistering agent. Neither of these methods is likely to command the easy acquiescence of the patient.

Warts. The wart virus seems to require a degree of cooperation from the human host. The common sites of infection on hands and feet suggest that only abraded or otherwise injured skin is likely to be infected. The rarity of warts on adult skin suggests that some kind of immunity to wart infection eventually develops with age. If common warts are left alone, the vast majority will disappear, although it may take some years for this to happen. If neither you nor your child is unduly alarmed by the wart, and if it is not in a place where it causes discomfort, the best treatment is no treatment at all. A wart that catches on clothing and bleeds, or a wart on the bottom (plantar) surface of the foot that hurts because it is walked on, or a wart that is distorting a fingernail or toenail—all these are candidates for removal. The reason to avoid therapy if possible is that none of the available options is very satisfactory. Freezing the wart with liquid nitrogen is certainly the fastest cure; unfortunately, it hurts, especially if the wart is large and even more if it is a deep, plantar growth. Lasers can be used to destroy warts, but the cost is absurdly high. Make certain your health insurance will cover it. Warts can also be attacked with blistering solutions; this ordinarily takes several treatments, is by no means painless, and does not always succeed. Home application of salicylic or lactic acid will eventually cure most warts, but the nightly ritual of soaking and scarring and medication is daunting. Many families give up long before the wart does.

A painless and really charming wart treatment is self-cure by visualization, a sort of self-hypnosis. It has been known at least since the 1920s that hypnosis can change the rate of healing of skin wounds, and there has been for centuries a plethora of traditional folk remedies for warts which seem to rely on suggestion. It should therefore not be too surprising that warts can be cured quite nicely by the patient herself. I should note that this treatment was devised and taught to me by a 9-year old. Peter had accompanied his friend to a hypnotist who was treating the friend's warts. He decided that he could accomplish the same thing for his own warts without any help, and he did. The technique is simple. 1) Get a timing device like a 2-minute egg timer. 2) Go to a quiet and private place where your little brother will not interrupt and make fun of you. 3) Look at the wart and imagine that it is becoming smaller and disappearing. Keep this up for 2 minutes; when your attention wanders from the wart, and it will, just resume visualizing again. 4) Repeat twice daily if possible. Families report several outcomes. The child who thought this was a dumb idea at the outset abandons the treatment within a few days. A few children give up after a week or two. The large majority of those children who were intrigued or excited at the beginning persevere; their warts generally disappear quite abruptly after 6 to 8 weeks. The sense of delighted self-mastery that these kids earn is wonderful.

Tinea Corporis (Ringworm). We all live surrounded by fungus spores, the microscopic seed-like bodies which will grow happily into active fungus colonies if given the right opportunities. As it happens, the surface of the human skin is a fairly hospitable environment for a variety of these little plants, so we sometimes find ourselves wondering what that round, dry, slightly red, and sometimes itchy patch of skin signifies. As a skin fungus infection matures, the central area may become less inflamed and flatter, and the edge of infection looks redder and somewhat ringlike, thus the common term ringworm. If the patch persists, grows, and is joined by a few other similar patches here and there, chances are good that we are carrying around some fungus or another. Cats, dogs, and people are frequent hosts to ringworm fungi; there is often the history of contact with an infected animal or close friend. Treatment of ringworm is slow but simple if only a few spots are present; there are a number of excellent topical fungicides like clotrimazole and miconazole. A really widespread infection is best treated with griseofulvin, an expensive oral antifungal given by mouth. Other oral antifungals are even more effective but also more toxic.

Tinea Capitis (Ringworm of The Scalp). Fungal infections of the scalp are common in school age children, especially among blacks and Hispanics. Ringworm of the scalp can look like round, bald areas with tiny broken-off hairs in the center, or like a scruffy form of dandruff, or it can resemble a bacterial infection with pus and swelling. The fungi live deep down in the scalp, so local treatment with antifungal medicines doesn't work; the antifungal drug griseofulvin has to be given by mouth for many weeks.

Tinea Pedis (Athlete's Foot). For some reason, the conventional medical teaching about tinea pedis has been that babies and small children don't get it. Unfortunately, the conventional teaching is wrong: they do. Nor is it true that athlete's foot infections are spread mostly in locker rooms or around swimming pools. Athlete's foot is just another instance of a situation where ubiquitous fungus spores happen to land in a place which meets their needs for growth. Fungal infections seem to thrive on feet which are kept warm and sweaty; the inside of a modern shoe made largely of rubber and plastics is fungus heaven. Add a pair of socks made of nonabsorbent synthetic thread, and it is a surprise that our feet don't rot off at our ankles. There are some kids who have very sweaty feet even in well-ventilated settings, and some families have a long tradition of chronic tinea pedis. These are the children most likely to have athlete's foot infections in infancy.

Not every itchy rash on the feet is a fungus infection. Tinea pedis will usually be most obvious as scaling or moist, red cracking of the webs between the toes, especially the third, fourth, and little toes. There may also be red, finely blistery, itchy spots along the edges of the sole. Chronic tinea may cause diffuse scaling of the entire sole, especially in older children. It is important to differentiate fungus infection from eczema and contact dermatitis of the foot. An eczema will usually involve the ankles or the top portion of the midfoot. A contact dermatitis will look like a superficial burn and will cover the portions of the toes and feet most exposed to shoe chemicals. The toe webs will be spared. Because host factors of diminished resistance and increased sweatiness are important, and because most children's footwear does not ventilate the foot, tinea pedis often recurs. Going barefoot, wearing sandals, choosing socks made of light wool or cotton, using absorbent foot powders—all these techniques may help to control the disease. Treatment with one of the modern antifungal creams such as clotrimazole (Lotrimin, Mycelex, or generic) or miconazole twice a day will lead to rapid improvement; several weeks may be needed for complete clearing. Some obsolete antifungals like undecylenic acid (Desenex) are still on the market despite their pitifully limited efficacy. Also to be avoided are antifungal powders or sprays; when you are treating an active infection, you need to use a cream.

Tinea Unguium. Toenail fungus infections are very rare in childhood. This is fortunate because the infected nails become thickened, yellow, and ugly, and because treatment is wholly unsatisfactory. If the nail is trimmed short and filed or ground down as thin as possible, you may achieve a modest degree of control by using an antifungal cream or liquid every day. As soon as treatment is stopped, the nail infection usually reappears. The same is true for systemic treatment with griseofulvin; the nails look great after 6 to 12 months of medication, but relapse after treatment is nearly universal. Oral itraconazole (Sporanox) works better than griseofulvin but it not infrequently causes liver injury and occasionally kills people, which seems like a heavy price to pay for pretty toenails. A number of new antifungal drugs, both topical and oral, are currently being evaluated, and some of them look promising. For the present, sometimes the wisest course is to do nothing, offensive as that may be to our sense of medical and parental omnipotence.

Tinea Versicolor. This superficial infection is caused by a peculiar yeast organism (Pityrosporum orbiculare, aka Malassezia furfur) which ordinarily sits around harmlessly on everyone's skin. Given the right conditions of heat, humidity, and an oily skin, it can grow vigorously and cause a rash. I've only seen it in preteens and adolescents, but it is said to occur in young infants as well. The rash is not very dramatic; rather faint, flat spots gradually increasing in size to blotches a few inches in diameter, slightly pink or tan at first and then often pale and depigmented, and sometimes a bit itchy. Since tinea versicolor tends to start on the back, it is easily overlooked and ignored even by its host. Initial treatment is easy: daily shampooing with the antidandruff shampoos selenium sulfide (Selsun, etc.) or zinc pyrithione (Head and Shoulders, etc.) for a week or two. Some antifungal creams also work well, but their cost becomes prohibitive since large areas are usually involved. The itching and pinkness disappear promptly but the depigmentation may persist until sun exposure occurs. The major problem is recurrence. The organism is ubiquitous, and some people's skins get infected again and again. A degree of control can be obtained by a routine of weekly or monthly use of any of these agents, at least during the warm seasons of the year when recurrences are most common.

Pityriasis Rosea is a fairly common skin infection that parents never seem to have heard about. It typically begins with a large, round or ring-like, slightly raised, and slightly scaly patch somewhere on the child's trunk. Everyone looks at this and says "Ah, ha ! Ringworm !" And they are wrong. A few days later, after you've bought the expensive antiringworm medicine which is not going to do any good, the rest of the rash appears. It starts as tiny, slightly raised bumps, mostly on the trunk; these develop into round or oval salmon-pink, faintly scaly patches, about ¼ to ½ inch across. There may be scores or hundreds of them. The rash may itch a bit, especially if the child is overheated. Usually there are no other symptoms except extreme impatience; the rash lasts for weeks and then creeps away, never to be seen again. Treatment is generally useless and quite unnecessary. I described this as an infection, and it most likely is, but the cause is actually unknown. How it spreads is a mystery; I've never seen pityriasis rosea spread from one person to another.

Psoriasis is a poorly understood disorder in which the normal processes of skin scaling are deranged. It varies in severity from trivial and limited rashes to exceedingly widespread and tenacious eruptions all over the body, and it may even be accompanied by joint inflammation. Even though it is not all that uncommon in childhood, I am always surprised by psoriasis, and I usually miss the diagnosis the first time I see a new case. In children, psoriasis often starts unimpressively, just a patch or two of moderately scaly, slightly reddened skin on the knees, elbows, or scalp. The characteristic, silvery-scaled, raised patches may not occur for many months. It may also start as a widespread eruption of little pink bumps that does not look at all like classic psoriasis. Sometimes psoriasis seems to be triggered by a strep throat. There are a variety of treatments that do a pretty good job of controlling this difficult disease, but management is tricky and sometimes complex. It is usually wise to seek the help of a dermatologist.

Contact Dermatitis, Including Poison Ivy and Oak. Kids' skin is really pretty tough and there are not a great many substances that are likely to cause contact irritations. Plants of the *Toxicodendron* (formerly *Rhus*) genus, popularly known as poison ivy, poison oak, and poison sumac probably cause the most trouble. Other causes of contact irritations include metal allergy from the nickel component of silver and gold jewelry, cosmetic reactions, especially from eye make-up, a variety of chemical irritations from footwear, and a kind of chronic eczema from dish-washing detergent. For most ordinary and mild cases, avoidance of the irritant plus treatment with 1% hydrocortisone cream will allow prompt healing.

Poison oak and poison ivy are variants of the same plant, and poison sumac is their first cousin; the problems they cause are identical. After the first exposure to these plants, the skin rather slowly develops a kind of allergic sensitivity, and a rash may appear a week or so later. With subsequent exposures, the allergic reaction usually develops much more promptly, typically within a few days but sometimes literally overnight. The reaction may be exceedingly widespread, prolonged, and severe. The folklore surrounding this disease is impressive and uniformly misleading. For example, it is widely believed that

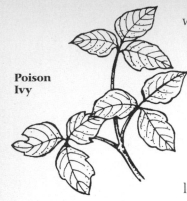

Poison Ivy

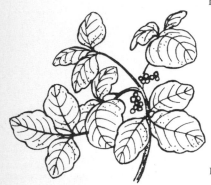

Western Poison Oak

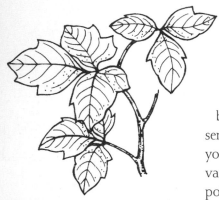

Southeastern Poison Oak

washing with various soaps can prevent rash. Unfortunately, the offending substance in these plants becomes fixed to the skin within minutes to hours. Soap and water will do a good job if used soon enough, but delayed bathing will not remove it. Watching the eruption occurring at more and more sites over a period of a few days leads to the mistaken notion that the patient is spreading it by scratching, or that the oozing blisters are somehow contagious, but this is not the case. It simply takes longer for the rash to appear in some areas than in others. Factors such as differing skin thickness, varying amounts of contact with the irritant oleoresin, and probably local skin sensitivity all effect the rate of development of the rash.

In a mild case the rash consists of small red flat patches, raised bumps, and raised scratches, few in number, and neither blistered nor oozing and weepy. A mild cortisone cream such as 1% hydrocortisone can be used several times a day; ½% hydrocortisone will probably be too weak to do much good. More severe cases can sometimes be managed with the most powerful cortisone type ointments (all of which require a prescription), plus an oral anti-itch medicine (hydroxyzine by prescription or diphenhydramine over the counter). However, severe cases tend to be quite widespread, and the amount of steroid cream needed becomes exceedingly costly. In these instances, it makes more sense to use oral prednisone for about one week, rarely a little longer. It is common practice to start treatment in this situation with an injection of a steroid drug. This is impressive to everyone; the shot hurts and it costs a great deal of money, so it must be useful. It is otherwise pointless and irrational, because the same medication given by mouth starts to work very promptly, does not hurt at all, and costs next to nothing. Even with the systemic use of prednisone, the patient will get some benefit from strong steroid creams and oral anti-itching drugs during the first few days.

Prevention is not easy. A new barrier cream (Stokogard) is claimed to give several hours of protection if it is applied before exposure. Hyposensitization treatments with orally administered extracts have not been impressively successful but are worth trying for the children with severe sensitivity and frequent recurrences. It is worth while teaching yourself and your kids how to recognize and therefore have a chance to avoid your local variety of *Toxicodendron*. Most helpful is the characteristic growth pattern of poison oak and poison ivy. The leaves are grouped in threes; western poison oak has wavy leaf edges, southeastern poison oak has jagged edges, and the edges of poison ivy are most often smooth. Poison sumac has a compound leaf

EVERYDAY PEDIATRICS FOR PARENTS

with 7 to 11 smooth-edged leaflets. The plants vary from vines to shrubs. In winter the bare branches look whip-like, with stubby little lateral branchlets.

Adolescent Skin

Acne. The treatment of adolescent acne starts when the adolescent wants it to. You may notice the first crops of blackheads or the first appearance of pimples, and you may gently and kindly point out to your teenager that the dread disease has struck, but nothing happens until the teenager himself decides to take action. This can take quite a while. Kids this age often do not want to admit embarrassing imperfection (of course, who does?) and facing the fact of their increasingly imperfect faces can be difficult. Eventually the unhappy victim of acne admits he has a problem; unfortunately, what happens thereafter bears only a glancing similarity to good medical practice. Acne therapy is basically in the hands of the peer culture and the advertisers of cosmetics. All this is regrettable, but that is how it is.

When the teenager does decide that the insights of medical science should be applied to his acne, provide the information needed for understanding by showing him the following pages.

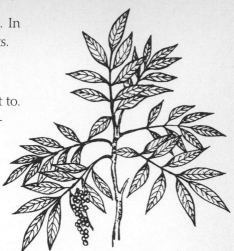

Poison Sumac

Acne: What Is It? Acne is a common disorder in which the oil glands of the skin produce an excessive amount of skin oil, and roughening occurs in the lining membranes of the tiny ducts that carry the oil to the surface of the skin. These ducts consequently become partly plugged by dried oil and debris from the duct lining. When a partial obstruction is right at the surface, a **blackhead** (open comedone) is formed. Where a complete plug forms, a **whitehead** (closed comedone) develops. The oil trapped within the duct is broken down into irritating fatty acids by the action of skin bacteria. This causes the formation of pimples which are basically small skin abscesses.

These processes tend to develop in adolescence when skin oil production increases in response to changes in sex hormones. The high sugar diet of the Western world appears to be an important factor in some people, although not in all. Specific skin bacteria play a role as well. Many women note that acne worsens at the beginning of their menstrual periods. Emotional stress also seems to cause pimple flareups. As adolescent development is completed in the late teens, the acne process tends to improve spontaneously; in most people, acne has disappeared by the early twenties, although it sometimes persists well into adult life.

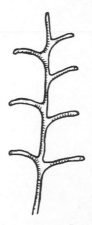

Poison Oak or Ivy branches in winter

What Can Be Done About It? The first thing to understand about acne is that, for the vast majority, it is a self-limited disorder which will last a few years; treatment *will not* cure it. The effect of treatment is to suppress the acne until it gradually cures itself. However, a very satisfactory degree of control can be obtained by present day therapy, properly used. Treatment must be tailored to the person, the person's skin, and the kind of acne. For example, a fair-skinned 13-year old girl needs only very gentle medication; the powerful agents used for severe acne would make her skin worse rather than better. A few years later, she might need much more potent medicine if her acne has increased in severity, as often happens.

How To Do It. What follows are some basic do's and don't's.

1. **Hygiene:** Simple face washing removes skin oils and helps keep oil pores open; warm water, soap, and a washcloth used twice a day can be very helpful, especially in mild acne. Frequent shampooing of the hair helps keep oil off the forehead. Avoiding hair gels, leave-on conditioners, and oily cosmetics helps, too. Sometimes antibacterial soaps like Dial, Safeguard, or pHisoHex are useful. *Scrubs, buffing pads, and abrasives are not helpful and often make acne worse; don't waste your time with them.* The reason they are not useful is because they remove only the outermost layer of skin, and the acne process occurs too far inside the skin to be squeezed off, picked off, or scraped off.

2. **Diet:** Although there has been much debate about the role of food, it is always worth experimenting to see if heavy sugar intake worsens acne. All one has to do is increase candy or soda pop consumption abruptly for a few days. If a large crop of pimples appears, try the reverse experiment of a low sugar diet for a few weeks. A few people find that foods high in fat like chocolate and peanut butter have a deleterious effect.

3. **Medication applied directly to the skin:** This encompasses a wide range of liquids, lotions, and gels which act by scaling off dead skin, opening pores, and exerting a drying effect. Sulfur, salicylic acid, and resorcinol are the mild agents used for less severe acne. These are not very effective for most people but some over-the-counter medications still include them. The mainstay of acne treatment for years has been benzoyl peroxide, a drug which works by interfering with the growth of skin bacteria, decreasing the concentration of free fatty acids, and inducing a mild scaling of the skin surface. Bars and washes are the least effective vehicles for benzoyl peroxide; lotions, available without prescription, are quite helpful; gels are

much more potent and potentially more irritating; some require a prescription. The water-based (aqueous) gels are less irritating then acetone-based products. The 2.5% or 5% strengths are usually used; the 10% is too strong for many people. Tretinoin (Retin-A) is a prescription–only drug which is closely related to vitamin A. It smooths the lining of the oil ducts so that old debris can be dislodged and fewer new plugs form. It must be applied carefully to minimize skin irritation; it also decreases the resistance of the skin to sunburn so it must be used cautiously during the summer months. Adapalane and tazarotene, two new drugs with similar mechanisms of action, are likely to become available soon. Topical antibiotics are helpful when the skin is irritated and infected around acne–plugged oil glands. Tetracycline, erythromycin, and clindamycin are all used. Quite commonly it is best to combine topical medicines, for example benzoyl peroxide or an antibiotic in the morning and tretinoin at bedtime.

4. **Other local skin treatments** include the use of a comedone extractor. This is a very small metal ring at the end of a handle. After the closed comedone (blackhead) is softened by washing the face with warm soapy water, the ring is pressed over the blackhead which pops out. This is a neat gadget for people with blackheads; ask your doctor to show you how and when to use it.

5. **Systemic treatments** are also available. Antibiotics taken by mouth for months to years suppress the growth of bacteria in the oil ducts and usually bring about a substantial decrease in pimples. This use of antibiotics is remarkably safe; side effects are rare and generally easily handled. Tetracyclines and erythromycin are the usual choices. Another vitamin A–like drug, isotretinoin (Accutane), is extraordinarily effective against severe acne which has not been controlled by other means. Unlike any other acne treatment, isotretinoin comes close to being a real cure. Unhappily, it has dangerous and unpleasant side effects including raised blood cholesterol, irritated eyes and lips, nosebleeds, dry skin, and some cases of cataracts, liver inflammation, and raised pressure within the skull. If it is taken during pregnancy, it has absolutely disastrous effects on the developing fetus. Clearly, it must be considered a drug of last resort.

What You Can Expect to Happen. Most people with acne find that they do best when they combine treatments: Hygiene, perhaps diet, local medications, and often a systemic antibiotic may eventually all be used. Balancing these agents takes time and attention, both from the patient and the doctor.

Many teenagers find it difficult to persist with a years-long undertaking like this in which improvement is slow and many changes of treatment may be needed. It is easy to give up, or forget to use the medicine, or try some magical and highly advertised cure recommended by a friend. However, the reward for perseverance is the clearest possible skin during adolescence and the least possible acne scarring to carry into adult life.

Chapter 27

Injuries and Poisonings

Raising kids means dealing with injuries. The world is a hazardous place even for the most careful adult, and, inevitably, it is even more dangerous for heedless, active, and inexperienced children. Therefore, the first word is prevention. Build a safe enough environment, and you will save everyone trips to the doctor's office.

We know a fair amount about the patterns of injuries in childhood. Boys tend to become injured more often than girls; lack of adult supervision increases the risk of injuries; any disruption in family routine, like illness, visitors, or moving to a new dwelling, is associated with an increase in accidents. The trick is to structure a fail-safe household, so that the inevitable lapses that could lead to disaster are contained. If the poisonous solvents are kept behind a latched cupboard door as well as high out of reach, Junior will not be discovered drinking the paint thinner when a visitor mistakenly leaves the door ajar. It is also necessary to keep in mind that most of our children inhabit multiple dwellings; the babysitter's house and Grandma's apartment require the same thoughtful attention as our own homes.

Be Prepared

The Boy Scout's motto is absolutely appropriate. You need to know what to do when an accident of any kind occurs. If the problem requires first aid, be prepared to give it. This may mean taking a Red Cross course, and it will certainly mean having first aid materials at hand. It also means having a clear understanding with your doctor about how medical help is to be sought. Should you call her office, or the local emergency room, or dial 911, and for what sorts of

EVERYDAY PEDIATRICS FOR PARENTS

problems? If there is a choice of hospitals, which has the E.R. best equipped for kids? Emergency rooms are worth avoiding if at all possible. They are increasingly overwhelmed with patients, the sights and sounds are often horrific, the waiting can be interminable, and the cost bizarre. In addition, many E.R.s are staffed by doctors with little pediatric training, and some do not even have the child-sized equipment the doctor will need. In short, E.R.s are a last resort for major problems, not your first choice for most injuries.

Post a list of crucial telephone numbers next to your phone so that everyone in the household will know who or where to call in case of an emergency. Include your doctor, poison control center, neighbors or other backup adults, and your work phones.

Home first aid materials may be purchased as a kit, providing the advantages of completeness and organization, so that everything needed is in one, easily accessible place. You can also make your own collection which should include the following.

EQUIPMENT:

• **Gauze pads, absorbent cotton,** and **cotton-wrapped applicator sticks** for cleaning wounds.

A liquid antiseptic cleanser is not really needed since ordinary soap works well.

• **Rubbing alcohol** can be used to clean uninjured skin but should *not* be put on any wound.

• **Wrapped adhesive bandages** (Band-Aids) in various sizes.

• **Gauze pads** in 2-inch and 4-inch squares for larger wounds.

• **Cotton gauze roller bandage,** 4 or 6 inches wide; the Kling bandage is excellent.

• **Elastic roller bandages** (Ace-type or self-adherent) in 2 or 3-inch and 4 or 6-inch widths.

• An **antibiotic cream** or **ointment** like polymxyin/bacitracin. Use these to keep dressings from sticking to scrapes and small burns.

• **Adhesive tapes.** The best all-purpose tape is "paper" tape because it sticks very well and does less damage to the skin. Heavier weight cloth or plastic tapes are sometimes useful to reinforce a bandage or help immobilize a finger or a toe.

• A **tourniquet** for emergency control of bleeding from a limb; this can be a 2-foot length of thin rubber tubing.

• **Bandage scissors.**

• A very fine-tipped **tweezers** or a small, sharp-tipped **penknife** for splinter removal.

In emergency situations, other materials may be needed such as splints or compresses, but these can be improvised on the spot.

MEDICINES:

• **Acetaminophen** Tylenol or any other brand, as a simple pain reliever.

• **Ibuprofen** or **aspirin,** when both pain control and relief of swelling and inflammation are needed.

• An **antihistamine** for allergic reactions. Diphenhydramine is a good one; it also has some sedative and anti-itching effects.

• **Codeine cough syrup.** Used in big doses, codeine is an effective pain killer.

• **Syrup of ipecac** to induce vomiting. Label this to read: To induce vomiting give 1 to 2 teaspoons to infants under 1 year, 1 tablespoon to all others; may repeat dose in 20 minutes if vomiting does not occur. Do not induce vomiting if the poison ingested was lye (Drano) or other agents which cause burning, gasoline or similar solvents. Call the doctor!

Injuries and Poisonings

251

Abrasions and Lacerations. When your child cuts or scrapes herself, it is natural to wonder "Does this need to be sewn up?" The answer may not be apparent until you have stopped the bleeding and cleaned up the wound sufficiently to see what has happened. **Stopping bleeding is the first step.** Direct pressure over the injured area, using a clean cloth if possible, will stanch the flow of blood most of the time. You may find that bleeding resumes as soon as you release the pressure; 5 or 10 minutes of continuous pressure may be needed. It may also help to elevate the injured part above the level of the body; this lowers the blood pressure in the veins, which are the usual source of most bleeding. Bleeding from a serious, deep laceration on a limb may be more easily controlled if a tourniquet is wrapped tightly around the limb between the wound and the rest of the body. *Uninterrupted tourniquet pressure is dangerous;* release it after about 10 minutes. **The next step is rinsing or washing the wound with water and, if possible, soap.** You really do not need disinfectant solutions; some of them are actively harmful to injured tissue (alcohol, for example), and some are simply no better than soap and water. Use cotton applicators, gauze, or absorbent cotton and soap to clean up. This is often the worst part of an injury; your child is screaming, you are about ready to faint, and you have no idea how much you should do and how much you should leave for the doctor or the nurse. As usual, there is no easy answer; early cleaning of a wound is a big help. If in doubt, call your doctor.

For small and cleanable abrasions, your ministrations will usually suffice. Once it is clean and the bleeding has stopped, bandage it with an appropriate sized dressing and a blob of an ointment or cream to minimize sticking of the bandage to the wound. Either a bland ointment like petroleum jelly (Vaseline) or an antibiotic ointment is fine. If you choose instead to leave the injured area open to the air, it will probably heal a bit more slowly, and it will collect dirt from time to time during the healing process. Of course, some children view bandages in the same way that dogs do, as challenges to be dispensed with as promptly as possible.

Small, gaping cuts can often be closed nicely with a bandage. We used to use "butterfly" adhesive bandages which are strips of tape the very central portion of which is covered in a nonstick material. These have been nicely superseded by the use of strips of paper tape. The intact skin on either side of the cut is carefully cleaned and dried (really dry; damp will not do), the edges of the cut are pinched together closely, and the tape is applied perpendicular to the laceration. Several pieces may be needed to secure even a tiny cut. If you tape

EVERYDAY PEDIATRICS FOR PARENTS

a cut, you cannot use any ointment in the area. Even the best paper tape will be defeated by soaking in these gooey preparations. If you got it clean in the first place, there is no need for an antibiotic dressing. Skin does a great job of killing bacteria if the dirt has been washed away. The paper tape method of skin closure is absolutely useless for cuts on mobile areas of the skin such as over any joint, unless the joint itself can be splinted in a fixed position. Nor can it be used near the mouth; the combination of saliva, food, and motion will destroy even the most cleverly applied bandage. Let your doctor take care of those.

Puncture Wounds. Any wound that pierces deeply into the skin through a relatively small hole is a puncture wound, and these are unexpectedly troublesome. They are often unimpressive in appearance, tend to bleed very little, are hard to clean, and are in some danger of being ignored. The problem is that whatever caused the puncture may have driven dirt, germs, or both deeply into the wound, thereby setting up the conditions for an infection. Heel punctures are common examples of this. A sneaker-clad child steps on a nail which drives through the rubber and fabric right up to the heel bone, and a low-grade bone infection slowly develops. (It does not matter whether the nail is new and shiny or ancient and rusty; a puncture is a puncture.) In the bad old days before the invention of tetanus immunization there was also the risk that tetanus spores would be implanted into the puncture, leading to an exceedingly unpleasant death from tetanus.

This story has a whole hatful of morals including 1) Make sure everyone in the family has up-to-date tetanus immunization. Really severe wounds may even require an additional dose of tetanus toxoid. 2) Wash every puncture wound as thoroughly as possible. This may require a a visit to your doctor's office where there is equipment to wash out the inside of the wound. 3) Heel punctures, especially through sneakers, should be brought to your doctor's attention.

Bites by Humans and Other Animals. It takes a few years to convince certain children that biting is an unacceptable form of interpersonal communication. Until that lesson is firmly implanted, these kids can be significant hazards to their families and friends. Happily, the bites of little children cause more anger than anguish. the skin is rarely broken, and the tooth marks fade in a week or so. Adults are often sorely and understandably tempted to bite back in an attempt to teach that biting is bad. I think this form of dental pedagogy should be eschewed if at all possible. Treat biting like any other infant felony with firm words, appropriate anger if that is what you are feeling, and unpleasant consequences like time-outs.

The bite injuries most often seen in older kids result during fistfights when a knuckle collides with the intended victim's front teeth. The teeth neatly incise through the skin down to the assailant's bone, leaving behind an inoculum of miscellaneous mouth bacteria, and a nasty infection flares up within a few days. Injuries of this sort need prompt medical attention. This problem can be prevented by using boxing gloves.

The significance of animal bites depends, not surprisingly, on the animal. **Cat bites** are most often small but deep punctures. The mouth bacteria of cats are a nasty lot so that infections are frequent and can be serious even when the bite appears unimportant. The peculiar infection called cat scratch disease can also result from cat bites; it is discussed on page 346 in Chapter 36. **Dog bites** involve tearing and crushing of soft tissues as well as punctures. Significant dog bites should receive medical attention, and prophylactic antibiotics are often appropriate. The tiny bites inflicted by pet mice, rats, and hamsters are mostly inconsequential; vigorous washing is usually all that is needed.

Rabies is a viral infection spread through exposure to the saliva of infected animals. Vast numbers of wild animals including skunks, raccoons, bats, foxes, and woodchucks have rabies which can spread to domestic pets. In the United States rabies vaccination of dogs and cats has resulted in reasonably good control of rabies, but in many countries bites by rabid dogs remain a serious health problem. The question of rabies exposure needs to be raised regarding every animal bite. Bites by the wild animals mentioned above are especially suspect; bites by wild rabbits, squirrels, and rats carry much less risk of rabies. Bites by a known, apparently healthy, and vaccinated dog or cat carry little risk, but if the biting animal is unknown, was acting unwell, or may not have been vaccinated, protective vaccination against rabies may be needed. Fortunately, the new antirabies vaccines and rabies immune globulin are effective and much safer than the old Pasteur treatment.

Splinters. Like everything else in childhood, splinters come in a wide variety of sizes. The tiny splinters that you discover in your children's feet after they have been running around barefoot on the wooden porch typically require nothing at all. They are exceedingly small, so superficially embedded that they don't even hurt, and eventually disappear without anyone's attention. At the other end of the splinter spectrum are the deep, massive, painful splinters which will obviously need a doctor's ministrations. The middle-sized splinters which you will be tempted to remove are best approached by the following method; it may be perceived by your child as threatening, but isn't. Wash the surrounding skin with soap and water. Wash a sharp-pointed small knife like a pocketknife with soap and water and rinse it with alcohol. If you don't have such a knife, clean a large needle. Have a tweezers ready to go. (Tweezers are useless unless the very tip ends come together tightly.) Use little picking motions with the knife tip or needle to unroof the end of the splinter nearest the surface of the skin. Proceed down the splinter as far as your patient will allow. Often it is possible to pop the splinter out with the knife or needle. If not, grasp it with a sharp-nosed tweezers or splinter forceps. Don't bother with the tweezers until you can get a really good grip on the splinter. When the splinter is removed, wash the area again, give your child a congratulatory kiss, and celebrate your success with a satisfied sigh of relief.

Sprains. Ligaments are the fibrous bands that connect bones or cartilages to each other; tendons are the fibrous structures that connect muscles to bones. Sprains are injuries in which some of the tiny fibers in a ligament or a tendon are torn but the ligament or tendon as a whole remains intact. It is not always easy to tell if an injury is just a sprain or whether the ligament or tendon is actually ruptured, and sometimes a visit to the doctor is really necessary. Failure to treat a torn ligament or tendon leads to significant disabilities.

FINGERS. Ball injuries are the most common cause of sprained fingers. A ball hits a finger and bends it so forcefully that damage to ligaments or tendons results. This is a situation where you really must be sure that nothing worse than a sprain has occurred because stable and strong finger joints are so important. **Chill the finger by immersing it in cold water for about 10 or 15 minutes.** Until it can be seen by your doctor, **immobilize the finger by bandaging it with adhesive tape to the neighboring finger,** with both fingers held in a gently curved position, as if holding a glass. *Do not splint a sprained finger straight out;* the curved position puts the structures of the finger in a normal, relaxed state. It is best to use several pieces of ½-inch wide heavy cloth adhesive tape, and the injured joint should be held firmly enough to discourage movement. If you are unable to get to a doctor, about 3 to 5 days of taping usually suffices, but it is wisest to have these injuries checked. Sometimes the sprain is swollen and painful enough to warrant the use of a mild pain reliever and anti-inflammatory like ibuprofen or aspirin for a day or so. (For more on the relative merits, problems, and uses of these drugs and acetaminophen as pain relievers, see page 262–64 at the end of this chapter.)

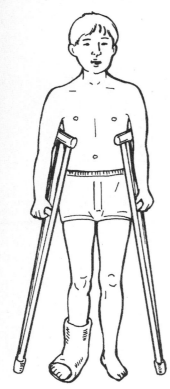

TOES. A stubbed toe is generally a sprained toe. Fortunately, these are next to never broken; toe bones are really tough. It is not usually necessary to immobilize a sprained toe, but it may help to wear a firm-soled shoe for a few days.

ANKLES. Most sprained ankles are straightforward and easily dealt with, but a severe sprain may hide a small fracture or even an torn ligament. This is why any moderately severe ankle sprain should be checked by your doctor. Lean on your kids to give their sprains enough time to heal before returning to full and unsupported activity because recurrent sprains can become a major dilemma. **Initial treatment requires ice, rest, elevation, and immobilization.** It seems to me that ice helps control pain and swelling if used promptly after an acute sprain; about 30 minutes of chilling is probably enough. I am unconvinced that fancy regimens of icing or alternating ice and heat do anything afterwards to speed healing. This is an area of folklore elevated to orthopedic mythology. Lying down as soon as possible with the injured extremity propped up on pillows will reduce the pain and help to control the swelling. During the days thereafter when healing is taking place, keep the ankle elevated whenever it can be arranged. An important part of the initial treatment is immobilization plus pressure over the injured tissues to minimize swelling and bleeding. A good way to accomplish this is to place a firm U-shaped pad under and around the ankle bone and hold it in place with an elastic bandage. Crutches, plus heavy elastic bandaging or adhesive strapping, plus gradual resumption of weight-bearing used to be routine for severe ankle sprains. Now, the use of air-filled or gel-filled "casts" has made it possible for walking to begin within a day or so. Crutches are now needed only rarely and briefly. Even children can be taught to use crutches properly. They must be held firmly, with the arms held straight, and the padded top of the crutches resting against the sides of the chest wall rather than tucked up into the armpits. This allows the body's weight to be borne by the arms, which is vastly more comfortable. For mild sprains it is sufficient to keep the ankle and foot firmly supported with an elastic bandage wrapped around in a figure 8 fashion holding the foot at a right angle to the leg. The bandage should not be so tight that the foot turns blue, and it can be removed during sleep.

Dislocated Radial Head (Nursemaid's Elbow). Should this be re-named "Au pair's dislocation?" This common childhood injury happens when a child is suddenly pulled or lifted by one hand, and it is particularly likely to occur if the child twists away at the same time. The end of one of the long

EVERYDAY PEDIATRICS FOR PARENTS

bones of the forearm (the radius) is attached at the elbow joint within a ring-shaped ligament; when this pulling and twisting occurs, the head of the radius is apparently pulled partly free of the ligament. What happens next is unclear. X-ray examination does not show any significant abnormality; perhaps the head of the radius traps a fold of the soft tissue lining the elbow joint as it tries to return into its proper place. The important point about dislocated radial head is to min-imize both diagnosis and treatment. All too often, these children are subjected to X-ray studies when simple clinical examination should suffice. Even when the story of the injury is unavailable, the picture of the sad-faced little child with her arm dangling limply at her side or held carefully by the other hand is close to diagnostic. Oddly enough, the child may think that the injury is at the wrist, but careful exami-nation reveals that the tender area is just below the elbow joint which nearly always clarifies the picture.

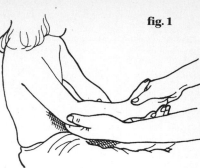

fig. 1

Reducing a dislocated radial head is ordinarily a task for a med-ical professional, but in emergency situations when you are far from any medical facilities, you may need to do it yourself. The crucial maneuver in replacing the radial head is turning the fore-arm to a palm-up position while bending the forearm. This can be done easily by grasping the child's hand in a handshake position, firmly holding the elbow with your other hand (fig. 1), and simulta-neously turning the hand, palm up, while completely flexing the elbow (fig. 2). At the conclusion of the movement the child's palm nearly touches her shoulder (fig. 3). It may require two or three such motions before the radial head slips back where it belongs and one feels and hears a click. An alter-native method used by some clinicians is to turn the hand up while straightening rather than flexing the forearm; this is apparently equally effective. After what seems to be a successful reduction, the child should be watched for 10 or 15 minutes. By that time, nearly every child will be playing happily and using both arms comfort-ably. Any immobilization or other intervention is wholly unneces-sary. Children often have more than one episode of nursemaid's elbow, so consider asking your doctor to show you how to treat the next one yourself. It is easier to learn from a demonstration rather than just reading about it in a book.

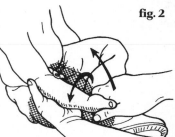

fig. 2

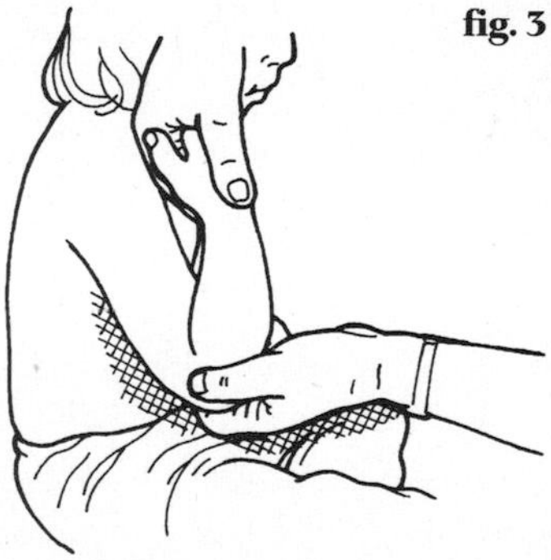

fig. 3

Other Dislocations. Reducing most dislocations is a matter of pulling on the extremity and then allowing it to slip back into its proper place. When the joint is a knee or a shoulder, this is a demanding task best left to medically trained people. However, finger dislocations can sometimes be replaced with relative ease, especially if treatment is instituted soon after the injury. The trick is to grasp the dislocated finger firmly and apply a firm, strong pull in the direction of the end of the finger. If the finger does not quickly pop back into place, give up the attempt. In any case of a dislocation, whether you have been able to reduce it or not, call your doctor so a decision can be made regarding medical follow-up.

Minor Burns. Burns are classified according to the depth of injury. **First degree** burns, which are superficial, affect only the topmost layer of skin, and appear red. Sunburn is a good example of a first degree burn. **Second degree** burns injure deeper structures of the skin, and cause blistering or loss of the top layer of the skin. Scalds often cause second degree burns. **Third degree** burns destroy the entire thickness of the skin. Fortunately, most of the burns sustained by children are first degree or superficial second degree in depth. **First aid for burns is a prolonged immersion in cold water;** about half an hour is needed for a burn of more than the most minor nature. Ice is not needed, although the numbing effect of ice water may be appreciated by some children. For most minor burns wash gently with water or a salt water solution (1 teaspoon salt to 1 quart of water), which stings less. If the wound is dirty, use soap as well. Then cover the burn with copious amounts of an ointment such as petroleum jelly or an antibiotic plus a gauze pad held in place by paper adhesive tape. If the burn is small and the burn site is unlikely to be bumped, open care without the gauze cover is a possibility. Frequent applications of one of these ointments will help protect the burned area while it is healing, but this is somewhat of a mess. Anyway, most burns hurt much less once they are protected by a substantial dressing. Unless a really heavy layer of ointment is used, the dressing will unfailingly stick to the wound. Change the dressing the next day before this happens, and redress as often as needed to keep the wound surface from further injury by the bandage. A variety of materials have been devised to allow healing without adherence. A simple plastic membrane (Telfa) works moderately well. The newer artificial membrane dressings (Omniderm, Duoderm, etc.) seem to be really superior in allowing rapid healing but they are exceedingly expensive; since these minor burns heal so nicely anyway it is hard to justify their use. The treatment of sunburn is different. Aspirin by mouth may help the inflammatory pain, and 1% hydrocortisone cream used 3 or 4 times a day may speed resolution of the burn.

The most important aspect of burns is prevention. Turn the water heater down so that the hot water is no more than 120°F. Get into the habit of keeping cups of hot coffee and bowls of soup out of reach when the baby is sitting in your lap, and practice turning the handles of pots away from the front of the stove.

Choking. See page 92 for discussion of the hazards of small objects and page 90 for the problems of finger foods. Ask your doctor or the local Red Cross for instruction in the Heimlich maneuver and other means to clear an airway. This is information every parent needs; *please don't put it off.*

Subungual Hematomas (Blood Under a Toenail or Fingernail).
Fingernail and toenail injuries sufficient to cause bleeding under the nail cry out for treatment. If the blood is not released, it continues to be painful for many days. Relief is obtained by placing a hole in the nail either with a special battery driven drill or by melting a hole with repeated gentle touches with a red-hot paper clip. This is not a home remedy for the faint of heart, but circumstances may warrant it. Partially unbend a metal paper clip, preferably a large one, so that one end sticks out. Grasp the unbent body of the clip with a pliers and heat the end red hot at the stove. Then quickly and gently, before it cools down, touch the red tip to the nail directly over the collection of blood. You will need to repeat these tiny touches several times, reheating the clip end between contacts. The hot clip will gradually melt a tiny hole through the nail. At the instant the nail is penetrated, a geyser of blood erupts and the pain is gone. If only a tiny drop of blood oozes out, make the hole larger. If you are sufficiently careful, the paper clip will not touch the nail bed. The blood will continue to drain slowly for hours, so apply a bandage to save the furniture. Your doctor would probably have used the little drill which looks much more scientific and perhaps less frightening, but the old paper clip method works just fine.

Epistaxes (Nosebleeds). An acute nosebleed may have an obvious cause, usually a blow to the nose, or be apparently spontaneous, in which case a cause must be sought. Low-grade nasal infection, dry air, high altitudes, and nose rubbing or nose picking (which can have an allergic basis) are the usual factors. Recurrent nosebleeds raise the possibility of an underlying bleeding disorder; if your child has more frequent nose bleeds than you can easily explain, he needs medical evaluation.

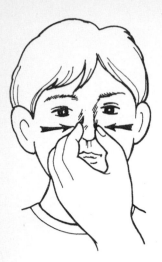

Treatment of most nose bleeds is exceedingly simple but rarely done correctly. In the vast majority of cases, the source of blood is the network of little veins within the mucous membranes which line the central septum at the tip half of the nose. This is the end part of the nose where the central structure is flexible cartilage rather than hard bone. Just apply direct pressure to collapse these veins. Do this by firmly squeezing between thumb and forefinger the entire end half, the cartilaginous part, of the nose. Bleeding will stop instantly if enough of the nose is compressed. If bleeding has not stopped you probably need to grasp more of the nose; pressure on the very tip does not help, nor does pressure up near the bridge. Use nothing but your fingers; tissues, handkerchiefs, or gauze pads just get in the way. Keep the pressure up without stopping for 5 to 10 minutes at least; it takes time for clotting to take place. If bleeding resumes when you release your pressure, try again for another 10 minutes. Keep the owner of the nose upright if possible. If he is lying down, blood pressure in the veins of his head will be a bit higher and the bleeding more copious. Ice applied anywhere on the head is supposed to cause constriction of the blood vessels in the nose; if someone else can hold ice on the nape of the patient's neck, this may be moderately helpful. Nosebleeds which cannot be controlled in this fashion need prompt medical attention; it is an easy way to lose a lot of blood.

Electric Shocks. Electricity is dangerous, and parents are rightly concerned about electric shock hazards to their children. All the more pity, then, that a substantial portion of that concern is focused on the least likely source of trouble, the wall outlets. Any number of homes are well equipped with outlet covers of diverse and ingenious design which allegedly keep inquisitive fingers out of the way of alternating current. The problem is that even the smallest finger is unable to penetrate deeply enough to make contact, unless you have supplied your child with a slender metal probe for assistance. There is nothing wrong with attempting to make outlets inaccessible, as long as attention is not diverted from the really nasty sources of electric shock, which are the cords that carry electricity and the appliances that use it. The cords are the worst hazard; they are all over the place, either permanently because the appliance is always needed, or temporarily when the appliance is in use. All that is required to deliver a tissue-destroying jolt is for the toddler to take an experimental bite through the insulation, or mouth the recipient end of a plugged-in extension cord. The resulting lip burns are serious indeed. So:

1. **Every electric cord should be fixed so firmly to the adjacent**

EVERYDAY PEDIATRICS FOR PARENTS

wall or floor or furniture that it cannot be picked up and chewed. This is a tough but important rule to follow. It is unsafe to leave electric cords under a carpet because gradual degradation of the cord could lead to an electrical short and a fire. Attaching cords to floors requires that they be out of the traffic pattern or covered by a rubber cord protector.

2. **Never leave an extension cord plugged in at the wall without the recipient end properly attached to the intended appliance.**

3. **Check the electric outlets in every room that has a wash basin or bath tub;** replace all standard outlets with ground fault circuit interrupters. The electric shock dangers of electric appliances are most severe when they are used near water. The best protection in these situations are the automatic ground fault circuit interrupters which cut off the electricity when an accident produces a misdirected flow of current. These should be standard with new construction but are unlikely to be present in old homes.

4. **Instruct all the tool users in your family regarding shock hazards.** The electrical dangers faced by older children include improper use of ungrounded electric tools in dangerous situations, for example, using an electric drill or electric hedge trimmer outside an a wet day.

5. **Make sure that your electric tools are double insulated,** or that they are always used with a three-wire, grounded cord.

Poisonings. Poison control is an area in which parents can accomplish a great deal. The three tasks are:

1. Rid the environment of dangerous substances.
2. Control access to those poisons which must be kept in the home.
3. Know what to do in the event that a child ingests a possibly toxic substance.

In order to do any of these tasks efficiently you need to know what is poisonous and what isn't. Among the most dangerous household poisons are **caustics** like **lye (Drano)** and **toilet bowl cleaners,** hydrocarbon liquids like **paint thinner, fire starter, kerosene,** and **gasoline, solvents** like **acetone, disinfectants** like **Lysol** and **Pinesol, liquid waxes** and **furniture polishes** like **lemon oil,** most **prescription drugs,** some **nonprescription drugs,** especially **iron,** and most **garden pesticides.** Some cleaning agents are toxic, including **borax, tri-sodium phosphate,** and **automatic dishwasher detergent.** Most other household detergents and soaps are safe. Cosmetics are generally safe, although the alcohol content of perfumes could conceivably cause some trouble. Garden plants are the focus of considerable worry, most of it unwarranted. There are large numbers of plants which are actually poisonous but so rarely available to children that they do not constitute much of a threat; tulip and daffodil bulbs are good examples of this. In every part of the country there are specific plants which do sometimes figure in poisonings; because these will vary with climate and terrain, it is not possible to provide a really useful nationwide list. Ask your doctor, the local poison control center, and plant nurseries what should be considered dangerous where you live.

1. **Get rid of every poison possible.** This means throwing out unneeded drugs, replacing liquid polishes with paste or foam formulations, discarding every solvent, caustic, and pesticide which is not absolutely needed, and disposing of all so-called disinfectants, none of which are of the least use in the home.

2. **Place the remaining poisons in securely locked cupboards, which are out of reach of kids of any age.** I know that this is difficult to accomplish. It is a lot handier to keep medicines next to the kitchen or bathroom sink; heaven knows they are harder to remember when out of sight. Do not trust child-proof caps on bottles. They are not child-proof at all, just child-resistant; the kids are slowed down a little. Of course it is more convenient to keep necessary chemicals like insecticides and charcoal fire starter out where you will be using them. But that's the point: If it is easy for the adults to get, it's easy for the kids to get, too.

3. **Every adult in the household, including babysitters, should understand how to proceed if a possible toxic ingestion occurs.** Ask your doctor whether to call her, the local E.R., or the local poison control center. Know where the bottle of **ipecac** is kept. Know when to use it and when not to. (Caustics like lye should not be vomited out because they will cause burning of the esophagus when they come up again. Hydrocarbon liquids like fire starter and gasoline can cause a chemical pneumonia if they are vomited.) Some physicians ask parents to keep activated charcoal at home to be used for those substances which should not be vomited. Unfortunately, the stuff is difficult to administer, so it is not much used except in medical settings.

Pain Relief. Doctors get so involved in the definitive treatment of injuries that pain relief is sometimes forgotten. Parents may need to make sure that this important aspect is taken into account. For run-of-the-mill injuries, pain relief can easily be managed with bandaging, immobilization of an injured part, occasionally with the use of ice, and simple analgesics. Aspirin is still a very useful pain killer. It has fallen out of favor in pediatric practice for two reasons: In large overdoses, aspirin is poisonous. This problem has been fairly well controlled by dispensing children's aspirin in small packages. The second reason for aspirin's unpopularity is the apparent connection between aspirin use and an uncommon but dangerous liver and brain disorder called Reye syndrome. Children who have been given aspirin when they became ill with chicken pox or influenza seem more likely to come down with this disease. Most pediatricians have concluded that the risks of using aspirin outweigh whatever advantages it has, at least for ordinary pain relief. My own view is that there are still situations where the virtues of aspirin should be kept in mind. The palatability of aspirin in the children's chewable form is a great help, especially with kids who reject acetaminophen. The anti-inflammatory effect is probably an additional help in burns and soft tissue injuries. If your child has already had chickenpox, and the influenza season of late fall and early winter is not in full swing, Reye syndrome ceases to be much of a consideration. Acetaminophen is just as good a pain killer as aspirin, although it is without any anti-inflammatory effect. In most situations this is wholly unimportant. Ibuprofen (Motrin, Advil, Nuprin, etc.) is a somewhat more powerful and longer lasting analgesic and it has a significant anti-inflammatory effect, if used in full doses. The rather expensive liquid form is available in concentrated form by prescription and in a more dilute preparation over the counter; generic tablets are relatively cheap.

Like other nonsteroidal, anti-inflammatory drugs, ibuprofen is more toxic than aspirin or acetaminophen, but this is rarely a problem for short-term use in children. Naproxen (Aleve) is another nonsteroidal anti-inflammatory which is now sold without a prescription. It has the advantage of prolonged action. Codeine is a great drug for pain. Especially when used along with aspirin or acetaminophen, codeine will control the discomfort of most severe soft tissue injuries, and even some fracture pain. The easiest way to give codeine to small children is in the form of liquid cough syrups like promethazine with codeine. These don't taste too terrible and are often already available in the home medicine cabinet. For older children, your doctor can prescribe aspirin with codeine or acetaminophen with codeine tablets. For severe pain from fractures and burns, morphine or similar narcotics are required. There is literally no risk of addiction when we treat acute pain from childhood injuries. If repeated doses are needed, they should be given before the pain returns. The idea is to keep the proper amount of the medicine in the blood stream all the time. This allows much more effective pain control with smaller doses of narcotic and avoids the pain which will otherwise occur after one dose has worn off and before the next has had time to take effect. There is no discernible virtue in needless suffering.

Chapter 28

The Management of Children's Illnesses

How do we define being sick? At first glance, this may seem a silly question; if you are sick, you know it, and the condition should not be all that difficult to recognize in someone else. But it seems to me that everyone actually has a personal definition of illness, and a quite individual sense of where the line is drawn between good health and disease. These standards are a complex product of culture, ethnicity, ease of availability and potential usefulness of medical care, and individual temperament. An office worker who awakens morning after morning with a backache is likely to decide that some kind of medical intervention is needed to cure his symptom. On the other hand, a construction worker may be more likely to define his morning discomfort as an inevitable part of life and ignore it. The ethnic and cultural rules of some groups define illness as a sign of poor personal discipline or weakness which must be denied as long as possible. These are families where the child's complaint "I'm sick!" is initially met with "No you're not; you're just a little tired," or "You just need something to eat." In other families, by contrast, illness is seen as a mortal threat; even small perturbations in health are defined as sufficient cause for a visit to the doctor. None of this is likely to be susceptible to change, nor need it be; it is just a fact of life that we all have our own thresholds, no matter how nuttily defined, for passing from health to illness.

If we apply these definitions to our kids in more or less in the same way we apply them to ourselves we are likely to be misled, because a child's reaction to illness is not the same as an adult's. In the first place, the infant and the young child has had little immunologic experience with the microbes of the world. During fetal life, antibodies against a variety of germs have flowed from the mother to her baby. After the baby is born breast milk also contains protective

EVERYDAY PEDIATRICS FOR PARENTS

substances. These provide valuable defense for many months during the baby's first year, but once the antibodies disappear, the baby becomes a happy hunting ground for every bug in town. A considerable number of these infections are caused by rather unimportant viruses which induce a nonspecific response of fever, general misery, loss of appetite, and a variety of symptoms in the respiratory and digestive systems. Some of them cause fleeting rashes as well. The neophyte parent observes the illness, takes the child's temperature and is appalled to discover a fever of 103° F. Knowing that this much fever in an adult would be worrisome, the parent appropriately arranges a medical visit. This is by no means a bad idea. This kind of fever and associated symptoms could be the beginning of a large number of exceedingly unpleasant diseases. However, when a knowledgeable physician has concluded the examination, he is likely to say that the baby has "a virus," or "the flu," or as one of my partners used to say, "a little bug." There are a whole basketful of these "little bugs," and every baby has to come into contact with each of them, get more or less sick, and develop the immune response that will protect him when the baby and the bug meet again. You will note that I said "more or less sick," and this variety of response to infectious agents is a fascinating phenomenon. There are healthy kids who hardly turn a hair with infections of this sort, and there are kids who get good and sick with absolutely every germ that comes down the pike. As far as I can see, this is about 90% luck; I don't think it is a matter of diet or how much sleep they get or how happy their home life might be; it is unexplainable variation.

Of course, the more often a baby is exposed to other babies and the germs that some of them are inevitably incubating, the more frequently infection and illness will result. This is especially true during the early years when the defense mechanisms against disease are still in the process of maturation. At the Berkeley Pediatric Group, our records of children's illnesses reach back over fifty years. Until day care for infants and toddlers became common in the 1970s and 80s, the average number of illness visits during the first year of life was literally less than one. After day care became the norm, the average number of visits increased to seven!

In any event, our children eventually meet a vast number of infectious organisms, they react with varying degrees of illness, and they get better most of the time with no help from parents, doctors, or drugs. One should not be too cavalier about infant illnesses, some of which are deadly. However, it is important to respect the power of the human body, even little bodies, to deal with the majority of everyday infections.

This leads to the vexatious question of how we should manage the not-very-sick child. The first step is arriving at a diagnosis. When I was a very young medical student, learning about the astounding number of ways in which the human body could become ill, I believed that our teachers knew pretty much what they were doing when they told us that patient A had disease X and patient B had disease Y. The patients we saw were often chosen as teaching subjects because they provided reasonably clear cut examples of one disease or another. The process of diagnosis followed a rational and understandable course, and appropriate therapy followed. But the more I learned, the less clear-cut the patients and the illnesses seemed to be. Imagine my chagrin when I eventually entered medical practice and found myself in a place with lots of gray, and precious little black and white. It wasn't that I was such a bad doctor; the problem seemed to be that most patients and most illnesses did not truly fit into ready-made diagnostic categories.

Diagnosis is the process through which the practitioner attempts to convert the undisciplined mess of the patient's symptoms into a definitive and accurate assessment. The neophyte's temptation is to call upon the entire storehouse of diagnostic tools to reach a convincing conclusion. The limitations of this approach are many; diagnostic procedures take time, money, blood (literally), may expose the patient to harmful substances like x-radiation, and often scare the hell out of him. Obviously, one had better approach diagnosis thoughtfully and with care. The longer I have been in practice, the fewer diagnostic tools I call upon. Eventually, one learns to trust one's clinical judgment and the use of the laboratory becomes less important in day to day pediatric practice; more looking at the patient, less looking at the lab tests.

Assume that the diagnostic procedures are completed, and the judgment has been made that the illness in question is an infection of minimal or modest importance. If the causative organism is probably a bacterium, the temptation to intervene by administering an antibiotic is strong. We know that the illness can be shortened, and we expect to minimize the risk of illness complications. Unhappily, we also know that using a drug exposes the child to a small but real risk of an adverse reaction. In the case of a few infections, we have some reason to believe that intervention early during an infection will blunt the specific antibody response, and thus leave the child less well protected by his own antibodies the next time the same germ attempts to invade. This is not a problem if the body has had a few days to recognize and begin to fight the infection on its own. Let me emphasize that the use of antibiotics does *not* suppress the body's immune systems in general. There has somehow arisen the notion that the human body has a general, all-inclusive, immunity-conferring mechanism that can be injured by antibiotics. In reality, our bodies have an impressive array of disease-fighting systems. Although in rare instances the use of an antibiotic may lessen the amount of antibody aimed at a particular germ, the other immune responses are unaffected. Another myth worth mentioning is the notion that the administration of antibiotics permanently suppresses the growth of the useful and necessary bacteria that live in our gut, allowing a terrifying overgrowth of nasty yeast germs. The reality is that our intestinal tracts are such warm havens for our friendly bacteria that they are never completely killed by antibiotics, and they rebound with alacrity when the antibiotics are stopped. When that happens, any yeast overgrowth is brought promptly under control by the competing bacteria.

In the case of infections likely to be due to viruses, the doctor's dilemma is somewhat different. He knows that the usual antibiotics will have no effect against viruses, but he will still be tempted to treat with them, hoping to decrease the risk of secondary bacterial infection. He may also be unsure of his diagnosis, and he may want to use an antibiotic on the off chance that the bug is a bacterium after all. Furthermore, he may be reacting to pressure from the child's family to "do something." It can be difficult for a parent to leave the doctor's office without the reassuring magic of a prescription in hand.

There is no proven formula to follow in this situation. If the family and the physician know and trust each other, watchful waiting while keeping in touch can be both sensible and tolerable. If neither familiarity nor trust characterize the doctor-patient relationship, the pressures to expose the child to excessive diagnostic and therapeutic intervention can be overwhelming. One popular solution is to fudge by suggesting useless but relatively harmless treatments. The doctor may be well aware that there is no such thing as a medicine which will "loosen" a cough (a so-called expectorant), but he may still tell the parent to obtain one of these fraudulent and nasty tasting syrups. He may know that bed rest is neither curative nor helpful for most illnesses, but he may be inclined to prescribe it anyway, just to give the illusion of offering medical guidance. I'm sorry if this sounds terribly cynical, but it is important to understand that the doctor truly wants to be helpful, and he also wants to be perceived as doing something useful. Parents are understandably anxious when their kids are sick, and they want to play a useful role in returning them to health. Having a medicine to administer, or a regimen of diet or rest or whatever to follow is reassuring.

This is one reason for the amazing popularity of herbal medicines and homeopathic cures. There are people who approach consumption as a science, who never buy a product without studying Consumers' Reports, who comparison shop fifteen brands of VCR, in short, modern adults who are skeptical about the marketplace. Yet an astounding number of these same folks will drift into a health food store and purchase a package of dried plant material on the advice of a clerk whose training in botany, therapeutics, and toxicology is not likely to be impressive. Neither seller nor buyer may be aware that plants can be quite dangerous, that mislabeling and contamination are real risks, and that mishaps due to the consumption of these products are common. It would even be desirable if there were some actual evidence of efficacy other than old wives' tales and the assurances advertised by the manufacturers. This herbal junk does not come under the control of the Food and Drug Administration unless the sellers make the mistake of claiming usefulness in the treatment of disease. The sellers know this and restrict themselves to vague promises of glowing health and fitness.

Homeopathic medicines at least have the advantage of utter harmlessness. By the nature of homeopathic compounding, there is little if any active material left in the sugar pills or solutions. The only possible side effects are likely to be the waste of money and the delay before real treatment is instituted if it is needed. When homeopathy was invented in the 18th century it was a weird theory but a safe one. Orthodox medical treatment in those days was somewhere between useless and highly hazardous. Doing nothing for an illness was often the safest and wisest choice and that is what Dr. Christian Freidrich Samuel Hahnemann advocated. He opined that medicines became more potent by grinding them up with one hundred times their weight of lactose (milk sugar), and then diluting them with water or alcohol and shaking them vigorously time after time. When you have mixed the one hundred–fold diluted drug with ten parts of water ten or fifteen times, you will have protected the patient nearly completely from the active ingredient. Considering that the drugs in use in those days were substances like strychnine and arsenic, it is hard to imagine a better approach. However, it is another question whether it still makes sense in an era when we actually know something about the actions of drugs and possess medicines which are truly useful.

How Doctors Think About Disease

The history of medicine is, to a large extent, the history of a search for patterns. For many millenia the tools of that investigation were nothing more than close observation. The shaman, healer, or priest or parent faced with a sick child had no laboratory to consult, no department of public health to advise about illnesses current in the community, no easily accessible body of knowledge about the interaction of agents of disease and their victims. Did a sick infant have measles or rubella or scarlet fever? It was only a few hundred years ago that physicians began to appreciate that an acute childhood illness with fever and a rash might be any of several different entities. In fact, we are still sorting out diseases, one from the other. Even in modern times, careful clinical study has led to the realization that more than one illness has been hiding under one name. At this point, the laboratory comes to the rescue by revealing the biochemical, genetic, or microbial differences that had previously been overlooked.

Happily for sick children and their doctors, enough is known to allow diagnosis most of the time on the basis of an accurate history of the illness plus a simple physical examination of the patient. For many illnesses, nothing more is required. For a minority of childhood illnesses, relatively simple laboratory studies are needed: a blood count, an analysis of urine, a throat swab, much less often an x-ray or more complicated lab studies. If a coherent pattern has not begun to emerge at this point, the neophyte physician begins to worry that he is confronted with a rare disease which is eluding his inexperienced eye. The lazy physician reaches for his prescription pad to order some kind of symptom-masking drug. The astute physician decides to retrace his steps to see what information he missed the first time around. He may also begin to wonder what part the patient's or the family's emotional life is playing. The old saying in medical training is that rare diseases occur infrequently. As a medical school aphorism has it, when you hear the thunder of hoofbeats, think "horses" rather than "zebras." The doctor who spends his time and his patients' money chasing zebras should be avoided.

In all fairness to the lazy physician mentioned in the preceding paragraph, sometimes the best course is to accept a certain imprecision of diagnosis. After all, if the illness is just a "little bug," why not say so and let it go at that? In fact, that is what we do much of the time, and it is often a good idea. The "little bug" category implies that the physician has judged the illness at hand to be of no great importance. No further diagnostic maneuvers are required and if any treatment is indicated it will be limited to symptom relief. It pains me when I hear this kind of illness labeled "the flu" because this is sloppy shorthand, and misleading to boot. Better to describe the illness as precisely as possible and admit that one does not know which of several dozen unimportant viral organisms might be involved. Even worse is "It's going around." The problem with this phrase is that it is most unusual for only one viral or other infectious disease to be "going around" in a community at any given time. Even during an epidemic of true influenza there will be a significant minority of other, fairly similar seeming germs in town. It is damned hard to tell one bug from another, and assumptions made on the basis that each new case will be a carbon copy of the last patient seen will lead to some stupid mistakes.

The role of the parent in the process of diagnosis will vary depending on all sorts of factors such as apparent severity of the illness, how long it lasts, and whether the family style is "Quick, call the doctor!" or "I'm sure we can handle this ourselves." Most parents find a comfortable path between undue anxiety and embarrassing dependence. They learn the skill of global observation and develop sensitivity to those basic cues of activity, appetite, skin color, and emotional state that spell out the severity of illness. They also learn to recognize the specific patterns of particular children. "He always vomits when he gets sick, no matter what is wrong with him." "She always says her throat hurts, even if what she really has turns out to be a stomach bug." "I know she doesn't have a fever but none of my kids run fevers when they are sick." Of course, given enough exposure to enough children, parents also develop impressive skills in recognizing a number of common childhood diseases. When the mother of five calls me to report that her youngest has chickenpox, chances are excellent that she is correct.

It is sometimes suggested that parents should learn to evaluate their children's illnesses by the decision-tree or algorithm method. This requires a step-by-step logical analysis of a child's illness, rather like following the diagnostic keys in a field guide to wildflowers. I am not sure why I have such distaste for algorithms; perhaps it is because I always have so much trouble with field guides, or maybe it is because I know that this is not how any experienced doctor actually thinks. Let's see: Dealing with bleeding. Step 1: If bleeding is bright red (see color chart), bleeding is arterial, turn to page 34. If bleeding is dark red (see color chart), bleeding is venous, proceed to step 2. Step 2: Measure blood flow (use metric measuring cup if available; if not, see conversion chart on inside back cover). If volume is 30 ml/minute or less, cleanse wound (see page 35 for best methods). If volume exceeds 30ml/minute, attempt to stanch flow (see page 36). Well, it is a possibility, but not very practical. It is probably just as useful to know a few important facts such as pain in the right lower quadrant may mean appendicitis, and a stiff neck plus a fever is always worth an immediate call to the doctor.

What should you do when the doctor's advice simply strikes you as wrong? The power relationship between patient and physician is never an even one. Presumably, your child's pediatrician knows quite a bit that you don't know, or you would not have sought her attention in the first place. So, challenging her is no easy matter for most parents. The most common way to deal with disagreements like this is to ignore the medical advice, tear up the prescription, and hope everything turns our for the best. Because most childhood medical problems are not fatal, and because the human body *can* heal itself, this approach often suffices. It is my guess that most parents never discuss their failure to follow the doctor's orders. If you still have a reasonable amount of faith in her, you will continue in her practice and not worry overly much about the disagreement. The problem with this kind of quiet, passive difference of opinion is that it may be based on inadequate information on the part of the parent. If the doctor's point of view had been expressed with more clarity or in more detail, perhaps the parent would have joined in her conclusion and followed her recommendations. This is one reason why open confrontation is a better idea. I do not underestimate the impediments to such a course. If the doctor is sufficiently arrogant, or busy, or unwilling to talk in plain English rather than medical jargon, a straightforward discussion about the merits of the case may be close to impossible. For parents who find that they are frequently at odds with their medical advisor, the best solution is to change doctors. Chronic strife between physician and patient is no great joy for anyone, and there is usually a certain degree of relief for both family and physician. As the old medical saying goes, there are lots worse ways to lose a patient.

Second Opinions. This is a subject which defies easy analysis. There are simply no rules for seeking a second opinion regarding the nature or management of an illness. From the point of view of the patient and his family, even a protracted and serious illness may be endured under the care of a trusted and confident physician. If it is clear that the doctor knows what she is doing, neither she nor the family may feel any need for consultation. However, an inexperienced or unsure physician may call for help early and often. Parents who are not completely sure about their child's doctor are also likely to want the views of another practitioner. I can't tell you how to proceed with this question except to quote a wise therapist, Shirley Luthman, who said simply that you had better go with your gut. **If you need a second opinion, tell your doctor, and discuss how best to get one.** It may be tempting to avoid an unpleasant confrontation by going to the second physician without telling the first one. This is a thoroughly bad idea. The second doctor will not have the advantage of prior access to the records of the problem; this is likely to result in wasted time and unnecessarily repeated tests. Later, when the first doctor eventually finds out about the consultation, she may well feel quite put out. Just bite the bullet, and ask for the consultation up front.

Observation or watching and assessing illness is in general a matter of global judgment involving mostly rather vague categories of behavior. The one seemingly precise measurement we tend to take is the child's **temperature.** At least, parents believe they should take it, but because temperature taking has always been in varying degrees difficult, parents often put off the actual act. The most common way to do this is to "measure" temperature with one's hand or lips pressed to the patient's forehead. The invention of the clinical thermometer came about because foreheads, lips, and fingers are all misleading. If you think the child may have a fever, or if you want to monitor an illness by watching the temperature, you simply have to use a thermometer.

Which thermometer to use? The old-fashioned mercury thermometer is accurate and cheap. It has the disadvantages of being breakable and slow, and it is hard to read unless you know to do it. About its fragility you can do nothing. Its slowness can be finessed by shaking the mercury column down just to 98°F (36.6°C) and no lower. It will take less time for the mercury to rise to its eventual resting point if it starts there rather than down at the butt of the device. It would be most unusual for you to want to measure how much cooler than normal someone might be. The trick of reading a thermometer is to hold the thermometer *horizontally*, the tip between thumb and forefinger, and rotate it slowly until the mercury column is visible. Thermometers have three sides: The opaque side will be out of sight, the numbers will be below, and the lines indicating gradations of two tenths of a degree will be above when the line of mercury comes into view.

Taking a temperature generally requires inserting the thermometer into a body orifice; skin temperature is lower than internal temperature by such a variable amount that devices like the fever-strips applied to the forehead are inaccurate. Rectal temperatures are undignified, and inconvenient in the presence of clothing, but we use them in early childhood because the kid can't bite the thermometer when it is placed this far from his mouth. A disadvantage of rectal temperature measurement is that a rectum full of stool is likely to be a bit warmer than the rest of the child because the teeming bacteria in the stool produce a small but measurable amount of heat. This has led to the incorrect notion that

EVERYDAY PEDIATRICS FOR PARENTS

one should subtract 1 degree (F) of temperature from a rectal reading: Don't do it. Just accept that rectal temps are somewhat more variable than one would prefer, but one cannot really know by how much. To take a rectal temp, hold the child on her belly across your lap or on a firm surface. If you are right handed, her head should be toward your left side, your left arm should press on her back to keep her from squirming, your left hand then spreads her buttocks and you insert the thermometer gently with your right hand. The tip needs to go into the anus about ½ inch. As you insert the thermometer twist it slowly back and forth to minimize friction with the mucous membranes of the anal canal; this twisting will make it possible to omit greasing the thermometer tip which adds a messy and unnecessary step and makes cleaning the device more difficult. As you are taking the temperature, watch the upward progress of the mercury and discontinue the procedure when the mercury stops moving; this should shorten the whole business, which everyone involved will appreciate.

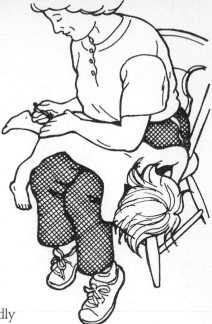

Oral temps also vary too much. Taken in the very front of the mouth, which may be the position chosen by the child, oral temps will be decidedly lower than a true internal body temp. Try to put the thermometer back along the side of the tongue. Food and drink taken a few minutes before the temperature reading may also cause some inaccuracy. For both oral and rectal temps, the longer the device is in place, the better, but even 1 minute will give an accurate reading if the mercury has been shaken down barely below normal. Temperatures can also be measured in the armpit, but this takes patience; one must have the arm held firmly against the body wall for many minutes to allow the normally lower skin temperature to equilibrate up to true body temp. Figure on about 5 minutes for babies and about 8 minutes for older people.

Alternative thermometers include electronic gadgets, some inexpensive and some very costly, which produce a temperature reading (rectally, orally, or under the armpit) within about 1 minute; this convenience is somewhat offset by the fact that the measurements are often grossly inaccurate. Another instrument reads the temperature from the ear drum. Maybe these devices will be worth using sometime during the coming millennium, but not at present. The other popular thermometer substitute is the sticky fever strip designed to be applied to the forehead. They are useful only in the unlikely event that you happen to be interested in skin temperature.

Having measured it, what does it mean? The notion that normal body temperature is 98.6°F (37°C) is simply incorrect. Body temperature varies during the course of the day. It is at its lowest point in the early morning hours; at 6 A.M. an accurately measured normal temp may be below 97°F (36.1°C) or as high as 99°F (37.2°C). During the day the body normally heats up to a maximum in late afternoon, but a range of 96.5°F (35.8°C) to 100°F (37.7°C) is found in perfectly healthy people. **A temp over 99°F (37.2°C) in the morning or over 100°F (37.7°C) later in the day should be considered to be abnormal.** If you take your child's temperature often enough, you will soon discover her particular pattern may be quite different from what you might expect.

Other aspects to be evaluated in judging the severity of illness are less quantitative than body temperature, but probably more important. **Activity, mood,** and **playfulness** are particularly revealing to a parent's eye. Each child has his characteristic level of activity, the mood with which he greets the events of his day, his enthusiasm for games and people. An unexpected deviation from this norm may alert you to a developing illness, and a return to the usual levels tells you that recovery is underway. **Appetite** nearly always diminishes or disappears when a child is sick, but because kids have such variable appetites even when in the best of health, variations in appetite by themselves give us limited information. Don't ignore the disappearance of interest in food, but don't read too much into it either. **Skin color** is controlled by the sympathetic nervous system which can react subtly and rapidly to the onset of an illness. This is not a foolproof sign, but an unaccustomed pallor is an excellent indication of something awry. **Abnormal stools** demand attention in more ways than one. Increases in frequency, volume, or wateriness, and changes in color and smell—all these require explanation. Decreased stool frequency may occur either because of decreased appetite, or secondary to inactivity, or as a side effect of medication. **Abnormal urination** is also worth noting. A decrease in urine flow may mean that there has been less fluid intake, or that the body has lost an undue amount of fluid by vomiting or diarrhea. An increase in urine frequency suggests urinary tract infection or the development of diabetes. **Pain** is a difficult symptom to assess in infancy and early childhood. It takes a few years before a child is mature enough to localize pain in a reliable way. In infancy pain can only be signaled in the most general fashion, largely by the baby's obviously distressful crying. Toddlers may have enough command of language to complain specifically of pain, but they are usually unable to indicate its whereabouts. They will often point to their abdomens, no matter the actual source of the trouble. In evaluating the significance of pain, parents inevitably develop a sense of how loudly a child is likely to complain under a variety of circumstances and learn to attend to the complaint which seems louder than expected. Other more specific symptoms such as coughing, wheezing, and vomiting point to specific illness problems and these will be discussed in the chapters that follow. The totality of these clues forms the parent's best guide to action. It is not just a matter of fever, or of appetite, or the absence of the child's ordinarily sunny disposition, but a summation of all these that leads to the phone call to the doctor's office.

Managing the Symptoms

Is it always wise or necessary to treat the symptoms of a child's illness? This question is neither as heartless nor as stupid as it may seem. Each complaint and the reasons for attempting to relieve it should be judged on the merits of the case; as I will try to make clear, there is no single, overriding rule to follow. Of course, every family will have its own particular criteria concerning the amelioration of discomfort.

You will probably find yourself powerfully affected by the desire to do something useful, to alleviate even mild discomfort, and to help put your offspring as quickly as possible on the road to recovery. This leads to a vast amount of pressure on the doctor to provide some kind of remedy. Into this breach the manufacturers of medicines have leapt, for better or for worse. The display counters of our nation's pharmacies groan under the weight of the products of their labors. So the blandishments of the hucksters, our parental anxiety, the cultural teaching that informs our thinking, and our own good sense all come together in the process of deciding what and how to treat. Well, no one ever told you that being a parent was simple.

Fever. Here is the most easily measured, the most obvious, the most objective symptom of childhood illness. Is it any wonder that we all want to treat it? In favor of treatment are several considerations: Fever is often associated with general malaise, headache, and a variety of nonspecific miseries. A temporary drop in fever is sometimes, although not always, associated with a decrease in those attendant symptoms. Furthermore, fever in the early years may be associated with fever convulsions, which are not particularly dangerous but are absolutely terrifying to the family. It is not actually true that fever convulsions can be prevented by treating the fever, but any parent whose child has had a fever convulsion will certainly want to try to avoid another. (For more detail, see Chapter 45 – Convulsions.) Fever also has the disadvantage of increasing the body's fluid losses and caloric requirements, and this often happens at a time when the child may have trouble taking adequate water and food. On the other hand, fever is a normal body response which clearly plays a significant role in fighting infection. There is evidence from experimental infections in animals indicating that vigorous use of fever-reducing medications makes some infections more severe. We do not have studies of childhood infections to confirm that this is the case in humans, but the evidence is suggestive enough to make us hesitate before automatically reaching for the bottle of acetaminophen. The other disadvantage of treating fever is that we are misled by the apparent improvement that may follow each dose; there are times when watching the natural course of a fever is crucial to making a correct diagnosis. My conclusion is that fevers should be treated only when the child is thoroughly miserable, and only when the parent is convinced that a real improvement in the child's malaise follows the administration of the medicine.

If we want to bring a fever down, we have two possible methods: externally chilling the child's body, or giving a medicine to change the body's own temperature regulating system. Chilling the body is best and most safely done by repeatedly sponging the naked child with tepid water. It takes a ridiculously long time to drop the temperature more than a degree, the child can reliably be expected to dislike and resist the procedure, and the temperature begins to rise as soon as the sponging has stopped. Immersion in cold water works faster, but it is a truly hateful experience for the subject and provides a stress which may be ill-advised and harmful. Combining external cooling with a fever-reducing medicine works better than external cooling by itself.

The medicines commonly used to reduce fever are acetaminophen, aspirin, and ibuprofen. **Acetaminophen** (paracetamol, Tylenol, Panadol, etc.) has been used for several decades. It is as effective as aspirin, works for about the same number of hours, and is quite safe in normal doses. Acetaminophen is acutely poisonous in large overdoses; chronic overuse of large amounts can also be injurious. An advantage of acetaminophen is that it comes in liquid forms as well as chewable and swallowable tablets. Unfortunately, the multiplicity of dosage forms leads to confusion because doses are typically described in terms of volume, and preparations differ in concentration. A 0.8 ml dose of baby drops provides 80 mg of the drug. If, by mistake, you use the same baby dropper to administer the more dilute syrup, 0.8 ml will contain only 25.6 mg, a dose which won't do much good. **Doses of this medication are best estimated on the basis of the child's weight. Give about 5 mg of acetaminophen for every pound of body weight for each dose. This works out to a dose of about 120 mg for an average 1–year old. Repeat doses no more than 5 times in 24 hours. Teenagers can take an adult dose, which is usually 325 to 650 mg, with a maximum of 4 gm (4000 mg) in 24 hours.**

Aspirin has been used for a century, and it was everyone's favorite fever reducer until recently when studies appeared to show that it sometimes caused a serious liver and brain inflammation (Reye syndrome) when given to children with chickenpox or influenza. A causal relationship between aspirin and this disease is suggestive but not proven to everyone's satisfaction, but most pediatricians are convinced enough to abandon the use of aspirin when other drugs can be used just as well. Aspirin's other disadvantage is that overdoses are poisonous; this used to be a big problem when the tasty little children's aspirin tablets were dispensed in large bottles. Adult aspirin tablets taste terrible, but children still manage to get poisoned if they get hold of a handful of Grandpa's pain pills. On the rare occasions when you might decide to use aspirin for fever or pain, the dose is the same as for acetaminophen.

Ibuprofen (Advil, Nuprin, Motrin) is the most popular and widely available member of a group of drugs called **nonsteroidal anti–inflammatory drugs (NSAIDs).** These agents relieve pain as well or better than aspirin or acetaminophen, and reduce fever as effectively and for somewhat longer periods after a dose. Some of the drugs in this class are so long-acting that once or twice a day dosing can be used for certain problems. Unfortunately, the disadvantage of the NSAIDs is an increased frequency of undesirable side effects, most often stomach irritation, and sometimes sleepiness, dizziness, and rashes. There are few good reasons for using ibuprofen or any other NSAID for fever, but they can be quite helpful for the control of pain and inflammation. **The dose of ibuprofen for fever control is 2 to 4 mg per pound of body weight per dose, with doses repeated every 6 to 8 hours. Use the 2 mg per pound dose to treat fevers under 102.5°F. For higher fevers use the 4 mg per pound dose. The usual adult dose is 200 to 400 mg.**

Pain. The control of pain has been discussed in Chapter 27, and there is only a little to add about pain in general. Pain in infants and young children has an added dimension that makes treatment more complicated, and that is the impossibility of explaining to the child the nature of the problem. The holding, rocking, soothing, tender, loving care that is lavished by the parent nursing a sick baby goes part of the way, but there's no escaping the child's unspoken question "What is happening to me, and why do I feel so awful?"

A time-honored though poorly understood method of pain relief is the application of heat or cold. The theory suggests that an inflamed area will feel better if it is gently chilled, thereby reducing blood flow and swelling. This works nicely with burns and sprains, but try it on a case of acute back strain and your patient may complain bitterly. In that situation, a hot compress or a heating pad may bring significant relief. Heat also seems helpful for some abdominal pain. A rather common event in childhood is a nasty, usually left-sided, belly pain that comes in waves. A heating pad, or better yet, a soak in a hot bath, is often effective in ending these episodes.

Certain pains in childhood are of special significance and demand medical attention. Headache in very young children is quite unusual, probably because they localize their pains so poorly. **If a toddler tells you his head hurts, pay attention.** A headache that awakens a child in the night or which is present when he awakens in the morning is a significant symptom. **Any pain in the genital area also needs attention;** this is particularly true for pain in the testicles which may signal a true surgical emergency. Abdominal pain that starts around the navel and then moves to another part of the abdomen is out of the ordinary and should be considered to be important. Pain which settles in the right lower quadrant of the belly strongly suggests appendicitis, another surgical emergency. The timing of pain can be quite suggestive. For example, a recurrent pattern of vague headache or bellyache occurring only on school mornings is practically diagnostic of emotional stress. Other symptoms such as vomiting, diarrhea, cough, and itching are dealt with in the following chapters on specific diseases.

Grossman's Laws of Drug Administration, otherwise known as **The Nine Commandments:**

1. *Give medicines as infrequently as possible.* At the beginning of an illness when everyone is worried and focused on taking care of the sick child it is sometimes possible to administer a medicine as often as 4 times a day; it is not easy to manage but it is within the realm of possibility. As the illness improves, parental concern lessens, and normal family chaos intervenes; it becomes more and more difficult to remember all those doses of medication. By the time the child has recovered, the medicine is being given

spottily if at all. It takes an abnormally organized family to complete an entire course of treatment without a hitch. So, when your doctor tells you that Susie's sinusitis will require 3 weeks of antibiotic, ask him to write his prescription with family reality in mind. Administration 3 times a day is more likely to be attained than 4, and 1 or 2 times a day is even better. If the treatment requires more than one drug, it is even more important that *both* are given at the same time if at all possible. It is pure fantasy to expect parents to give drug "A" 3 times a day after meals and drug "B" 4 times a day on an empty stomach.

2. ***Medicines should be taken at convenient times of day, which usually means mealtimes, upon arising, or bedtime.*** These are the nodal points of the day, and they serve as semiautomatic reminders. How can a parent, or anyone else, be expected to remember to give medicines at 3 in the afternoon, let alone 3 o'clock in the morning? Unless the child awakens in the middle of the night needing her medicine for symptom relief, let her sleep! There are indeed illnesses where it is necessary to give medicines around the clock, but they are most uncommon.

3. ***Make sure that the medicine is in the most palatable form.*** Doctors sometimes overlook this important law, so it is worthwhile to mention when medication is prescribed. (I learned about this in medical school from a wise physician, Dr. Otto Guttentag. His advice can be stated as **Guttentag's Law: *Doctors should never prescribe a medicine until they have tasted it themselves.*** The larger meaning of his teaching is that physicians need to put themselves in the patient's place in order to understand his experience.) Liquid medicines should be concentrated so that a small volume per dose is possible. For babies and small toddlers, it is helpful if the volume of the dose can be kept down below ½ teaspoon (2.5 ml). It can take forever to get an entire teaspoon down a sick 1-year old. Using a medicine dropper or a small cup may help. Taste is even more crucial; some medicines vary in flavor from brand to brand, and it may be worth paying more for the good-tasting one. Bitter medicines are a terrible problem. Bitterness is a flavor that resists disguise, and kids don't like it. Mixing a bitter drug with cold applesauce, chocolate syrup, or ice cream often works reasonably well. Chewable tablets can be used for children who have not learned to swallow tablets.

4. ***Make sure that prescriptions are dispensed in multiple bottles if the child spends time in multiple places.*** If a child recovering from an ear

infection is in day care when her midday dose of amoxicillin is due, her chances of getting her medicine will increase if a bottle of the stuff stays at the day care center. No one will have to remember to bring it every morning, and no one will have to remember to return it home every night. You know how long that unbroken routine could be expected to last. If she is spending the weekend with Dad, a separate little bottle will be advisable for his house, too. Tell the druggist.

5. **Teach your kids to swallow tablets.** This is a skill at least as important as kicking a soccer ball, or skipping rope, and requires less instruction and practice. The following methods can be used with children of 4 or over.

    a. Take a sip of water and hold it in your mouth; don't swallow it yet! Tilt your head back as far as you can. Toss a small, smooth, tablet-shaped candy (like an M&M) into the puddle of water in the back of your mouth, and swallow. If this doesn't work the first time, eat the candy and try again.

    b. Fill a clean, small mouthed soda pop or beer bottle with cold water. Place a small, smooth, tablet-shaped candy on your tongue. Drink rapidly from the bottle; the tablet will be washed down by the water.

6. **Don't neglect the rectum.** There are children whose resistance to taking medicines by mouth is awe inspiring; well, perhaps awe is the wrong word, but it is certainly impressive. There are also children who are vomiting so frequently that the medicine does not stay down long enough to be absorbed. In these instances, ask the doctor to give the medication by injection if that is possible, abandon the attempt to medicate, or give it rectally. This is a preferred route of administration in Europe, but it is decreasingly popular here. The disadvantages include slow or erratic absorbtion if the medicine is inserted into a rectum full of stool, and lack of information about completeness of absorbtion even when it is given into an empty rectum. Despite these and aesthetic drawbacks, rectal medication is sometimes worth a try. Skillful pharmacists used to make up all sorts of medications into rectal suppositories, but this seems to be a dying art. If the medicine only comes in tablet form, and your neighborhood druggist won't or can't manage suppositories, ask him to grind up the tablets and put the resulting powder into large empty gelatin capsules. Alternatively, you can take medicines that come in capsule form and use them as suppositories. Before inserting the capsules, prick them several times with a needle to increase the speed of dissolution. Make sure you push the capsule or suppository well up into the rectum; you should have the sensation of it falling into an

empty space. If it is left in the anal canal, too near the outside, the child can easily expel it.

7. **Be wary of generic medications.** Most generic medications are just fine, but some are not the same as the fancy proprietary brands. If a medication that has worked in the past unexpectedly fails, it may be because the generic substitute is not what it should be. Sometimes this is a matter of inadequate quality control, sometimes it is because the generic is formulated differently in particle size, or type of tablet coating, or type of liquid in which it is dissolved or suspended.

8. **Do not leave your doctor's office without written instructions.** I'm not trying to be insulting, but there is no way that you or any other worried parent is going to remember everything the pediatrician tells you. When you have had a sleepless night trying to cope with a miserable child, and you are attempting to get her clothes back on at the same time that you are listening to the doctor tell you in impenetrable medical jargon that she has Tertiary Coreopsis for which three medicines need to be given, don't expect to get anything straight. Ask her to write it all down.

9. **If a treatment fails, ask yourself if it was actually given.** Did the other adults who were supposed to give doses of the medication forget? Did Grandma decide that her home remedy was preferable and substitute it? Did the teenager who demanded to be in charge of her own illness pour the nasty tasting stuff down the sink? (Just asking.)

Rest. Rest is a time-honored treatment for all sorts of human ailments. Unfortunately, it is rarely useful and often harmful. I know that this is heresy, and I don't want to upset anyone, but let's look at the facts. To begin with, a brief examination of the advantages of rest. The first advantage is comfort. An acutely injured body part is likely to hurt terribly if it is moved; rest feels good, and the body's wisdom in encouraging immobility in this fashion needs to be heeded. Time is required for bones to knit and tissues to start regenerating, so we splint a sprained ankle for a few days and keep a broken arm in a cast for a few weeks. Second, many illnesses are accompanied by exhaustion, weakness, miscellaneous miseries, and a complete lack of interest in anything but sleep. If you feel truly terrible, rest is great. This concludes the list of reasons to rest when unwell. You will notice that in these cases the message from the body is "Rest!" in no uncertain terms.

The disadvantages of rest may be less obvious but they are equally important. First is the process known as disuse atrophy. When we rest a muscle or immobilize a bone, useful tissue immediately begins to be lost. This is dramatically obvious when the cast is taken off a fractured leg, and the muscles are revealed to have lost both size and strength. It will take months or even years to regain the prefracture state. Second are the metabolic changes, that is to say, changes in the function of various body organs, which may be induced by excessive rest. I became acutely aware of this when I contracted hepatitis during my internship. My doctors ordered me to rest in bed for weeks, and during this enforced convalescence I naturally read up on hepatitis. I discovered that a large and careful study of soldiers with hepatitis had proved that bed rest prolonged their illnesses. The soldiers who were encouraged to move about and exercise recovered faster! I don't know how many other illnesses are adversely affected by rest. However, we do know that rest lowers heart output and blood flow and decreases the depth of breathing, and these changes are surely not helpful. In the not too distant past, patients rested in bed for many days after surgery, and they often developed blood clots in their legs and infection in their lungs precisely because of their inactivity. Now we roust them out of bed, walk them around, and make them practice deep breathing, and they have fewer complications and recover faster.

My conclusion is that rest, like every other good thing, can be overdone. If a sick child feels like resting, fine; if he doesn't, there is no virtue in forcing him to stay in bed. As usual, a mixture of attention to the child's wishes plus sound parental judgment is required.

Food and Liquids. A recurrent theme in this book is the complexity of our feelings about feeding our kids. Many of us define ourselves as parents in terms of feeding. The development of independent behavior by our growing children gradually forces most of us to move on to broader, less domineering, and more collaborative definitions of our roles. But when illness strikes, we tend to be thrown back to the old patterns. Our children seem helpless and dependent, and we rush to aid them with chicken soup and bowls of ice cream. There is nothing terribly wrong with this response as long as we keep in mind that food is not actually curative.

What do we need to know about the requirements of the child's body for food and water during an illness?

1. **Amount of food.** Fever increases the body's use of fuel, so calorie consumption may go up a bit. But illness usually decreases activity, so calorie consumption may also go down. Illness is also likely to decrease appetite, and some illnesses make it harder to eat because of discomfort, so calorie

EVERYDAY PEDIATRICS FOR PARENTS

intake is limited. Net effect on calories: not very important in the short run for the child who is otherwise in generally good health. The child will eat less, lose a little weight, and regain it when she recovers. For the child with a serious ongoing health problem, weight loss during acute illnesses is a different matter, and these children may need dietary supplements to help keep their weight loss in bounds.

2. **Type of food.** Some illnesses limit the acceptability of certain foods. A sore throat or canker sores in the mouth may preclude pretty much everything except soups, smooth cereals, milk, and ice cream. An upset stomach may rebel at anything other than sweet juices and clear broth. A diet full of hard-to-digest raw vegetables, whole grain cereals, and other sources of fiber will increase the number of stools for a child with diarrhea. And, in general, the decrease in appetite characteristic of most illnesses will suggest the wisdom of offering those foods known to be most favored by the child. I should also mention that many families have their own tried and true beliefs about what foods can be given to sick children. This may be as simple and straightforward (and mistaken) as the old saying "Feed a cold, starve a fever." I recall fondly that when my brother or I were ill, my father would always prepare a Hungarian specialty, wonderfully curative caraway tea. Some folk remedies are imbedded in complex systems which classify illnesses along theoretical lines. The Chinese define the patients, their illnesses, and foods as "hot" or "cold," and proper diet follows from appropriate matching. Latin Americans have a similar system. The significance of all these dietary therapies is in the interplay of the parent's need to help the child and the child's response to these evidences of parental love. Medicines can have placebo effects, and so can foods.

3. **Water requirements.** This is a subject chock-full of misunderstandings and nonsense, a substantial portion of which is the fault of the medical profession. We have been guilty of telling people to "push fluids" to loosen chest secretions in patients with bronchitis or asthma (it doesn't work) or to flush out jaundice in newborn babies (that doesn't work either) or to go to bed and drink tea and juices to get rid of a bad cold (equally useless). What is really known about the requirements for fluids during illness is this: Fever, vomiting, and diarrhea increase fluid loss. The response of our bodies is to signal us through thirst to increase our liquid intake and to conserve fluid by decreasing the output of urine. Most of the time this is all that is needed, but if vomiting precludes a satisfactory intake of fluid or if

the fluid losses of diarrhea are too great to replace, we can become dehydrated. This is rarely a problem with older kids or adults, but it can be disastrous with babies and small children who have a much smaller reserve of body fluid. The moral is simple: Quit worrying about dehydration in ordinary everyday children's illnesses except those with continued vomiting or diarrhea. Nobody gets dangerously dried out with one or two episodes of vomiting or diarrhea, and nobody gets dehydrated from a bad cold or an ear infection, even though they don't eat or drink much for a day or two.

What follows from these observations is that we can tailor our offerings of food and drink to our sick children in accordance with the understanding that our goal is their comfort, rather than their cure. The child with the really nasty illness needs to be under his doctor's care, and she can advise you about any special dietary requirements. For the rest of the everyday illnesses, the combination of common sense and family folk wisdom will do very well.

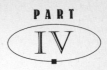

Introduction

Infections

There are hundreds of agents of infection that cause human disease—viruses, bacteria, Rickettsia, fungi, yeasts, worms, flukes, protozoa, amebae, and insects. The great majority of the infections suffered by American children today are caused by the relatively familiar microbes known as viruses and bacteria. This is not true everywhere; parasites and protozoa are still major causes of serious disease, especially in the developing world. For our purposes, I'll limit this chapter to some of the infectious problems that American children are most likely to acquire.

Viruses are exceedingly small, submicroscopic bits of genetic material, DNA or RNA, that invade living cells and alter their function, forcing them to produce endless numbers of new, identical, virus particles. The interaction of virus and the invaded host produces the symptoms of the illness. Diseases caused by viruses have been familiar to humanity for a long time; the possibility that invisible infectious agents could cause these illnesses was suspected but not proven until this century. The development of the powerful electron microscope made it possible to visualize viruses; laboratory techniques of growing viruses and measuring the response of the patient to viral infection have resulted in a rapid increase in our understanding of these germs. Viruses vary from the rather benign varieties that cause the common cold to devastating species like those that produce rabies or AIDS. Viruses have not been easy to attack with medicines. The antibiotics which so often can be used to cure bacterial infection are without effect on viruses. Antiviral antibiotics have been sought with diligence but only limited success. Acyclovir, used against herpes and chickenpox, amantadine and rimantadine against influenza, and ribavirin against respiratory syncytial virus are examples of this small group of drugs, most of which are not particularly satisfactory.

Bacteria are single-celled organisms, larger than the viruses, and visible with the aid of an ordinary microscope. Bacteria were first seen by Antony van Leeuwenhoek in 1676; it took nearly two centuries of further study to prove that these tiny organisms were capable of causing disease. The various varieties of bacteria cause a vast array of illnesses ranging from trivial skin infections to potentially deadly conditions like meningitis and tuberculosis. The development of anti-infective agents has had its greatest successes with bacterial diseases. The first modern drug of this type, salvarsan, which cures syphilis, was invented a century ago. The more familiar antibiotics like penicillin, discovered over sixty years ago, proved to be able to control a host of bacterial infections.

The old fashioned disinfectants like phenol and iodine, which had been the major germ killers of an earlier era, were nearly as poisonous for human tissue as they were for germs. In happy contrast, the antibiotics are exceedingly toxic to the germs against which they are used but have very little toxicity for the human being who is host to the infection. Antibiotics are not without risk to the person who takes them, but, used in ordinary amounts, the risk is small and the rewards in terms of lessened death and disease makes their use worthwhile.

One type of antibiotic side effect is dose related, that is, the more of the drug you take, the greater the likelihood of the undesired effect. Examples of this are the stomach irritation and pain caused by erythromycin and the staining of young children's teeth caused by tetracyclines. There are also allergic reactions which can occur after even minute doses of an antibiotic to which one has become sensitized by prior use. The importance of all this is that people often mistakenly believe themselves to be allergic to an antibiotic when in fact their adverse reaction was not allergic, and it would be safe for them to use the drug again. The most pressing problem with current antibiotic use is that so many common bacteria have evolved the ability to withstand some or all of our usual antibiotics. In general, the more an antibiotic is used in any community, the more the susceptible forms of bacteria are killed and the remaining forms become increasingly resistant. This is the best reason for limiting antibiotic use as much as possible, because these resistant organisms pose an increasingly serious threat.

Contagion: How Infections Spread. In order to carry out the genetic command to be fruitful and multiply, germs often must leave one happy home in search of another. This can happen if they overreach themselves and kill their current host, or if the competition of other organisms prevents as large a population explosion as they have in mind. Person-to-person contact spreads germs by way of infected body secretions or products. Viruses or bacteria growing in the respiratory tract are present in nasal mucus and in droplets coughed up from the lower air passages. These waft easily through the air from host #1 and get inhaled by hosts #2 and #3, and so on. This mode of transmission occurs most efficiently in enclosed spaces crowded with susceptible new hosts. Alternatively, after host #1 wipes her nose, the viruses may pause briefly on her fingers before being transferred by way of a handshake or a stuffed animal or a shared bagel to host #2. Germs growing in the intestinal tract have equally easy access to new homes. Present in untold billions in the stool, they hitch a ride on the hands of whomever changes a diaper or wipes a bottom. It is then only a hop, skip, and jump to the mouth of the next victim by way of hands, food, or toys. Some disease causing organisms live exclusively on or in the skin and spread by direct skin-to-skin contact, or through shared objects like clothing, bedding, or toys.

There are also numerous organisms that spread from animal-to-person. We can get Salmonella infections from the feces of turtles, ornithosis from the respiratory secretions of parrots, and fungus infections of the skin from cats and dogs. Food and water are excellent vehicles for the spread of infection. The germs of tuberculosis, brucellosis, and other equally nasty diseases can spread through unpasteurized milk. Salmonella contaminates eggs; meat can harbor bacteria and tapeworms.

Some germs move from one host to another through intermediaries. For example, the malaria parasite is spread from patient to patient by the bites of Anopheles mosquitoes. Sometimes the human patient is the end of the line for a germ. The bacterium that causes Lyme disease lives most of its life in a certain mouse; then the mouse is bitten by a deer tick which in turn transmits the germ to a human. This is nearly always a dead end for the Lyme organism except in very rare instances where a pregnant woman's infection can reach her fetus.

Controlling Contagion. It is probably depressingly clear that germs have a wonderful variety of methods to find their ways onto and into human bodies. We may as well learn to live realistically with that fact. There are a limited number of measures we can take to protect ourselves and our children. **1) Use soap and water generously on contaminated people and objects.** Many common gems can be destroyed or washed away with ease. Disinfectants are practically never necessary except in special circumstances like the preparation of skin before a surgical incision. **2) Indoor spaces full of potentially contagious people are excellent sources of germs.** If the Sunday morning infant day care group at your church is full of sniffling babies, you may decide to forego the experience. **3) Know your enemies.** If your local sources of eggs carry salmonella, make sure the eggs are well cooked. When your daughter asks for a pet turtle, refuse. Don't buy unpasteurized milk anywhere. If you live in an area with Lyme disease, check your kids' skin for tiny ticks. **4) Immunizations work.** Make sure that your whole family is protected.

The chapters that follow cover the most common infections to which children growing up in our country today are susceptible. Each is briefly described, and if an illness has a characteristic pattern or course, I mention it so you will have a general idea of what to expect. The treatment and preventive measures, if any, are noted. Chapter 37, which can easily be mistaken for a sermon, deals with the general question of immunizations.

Chapter 29

Infections With Fever and Rash

Scarlet Fever is an infection caused by a bacterium, the **group A streptococcus** (aka Streptococcus pyogenes). The child with scarlet fever becomes abruptly sick with fever, often a headache and bellyache, and a sore and usually dramatically red throat; in short, the typical beginning of a strep throat. Sometime within the next 2 days a fine, red, rough feeling rash appears; the rashy skin develops the texture of fine sandpaper. One old-time pediatrician used to say he could diagnose scarlet fever with his eyes closed by touching the child's forehead. The rash begins on the neck or trunk and may spread over the whole body. It may be less noticeable on the face, and the area around the mouth is often spared. The severity of scarlet fever varies; some children are miserably sick for days, others hardly seem ill at all. After a few days the body's defense mechanisms overcome the strep, the symptoms slowly disappear, and the rash gradually fades.

The group A streptococcus can cause a variety of other infections, generally without any rash. Ordinary strep throat is most common; it is discussed in detail in Chapter 30. Some strep infections cause kidney inflammation (glomerulonephritis), or heart inflammation (rheumatic fever), and a few particularly dangerous ones involve the destruction of muscle and skin tissue. Oddly enough, certain forms of strep infection, including scarlet fever and rheumatic fever, have become less common and less severe during the past century. This is a prime example of one of medicine's most persistent puzzles: why diseases appear, wax, and wane. In this instance, we have hardly a clue. There seems to be no reason to credit either medical science or public health measures. The decline in the virulence of the streptococcus occurred long before the antibiotic era, and during a time in the early twentieth century when living standards were often abysmal.

This is a highly contagious illness; the patient may have spread the strep germs for days before becoming ill, and he will continue to be contagious until about 1 day after adequate antibiotic treatment is started. If untreated, he will probably continue to spread strep germs for many days. Those in contact with a case of scarlet fever may get a strep throat without the rash, or full-blown scarlet fever, or a barely inapparent respiratory illness, or become carriers without symptoms, or get nothing at all.

Treatment with an appropriate antibiotic, usually a penicillin, cures scarlet fever and other strep infections. The course of the disease is shortened, the severity is lessened, and the risk of developing complications is lessened. This is an illness well worth treating with an antibiotic.

Chicken Pox (Varicella) is an infection caused by the varicella-zoster virus (VZV), a member of the herpesvirus family. All these names are important, in part because they tend to cause some confusion. The herpesvirus family is a substantial group of germs that cause a wide variety of illnesses. The family includes herpes simplex which causes a sexually transmitted disease, cold sores, and a severe, generalized infection in infancy; Epstein-Barr virus, which causes infectious mononucleosis; human herpesviruses 6 and 7, which cause roseola, among others.

When humans are first infected with the chicken pox virus, we develop a generalized infection; it is not just in our skins. The first sign of the illness is usually a scattering of tiny red bumps on the neck and upper trunk. These turn into equally tiny water blisters, less than an ⅛ inch (a few millimeters) in size; the blisters are thin-walled and easily broken. The rash spreads from head to foot over 2 or 3 days, new spots appearing for as long as 5 days; it itches terribly, and then gradually dries up. It may take a couple of weeks to disappear. The chicken pox spots may also develop on mucous membranes, especially in the throat. The other main symptom is fever. There can be complications of including pneumonia and brain inflammation, but these are rare. Reye syndrome, an inflammation of brain and liver, can occur. This is thought to be more common if the child has been given aspirin during the illness; see the discussion concerning this in the section on treating fever in Chapter 28. Quite a few children get secondary bacterial infections of the skin, probably because they scratch the itchy sores. If a pregnant women gets chicken pox early in her pregnancy, the fetus may be injured. If she gets it near the time of the baby's birth, the baby may get a very severe case. Chicken pox is likely to be a much more severe disease if contracted in adult life, and it is especially dangerous for people with impaired immune systems such as patients receiving certain anticancer treatments or cortisone-like drugs.

Chicken pox is contagious 1 or 2 days before the rash appears and remains contagious for about 5 days of rash. The rash itself is not the source of the contagion; it is an airborne infection, spread from the nose and throat. This is a highly contagious illness; anyone who is not immune and who is exposed has an excellent chance of coming down with chicken pox in 10 to 21 days. Prolonged exposure, especially indoors, increases the likelihood of contagion and may increase the severity of the illness. This is commonly the case when sibling #1 comes down with chicken pox, and sibling #2 spends lots of time with him during the long period of contagiousness.

Treatment is generally limited to relief of itching. Old fashioned calamine lotion is basically useless; don't bother with it. Local applications of baking soda made into a wet paste, or various commercially available anti-itch lotions can help. A prescription lotion called crotamiton (Eurax) is excellent. Cool baths in water with a handful of baking soda mixed in are temporarily soothing. Anti-itch medicines taken by mouth are especially useful at night when sleep is likely to be disturbed by the itching. Hydroxyzine by prescription or diphenhydramine (Benadryl, etc.) over the counter are excellent. A new treatment for chicken pox is the antiviral antibiotic acyclovir. If it is started within 24 hours of the first appearance of the rash, it will cause a modest decrease in the amount of rash and the duration of fever. This is a wonderful drug for the treatment of anyone abnormally susceptible to chicken pox but it is largely a waste of time and money for healthy kids. If any of the pox becomes swollen, sore, heavily scabbed, or drains any pus, it is probably infected with skin bacteria and should be treated to minimize scarring. Call your doctor.

It is now possible to immunize against chicken pox with a vaccine made from live but weakened (attenuated) chicken pox virus. For certain patients with deficient immunity this vaccine appears to be valuable. However, for most children the use of the vaccine must be considered in the light of two unanswered questions. Every vaccine confers the greatest degree of immunity during the first few years or decades after it is administered. 1) How long will the immunity induced by this vaccine last? Are we in danger of raising millions of kids who will lose their immunity sometime during adult life and become susceptible to really serious infection with this virus? Repeated doses of chicken pox vaccine might be required to keep immunity at an adequate level, and this is an expensive and impractical prospect. 2) What will happen a few decades down the road to the latent infection which this live virus will confer on its recipients? We know that the normal, "wild" strain of chickenpox virus lives forever in some of our nerve cells after we have a case of chicken pox; it may later become activated and cause the disease called zoster (also known as shingles and as herpes zoster). What will the vaccine version of this virus do? So far, we have precious little information about the second issue and none at all about the first. As far as I can see, the wisest thing for parents of young children to do is expose them to a nice, fresh case of chicken pox at any age after early infancy. Keep in mind that there is no convenient time to do this, there are only more or less inconvenient times, so get the disease out of the way in early childhood if you can. For older teenagers and adults who have not had the good fortune to have had their chicken pox and been done with it, taking the vaccine probably makes some sense. This advice may have to be modified after we have a few more decades of experience with the vaccine.

Measles (Rubeola). In the old days before measles vaccine, parents and doctors alike tended to underestimate this disease. I suppose it was the contempt bred of familiarity, because we surely were familiar with the illness. Every child got measles, and became thoroughly sick with a drippy nose, sore, red eyes, a dry cough, lots of fever, and finally, after about four days, a red, flat or slightly raised, patchy rash starting on the neck and spreading all over the body. Measles all by itself makes even healthy children decidedly sick. When it occurs in malnourished or immune-suppressed children it can be fatal. Measles can cause a variety of complications when the virus invades brain, heart, lungs, and other tissues. Much more commonly, secondary bacterial infections add to the child's misery; most often these are ear and sinus infections and pneumonia. In short, measles is no minor annoyance; it is a big disease and deserves respect.

The measles virus is in the same family as the viruses causing distemper in dogs, cattle plague, and an illness in seals. It is spread by coughing and sneezing. The incubation period from exposure to illness is 8 to 12 days. The contagious period begins 1 or 2 days before the patient has any symptoms and continues until about 4 days after the rash has started.

Treatment is generally symptomatic unless there are secondary bacterial complications. A decongestant like pseudoephedrine (Sudafed, etc.) for the nose, a cough suppressant like dextromethorphan (the only effective ingredient in over-the-counter cough syrups), and possibly acetaminophen for the fever are about all one can offer. A somewhat darkened room may help when the eyes are most inflamed and light sensitive. High doses of vitamin A are used in those parts of the world where children are severely malnourished. There is no evidence supporting the use of extra vitamin A for most normal American children, but those with a variety of serious health problems and the very young with bad cases of measles may benefit.

Live, attenuated, measles virus vaccine has made this a disease of the past for most children in our country. This is a great vaccine, extremely effective and well tolerated. If a child has been exposed to measles before being vaccinated, a dose of human immunoglobulin (gamma globulin) can be used to modify or prevent the disease.

Rubella (German Measles, Three–Day Measles). Here is another disease which is now largely of historical interest in the United States. Rubella in babies and children is typically a mild and unimpressive disease. It is of importance because it causes severe fetal abnormalities or fetal death if a woman contracts the disease during the first part of pregnancy, especially during the first three months. "Rubella babies" are often deaf, blind, and retarded. This was the impetus behind the successful search for a vaccine.

The illness starts with swollen and somewhat tender lymph glands behind and below the ears. There may be mild cold symptoms, low fever, and a general sense of being unwell. Older girls and women may have sore or swollen joints. After a few days a rash of discrete, red, flat, or slightly raised little spots appears on the face and then spreads down the body and out to the extremities; by the time it gets to the hands and feet it has usually faded from the face. The popular term "three-day measles" refers to the length of time the rash tends to last.

The rubella virus spreads from the nose and throat secretions of people infected with the germ. Many people exposed to rubella virus develop an infection without any symptoms at all, but they may be a source of the virus for others. The incubation period is 2 to 3 weeks. In patients who are developing the disease, the virus is most contagious from about 5 days before the rash appears until nearly 1 week after it is first seen.

Treatment is not needed except perhaps acetaminophen for the fever and sometimes an anti-inflammatory for the joint soreness.

The rubella vaccine has made this an avoidable disease. The vaccine is effective, provides lasting immunity, and rarely causes side effects. In the developing world where the vaccine is not yet in widespread use, rubella remains a common illness and cases of severe fetal damage from congenital infection continue to occur. Unimmunized children and adults who have had neither the illness nor the vaccine are at risk during travel in these areas.

Roseola (Exanthem Subitum; Herpesvirus 6 Infection). This is one of my favorite childhood diseases. If this sentence strikes you as bizarre, you must consider that the pediatrician's point of view is bound to be different from that of the parent or the child. As a pediatrician, I like roseola because it is a brief, often puzzling, but nearly wholly harmless illness that resolves in a clear-cut fashion, providing relief for patient and family and a satisfying diagnosis for the doctor.

It was first recognized as a distinct entity late in the nineteenth century. Prior to that time, doctors did not clearly differentiate roseola from the other acute childhood infections with rashes. Although we have been certain for many years that it is due to a virus, the agent that causes it was only recently isolated. This turned out to be another member of the family of herpesviruses, namely herpesvirus 6; herpesvirus 7 probably also causes an identical illness.

Roseola is an infection of older babies and young children, nearly always under the age of 3 years. The child becomes feverish but does not usually act particularly ill. The fever rises abruptly to alarming heights, not infrequently as high as 105 or 106° F (40.5 to 41°C), but no obvious excuse for all this heat presents itself. The child often persists in playing happily, eating reasonably well, and generally refusing to act as sick as the fever suggests she should. An observant parent may note a modest amount of swelling of the eyelids and the adjacent areas of the cheek. Often the baby will have a mild diarrhea, and sometimes there will even be a fever convulsion. If the child is examined by her doctor, a rather red throat and somewhat red ear drums may be found. (This often leads to the misdiagnosis of an ear infection.) After 3 or 4 days, the fever drops, and a faint, pink, nearly flat or just barely raised rash abruptly appears on the trunk; it is often first noted in the diaper area. (The rapid and unexpected blossoming of the rash is the reason for roseola's other medical name, exanthem subitum, which means sudden rash.) The rash may spread to the extremities but not usually to the face. It lasts anywhere from a few hours to about 2 days. Oddly enough, many of the children act less well during the end of the illness when the rash has already bloomed and the fever has gone.

Since the discovery of herpesvirus 6, studies have shown that it is actually one of the commonest causes of acute, feverish illnesses in infancy. The large majority of these illnesses are not accompanied by a roseola rash, and because virus studies are rarely done, these illnesses come and go without a specific diagnosis being made. They comprise a substantial portion of the infections that we have generally ascribed to "a virus," without having known which virus it was. Children are born with excellent immunity to herpesvirus 6, having absorbed specific antibodies from their mothers during fetal life. This immunity rapidly wanes, and within a few months babies are susceptible to the germ. By the age of 3 years, nearly every child will have had a herpesvirus 6 infection, with or without a roseola rash. Like the other members of the herpesvirus family, this virus remains permanently in our bodies, inactive and harmless unless there is a serious disorder of immunity, like AIDS.

Before the viral cause of roseola was discovered, one of the puzzles of the illness was its failure to spread in families; second cases in exposed siblings rarely occur. Now it has been discovered that the virus does not move from case to case; instead it comes from adults who carry the virus and shed it into their saliva or respiratory secretions from time to time. The period between exposure and illness is about 9 days.

Treatment of roseola (or any other herpesvirus 6 infection) is directed against the fever, if it seems necessary. This is a fine example of a fever which rarely requires any attention at all. If a blazing hot toddler is racing around the house playing happily, the message is "Leave her alone; her body knows what it is doing."

No vaccine against roseola exists, nor is one needed.

Slap–Face Fever (Erythema Infectiosum; Fifth Disease). This is a quite common infection which is not very well known, probably because of the mildness of most cases. The usual story is that the child (or on rare occasions the adult) is noted to have bright red cheeks, rather as if he had been slapped. Sometimes there is a preceding or accompanying low fever and perhaps a sore throat, but most often the patient is unaware of any illness. The face rash is often followed by a pretty, pink, lacy-patterned rash on the outer areas of the extremities. All these rashes tend to come and go; sunshine makes them temporarily brighter. The rashes last from a few days to a few weeks. That is all there is to it for most patients, but a few people, especially older girls and women, may get an arthritis which can sometimes be persistent. The infection can also trigger acute anemia in people with a variety of blood and immune disorders. If the disease occurs early in pregnancy the fetus may be harmed.

Parvovirus B19 which causes slap-face fever is probably spread through nose and throat secretions during the days before the rash appears; by the time the disease is recognized, the patient is no longer likely to be contagious. Patients who develop anemia from this infection remain contagious for many more days. The majority of people who become infected with this virus do not get slap-face disease; they either remain completely free of symptoms or have mild respiratory or digestive upsets.

Slap-face fever requires no treatment.

There are no preventive measures. The majority of adults are immune.

Hand, Foot, and Mouth Disease. This is a fairly common infection which has probably been around for millenia but has only been recognized as a specific disease for a few decades. The patients are young children who are mildly ill with sores in the mouth (mostly on the tongue and the insides of the cheeks), a little fever, and an absolutely distinctive rash. The rash consists of tiny, firm blisters just deep enough within the skin so that they do not seem to reach the surface. Unlike chicken pox blisters, they cannot be broken by scratching or rubbing. They tend to cluster on the palms and soles, but may be anywhere on the extremities and buttocks. There may be no more than a few of these skin spots.

The causative organisms are the coxsackieviruses A16, A10, and A5. These viruses spread by way of fecal contamination from child to child. Child #1 recovers from her illness and returns to nursery school, still excreting virus in her stool; she scratches her buttocks, picks up a batch of coxsackievirus on her fingers, and transfers some to her peanut butter sandwich which is torn from her grasp and eaten by hungry and ill-mannered child #2, who gets sick a few days later.

The only part of this illness that may need treatment is the sore mouth. For children old enough to suck on hard candies, one may use the local anesthetic benzocaine in the form of a flavored troche. (A troche, pronounced tro'key, is a medicated hard candy; also known as a lozenge.) It helps a little. Ice cream and cold drinks are generally tolerated even when the child's mouth is too sore to handle most other foods.

There are no preventive measures since virus-laced materials are bound to find their way into the mouths of the young, and there is no vaccine.

Viral Exanthems. Many of the other common illnesses marked by fever and a rash are simply, if not helpfully, termed viral exanthems. The study of virus infections has always been difficult, time consuming and expensive, and many of these illnesses are not much more than minor annoyances for a healthy child. To determine which of an assortment of viral agents is causing an illness would typically require copious blood specimens both early and later in the illness, throat washings, and stool specimens. This is an expensive and laborious business, and it can take weeks to get an answer, by which time the patient is usually well and the illness episode forgotten. It is obvious that neither patient nor doctor is likely to have much enthusiasm for chasing such wild viral geese. So, a considerable number of illnesses continue to be lumped under this heading, which is a wastebasket diagnosis for the minor childhood infections with rashes which do not fit into the well-delineated syndromes like measles, rubella, etc., described above.

These are the "little bugs" which will rarely require much attention. It is not really possible to say when a child afflicted with one of them becomes contagious, nor when his contagiousness ceases. Furthermore, there is no way of knowing precisely how these illnesses spread, nor how long they take to incubate in a new host. It is a good bet that kids who are about to come down with these bugs are contagious a day or so before their symptoms appear, and they may well be contagious until their fevers and rashes are gone, but that is not much more than a guess.

Treatment is seldom needed; the rashes don't ordinarily itch and the fevers don't amount to much. Most adolescents or adults with "little bugs" will feel unwell enough to appreciate some extra rest, but this may not be the case with children. Sick kids will often feel grumpy and miserable but resist naps or earlier bedtimes. There is no sense fighting about this; the patients will get better just as fast with or without extra sleep. It is a waste of time to push fluids for illnesses like these; since the children are not losing fluids by vomiting or diarrhea, they are in no danger of becoming dehydrated. Since these are viral illnesses, antibiotics are unnecessary and useless.

Chapter 30

Infections of The Eyes, Ears, Nose, and Throat

Conjunctivitis is infection or irritation of the lining membrane covering the white of the eye and the inner surfaces of the eyelids. As the newborn infant traverses his mother's vagina on the way out his eyes are exposed to whatever germs happen to be living there at the time. After he is born, the conjunctivae may be colonized by a variety of organisms that normally live on the skin or in the nose. As if all this were not enough, he may also have his eyelids held open and silver nitrate, a rather irritating antiseptic, dropped in. No wonder so many babies develop conjunctivitis.

Mom's vaginal germs are really the only major problems. The irritation caused by silver nitrate clears up spontaneously. Most often it can be avoided altogether by using less irritating antibiotic ointments like erythromycin or tetracycline instead. Any infections caused by the usual skin and nasal germs are easily treated. But there can be some really bad actors living peacefully in vaginal tissues. A long forgotten episode of a sexually transmitted disease like herpes, gonorrhea, or chlamydia may have left behind organisms which cause the woman no symptoms at all but are quite capable of infecting her new baby. This is the reason that a red eye or an eye oozing pus in the first week or so of life requires careful evaluation. This is also the reason that it is absolutely crucial to use a prophylactic antibiotic or antiseptic in every baby's eyes after birth. These agents prevent gonorrhea of the eyes which causes blindness if untreated or treated too late. Unfortunately, they work less well against chlamydia and they are useless against herpes; early and vigorous treatment is needed for those infections.

After the newborn period, **conjunctivitis (pink eye)** has somewhat different causes. A variety of microbes can infect the lining membranes of the eye. Most of these cases are viral. **Viral conjunctivitis** may be part of a more general respiratory infection, with cold or cough or sore throat. On the other hand, these infections may be quite localized, causing only red, sore eyes weeping tears, mucus, or pus. Sometimes quite impressive outbreaks of this sort can sweep through a nursery school or a summer camp. It can be difficult to differentiate conjunctivitis caused by viruses from conjunctivitis caused by bacteria. The viral cases will nearly always heal spontaneously, while the bacterial cases can be cured with antibiotics. We often end up advising the use of antibiotic ointments or eye drops even though we don't really know whether they will do any good. Since they are quite safe, it seems like a reasonable approach. Sometimes it is a waste of parent's money, effort, and patience, but often it helps to speed the return of an infected and contagious child to normal activities.

Bacterial conjunctivitis, like the viral cases, can be an isolated event affecting the eyes and nothing else, or it can be part of a larger respiratory infection. In either case, the germs involved are the usual bacteria of ear infections and sinusitis. The most common sequence is a viral cold, complicated by secondary bacterial invasion. Any time pus appears in one or both eyes during the course of a bad cold, suspect a coexisting ear infection, even if your child fails to complain about her ears. Certain bacteria have a habit of invading up the eustachian tubes into the middle ears at the same time their litter mates are finding their way to the conjunctivae. If the conjunctivitis is an isolated bacterial infection, treatment with eye drops or ointment will suffice. If the infection is wider spread, a systemic antibiotic is a good idea.

An unusual cause of conjunctivitis is **sunburn.** This is a condition limited to children who ski during bright spring weather or spend long hours aboard small boats. An exceptionally painful burn may result from prolonged exposure to sunlight reflected off snow or water into eyes unprotected by dark glasses. Cortisone-type eye drops are usually prescribed, and aspirin or an anti-inflammatory agent like ibuprofen is given by mouth.

How to Use Eye Drops and Eye Ointments. Nobody likes having stuff put on their eyes, kids least of all. If you must use eye medications, eye drops are certainly easiest. They do have the disadvantage of adhering less well to the eye tissues than ointments, so that more frequent use may be required. An easy way to use eye drops is as follows:

- With the child lying flat on her back, have her close her eyes.
- Place several drops of the eye medication at the inner corner of her closed lids.
- Have her open her eyes; the drops will flood across her eye without effort and without the sensation of a large wet object falling out of the sky.
- For the child unable to cooperate, try a variation of the headlock method used for nose drops (see page 301) Then:
- Trap her flailing arms as best you can with your forearms, elbows, and chest. (An extra pair of adult's or even an older child's hands is a major help.)
- Pry her eyelids apart with one hand and squirt in the eye drops with the

other. Since she has undoubtedly been crying and her eyes are wet with tears, holding her lids apart may be a good trick. The use of bits of facial or toilet tissue under your fingertips to increase traction on the lids may help.

Eye ointments will be useful only if you can manage to get them *inside* the lids; smearing them on the outside of closed eyelids and expecting the medicine to migrate inside is unduly optimistic.

The requirements for success with eye ointment are these:

- The eyes must be open and the lower lid held down.
- Apply a very generous ribbon of ointment completely across the inside of the lower lid as close as possible to the eyeball. (Careful! You do not want the tip of the ointment tube to touch the eye!)
- Keep holding the eye open until the ointment melts from the warmth of the body, allowing the medicine to spread over the eye and giving it a chance to soak in. (This will take a minute or more. If you do not do this, the child will close her eye immediately and forcefully, pushing the ointment out onto her cheek where it will do no good at all.)

The descriptions above may suggest the wisdom of treating conjunctivitis by giving the antibiotic by mouth and thereby avoiding a screaming, sweating battle three times a day. However, it does seem like a shame to saturate 30 pounds of child with a systemic antibiotic when all you really want to do is treat about 1 square inch of conjunctiva. Well, both parents and pediatricians sometimes choose a tactic on purely pragmatic grounds; whatever works.

Other Infections Around the Eyes. When bacterial infection manages to get into the deeper tissues of the eyelids or into the area around the eye itself, quite serious consequences are possible. This may happen as part of an untreated sinus infection, or as the result of a penetrating injury. If the infection is confined to the outer layers of these tissues, it is termed a **preseptal** or **periorbital cellulitis.** Children with this infection have tender, reddened swelling under or around the eyes. They are likely to be feverish and act ill. Treatment with high doses of antibiotic by mouth or by injection is necessary. If the infection is present in the innermost tissues of the eyelids and around the eye itself, it is termed an **orbital cellulitis.** This infection is marked by extreme eye pain and by swelling around and behind the eye in the orbital cavity. Orbital infections threaten both vision and life; they require intensive treatment in the hospital.

Infections of the upper respiratory tract are the most common diseases of American children. Most of the time these episodes are unimportant and parents should expect them to disappear with little or no formal help from the medical world. Home remedies, or no remedies at all, are sufficient. All too often, however, children are dosed with largely useless drugs that are alleged to reduce the children's discomfort and bring back smiles to their faces. This is unfortunate but understandable; we do want our kids to feel better as soon as possible so that we can all get back to the more important parts of our lives. In particular, parents face the dilemma of deciding when the child is sick enough to stay home (with an adult who needs to be at work), or well enough to go to school. Who has not succumbed to the temptation to feel his child's head for fever, give him a dose of decongestant, and send him sniffling off to catch the school bus?

Guidelines in this situation are nebulous at best. Safe assumptions include the following:

1. A brand new respiratory infection *is* contagious.
2. Most mild common colds are contagious for at least the first 3 days, and probably for about a week.
3. Respiratory infections with a fever should be considered to be contagious until the fever has been absent for 24 hours.
4. Illnesses being treated with an antibiotic should be considered to be contagious until at least 24 hours of therapy has passed, and the fever is gone.
5. Sometimes a child should stay home past the period of fever and contagiousness just because she feels too rotten to cope with school.

Common Colds. There are literally over 100 different viruses capable of causing the vaguely defined illnesses we call common colds. This means that the term carries little specific meaning because each of these viruses can initiate a somewhat different response in each host. Between the variations in germs and the variations in patients, there is ample room for confusion about what is a common cold and what is something else.

Let's agree that a common cold is an upper respiratory tract infection characterized by nasal drainage and stuffiness, and differing degrees of sore throat, cough, headache, low fever, and mild misery. The nasal discharge starts out as thin, clear mucous, and gradually becomes thicker and more opaque, often ending up as green or yellow pus that slowly disappears. The duration of the cold is 1 to 2 weeks; anything longer than that suggests that a secondary bacterial infection has supervened. It may be difficult to distinguish an ordinary cold from an acute nasal allergy, especially early in the illness. Allergic reactions tend to be accompanied by annoying nasal itching, and it is often possible to identify a specific allergic trigger, such as contact with a cat or exposure to particular plants

EVERYDAY PEDIATRICS FOR PARENTS

or foods. During an allergic reaction, the nasal mucous membranes often have a pale and swollen appearance; a simple microscopic examination of nasal secretions is also an aid to diagnosis. If your child seems to have an undue number of colds, a visit to the doctor may clarify the situation.

It generally takes only 2 to 4 days after exposure to come down with a cold. Contagiousness is probably greatest early in the cold and is gone after about 1 week. However, because so many different viruses cause colds, it is impossible to be precise about the incubation period and time of infectiousness. Colds are probably spread both through the air and by way of contaminated objects including sneezed-upon and blown-upon hands.

Treatment is best summarized by the old folk wisdom that if you treat a cold it will be better in 14 days, but if you let it alone it will last a fortnight. There are some symptom-relieving treatments that help a little, but most of what we do for our kids' colds is a waste of time. Everyone wants to use **decongestants,** and the idea that we can shrink the mucous membranes and let some air in and out is surely attractive. The problem is that an effective decongestant paralyses the tiny cilia in the nose and sinuses; it is their task to clear secretions and they can't do it when they are in pharmaceutical bondage. Pseudoephredrine is the least toxic of the oral decongestants; it may decrease appetite a bit and sometimes causes sleeplessness, but these side effects are less than those caused by phenylpropanolamine, the other popular drug. **Antihistamines** may help as they tend to dry nasal secretions, and have a sedative effect at night, but avoid them if possible.

Decongestant nose drops often work powerfully for an hour or two, but it is nearly always a mistake to use them; they sting, there is often rebound worsening when a dose wears off, and they stop the cilia in their tracks. **Cleansing nose drops** can help small infants especially. **Use a home-made solution of 8 ounces tap water, ¼ teaspoon salt, and ¼ teaspoon baking soda.** Hold the baby on your lap facing you, then lay him down on his back and hold his head bent back a bit between your knees. Hold his hands in one of your hands, and with the other hand use a medicine dropper to drip several drops of the solution slowly into each nostril. It will wash down the back of his throat, carrying a considerable amount of mucus with it, and he will be able to nurse or sleep and breath better for awhile. This solution does not sting and has nothing in it to harm his nasal tissues. Commercially available saline drops work just as well at several hundred times the price.

Cough suppressants can help the cold that is marked by a frequent, sleep-disruptive cough. Dextromethorphan is really very good; you may need to use somewhat larger doses than the amount suggested on the bottle. Codeine is a powerful cough suppressant which has the added advantage of being sedating. It has the disadvantages of causing constipation, especially if used often, and it can cause nausea and other unpleasant symptoms in certain susceptible people. No matter what kind of cough suppressant you use, try to obtain one without the ubiquitous so-called **expectorant** guaifenesin. This is one of those peculiar drugs which has long been known to be essentially useless but refuses to go away. Its persistence is partly due to the enduring but baseless idea that it would be a good thing to increase the volume of sputum coughed up from the lungs. There is no evidence that guaifenesin has any place in the treatment of the common cold, or anything else, for that matter, and it tastes bad to boot. The place of **vitamin C (ascorbic acid)** in the treatment or prevention of colds continues to be argued. Linus Pauling's initial claims that massive doses of several grams of C prevented or aborted colds led to a great deal of enthusiastic huckstering and a few careful clinical studies. As best I can make out, most of the experimental subjects showed little or no effect of vitamin C. However, there did appear to be a small group of people who seemed to get a modest amount of improvement. Many families in my own practice have tried vitamin C either as a winter-long prophylactic or as an attempted cure when a cold erupted. The large majority (including my own family) eventually found it useless and gave it up, but a few parents remain convinced that they can cut down family colds with enough vitamin C. If you decide to experiment with it, use plain vitamin C (ascorbic acid) just as Linus Pauling did; don't waste money on organic or chelated or otherwise tarted-up versions. Vitamin C is just vitamin C.

Devices to blow moist or hot or cold air at the patient or into his room do nothing for the common cold except to complexify treatment and ruin the wallpaper. One recently marketed little machine blows very hot air directly up the patient's nose. It makes his nose hot but, unhappily, that is all. Vaporizers and humidifiers seem helpful in laryngitis and croup (see pages 318–20) but have no effect on colds.

Antibiotics. Some colds are complicated by a superimposed bacterial infection. This is signaled by the persistence of cold symptoms for more than about 2 weeks, especially when the nasal discharge remains bright yellow or a rather fluorescent green. The bacterial infection may be a rhinitis, that is to say, limited to the nose itself, or a sinusitis, extending into the

Eustachian Tube

Adenoid

Tonsils

EVERYDAY PEDIATRICS FOR PARENTS

adjacent sinuses around the nose, or otitis media, infection in the middle ear space. The nose, sinuses, and middle ears are all effectively one continuous space, so infection in one area is often joined by infection next door. The tonsils and adenoid are masses of lymph tissue in the nose and throat. The tonsils are in the back of the throat at either side and the adenoid is out of sight, up above the tonsils in the back of the nose. Neither tonsils nor adenoid are likely to become infected from an ordinary cold. It can be difficult to know when to seek medical attention for symptoms that hang on after the cold should have disappeared. Both doctors and parents would like the child's body to have the chance to throw off the infection by itself, but if that does not happen, the dragging on of infection can have decidedly adverse effects. Chronic infection in these areas can do long-term damage. You do no favor to your child to let her have a drippy, green nasal discharge all winter long.

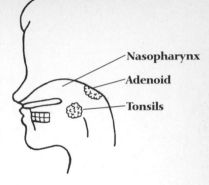

The attention paid to **diet** while treating the common cold is touching evidence of how much we want to feel that we can do something useful for our pitiful, sniveling children. Devotees of fruit juice cures, chicken soup (also known as Jewish penicillin), and the like remind me of the favorite prescription of one of my old medical school teachers. His Two-Bottle Treatment was as follows: Obtain a bottle of bourbon or scotch and place at the foot of your bed. Every 15 to 30 minutes, arise and drink a small glass of the whiskey of your choice. When upon arising you see two bottles, lie down and sleep off the cold. This is probably never going to get past the FDA, even for adults, but it clearly expresses the impotence of either doctors or parents to cure colds.

It may be apparent from this discussion that prospects for a common cold vaccine are dim; there are too many viruses involved. Environmental efforts at prevention seem headed for defeat. Any child who is around other little children is going to share their germs, and the germs of the adults as well, for that matter. Antibiotics clearly have no place in preventing common colds. There are a few children who so regularly get a secondary bacterial infection with every cold that they are started on an antibiotic at the first sign of a sniffle; this may prevent an ear infection but it can't stop the cold itself.

Sinusitis. It is not easy to think up any very convincing reason why we have been outfitted with sinuses. These hollow structures surround our noses, filling up the bony protuberances of our cheeks and the lower, central part of our foreheads. Having these spaces filled with air instead of solid bone undoubtedly lightens the weight of our skulls. It also provides gainful employment to physicians specializing in diseases of the ears, nose, and throat. The disadvantages

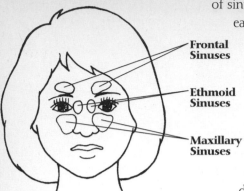

Frontal
Sinuses

Ethmoid
Sinuses

Maxillary
Sinuses

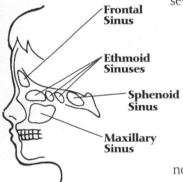

Frontal
Sinus

Ethmoid
Sinuses

Sphenoid
Sinus

Maxillary
Sinus

of sinuses are legion: Sinuses are often the site of allergic reactions, they are easily infected, and some sinuses have such small openings that they are easily plugged up by any inflammatory process. In short, sinuses were an evolutionary option the human race was ill-advised to choose.

When we have a cold, the tissues lining the nose and the sinuses becomes inflamed and swollen. Most of the time, our bodies fight off the invading viral agents, and everything settles back to normal existence. But not infrequently, the ordinary bacteria that usually live quietly in our noses begin to grow and invade the virus-damaged tissue, and we have a bacterial sinus infection. The symptoms of sinusitis may include fever, headache or face pain, nasal congestion, thick and gooey nasal discharge, and a cough due to the drainage of mucus down the back of the throat. The infection can vary from rather trivial to quite severe, and from annoyingly chronic to dramatically acute. The sinuses are only partially developed in babies and small children, and it is relatively unusual for doctors to make the diagnosis of sinusitis until middle childhood. I am not sure whether this is due to the technical difficulty of making a firm diagnosis in smaller kids, or because the partially developed sinuses are more easily kept open and draining.

Treatment of sinusitis is generally easy since the causative bacteria are susceptible to ordinary, orally administered antibiotics. It does seem to take longer to cure than most other bacterial infections; 3 weeks of treatment is not unusual. Other measures such as decongestants and nose drops are best avoided for the same reasons noted in the preceding paragraphs on the treatment of the common cold. As usual, the hardest question concerning sinusitis is when to treat. At what point does one decide that the green goo coming out of the child's nose constitutes a real sinus infection meriting a course of antibiotic? This is easily decided if the child is obviously sick because of the infection. The situation is less clear with the child who is only mildly ill. Left alone, most of these kids eventually cure themselves, but some of them stay infected, and the resulting damage to sinus tissues is probably the reason that so many adults have chronic sinus disease.

Infections of The Middle Ear (Otitis Media). First a word about anatomy and medical terms. Think of the ear as a structure having 7 parts. The **outer ear** poses few medical problems besides cuts and bruises and occasional irritation from earrings in pierced ears. The **ear canal** is the site of swimmer's

EVERYDAY PEDIATRICS FOR PARENTS

ear infections and impacted wax; we'll get around to it later. The **ear drum** or *tympanic membrane* is the tough, thin membrane which separates the ear canal and the middle ear. Sound waves impinging on the ear drum are transmitted through the **middle ear,** a small, air-filled space. Three small bones, the **auditory ossicles,** form a chain crossing the middle ear. Further inside the skull is the **inner ear** which contains the nerve structures for balance and for hearing. A seventh structure, the **eustachian tube,** is a muscular tunnel connecting the middle ear with the upper, back part of the nose and throat cavity. This allows us to equalize ear pressure in our ears, for example when we change altitude in an airplane.

The common, everyday ear infections which are the bane of existence for countless kids are infections in the middle ear, otherwise known as otitis media. There are subvarieties of otitis based on acuteness or chronicity, presence or absence of a perforation in the ear drum, and stickiness of middle ear secretions, but all the them are problems of infection, swelling of lining membranes, and plugging up of the eustachian tube. Ear infections have doubtless been part of human life for ever, but we seem to be living in a time when they have become increasingly common. This it is due in part to the crowding together of very young children in day care settings before they have had time to develop much in the way of immune mechanisms. It is also related to the decline of breast feeding; we know that breast fed babies are decidedly less prone to ear infection. And is due to the physician's increased skill at diagnosis. To discover an infected middle ear in a frightened, squalling, sick, and combative baby requires having the knowledge and the equipment to get a good look down a narrow, curving ear canal, which is usually partly or fully occluded with ear wax, in order to inspect an ear drum that is only about ⅛ inch across. Not too many years ago, we physicians attempted to do this with the aid of a small, hollow, conical ear speculum through which we tried to shine some light, reflected from a mirror worn around our heads. When I was taught to do this in medical school, I soon discovered that wearing a head mirror made me feel like a real doctor, but the task of actually seeing anything deep in the recesses of an infant's ear bordered on the impossible. Even getting the wax out of the way is a major undertaking. Back in those literally dark ages we did have otoscopes with feeble electric lights and magnifying lenses, and that was an enormous

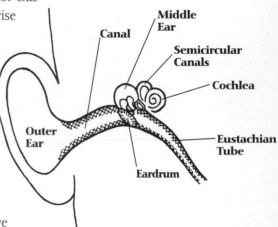

Middle Ear

Canal

Semicircular Canals

Cochlea

Outer Ear

Eustachian Tube

Eardrum

help. With perseverance, a parent or a nurse to hold the child in a grip of steel, and some creative imagination, one could often if not always convince oneself that the ear drum had been inspected in its entirety. In the last few decades, our electric otoscopes have become vastly better and brighter. We have learned to use sealed-end otoscopes which allow us to puff air into the ear canal and study ear drum motility. In addition, we have fancy devices called tympanometers which bounce sound waves off the ear drum and give us additional information about the middle ear. Small wonder, then, that we are more often able to straighten up after peering into a child's ear and announce with some sense of certainty that the ear is, or is not, infected.

What causes an ear infection? The usual sequence seems to be the acquisition of a common cold, which plugs up the eustachian tube; secretions pour into the middle ear, and the cold viruses, aided and abetted by the normal, resident bacteria, infect the middle ear space. The relative contributions of bacteria and viruses to the actual infection are the subject of endless study and debate. It is possible to find bacteria in an infected middle ear, and quite often viruses as well, but the only way to do this is to puncture the ear drum with a long hollow needle and culture the middle ear fluid. This is technically difficult, inevitably painful, quite expensive, and probably not a nice thing to do to the ear drum; for all these reasons, diagnostic ear drum puncture is rarely used to study an individual case. Enough studies have been done so that we have a general idea about which bacteria are likely to be implicated and which antibiotics are likely to be effective. So a rational basis for treatment exists.

When an older child develops an ear infection he will let you know about it because it hurts. A very mild infection may cause not much more than the sensation of a plugged up ear, but this is unusual. Younger children are not so forthcoming with such useful and precise diagnostic information. The only suggestions may be excessive fussiness in a child with a common cold, or a degree or two more fever than you would ordinarily expect. Subtle hints include the child who seems to lose his balance too easily (because the middle ear infection stirs up his inner ear balancing mechanisms), or the child who tugs at his ear lobe and whines. Some children never have any obvious signs of discomfort from ear infection; you may notice that your child seems to be hearing less well than usual and upon examination the doctor finds an old, low-grade infection. A surprising number of ear infections turn up at well child examinations without any history of a preceding illness. The first sign may be the doctor's statement "He has an otitis we need to treat."

EVERYDAY PEDIATRICS FOR PARENTS

But do we actually need to treat middle ear infections? After all, children managed to get over them before modern medicines came along. Why not just wait them out? Well, several reasons. First, not all children got better. Some of them got ear infections which lasted all their lives. One of my partners recalls his practice in a rural area of New Hampshire a half century ago where he saw older children and adults who had acquired their chronically infected ears in the preantibiotic era before World War II. There was even a term for the condition of endlessly draining ear pus; the locals called them "beeling ears." Untreated, persistent ear infections also cause permanent hearing loss. In the developing world today some degree of impaired hearing is present in one quarter of the population, and this is largely the result of otitis media. The other risk of untreated ear infection is extension of the infection into the mastoid bone behind the ear. Acute mastoiditis and the required mastoidectomy surgery have now nearly disappeared in our country. Severe middle ear infection can also seed bacteria into the blood stream, and invade into the adjacent lining membranes of the brain. The World Health Organization (WHO) reports that over 50,000 children die every year because of otitis media and its complications. Second, ear infections make you sick. They hurt, they impair hearing until they are cleared, and the child or adult who has an ear infection is an unhappy soul. Anything we can do to shorten them is worth considering.

The mainstays of therapy for otitis media are antibiotics. Which one, how much, and for how long depend on the likely bacteria and their usual patterns of sensitivity to antibiotic attack. Resistant strains have emerged among many of the ordinary germs that cause otitis, and this has meant that the old faithful antibiotics like penicillin and amoxicillin sometimes fail. When your child's doctor prescribes a drug, he will take into account these sensitivity patterns which vary from community to community and from year to year. He will also consider your child's history of infections and his past reactions to antibiotics. This raises the question of allergy to drugs in general. Particularly during childhood, many illnesses are marked by rashes. If a child happens to be taking an antibiotic and a rash appears, it is easy but often wrong to attribute the rash to the drug. *Perhaps* they are related, but frequently the rash is the direct effect of the illness itself, and the antibiotic is blameless. Sorting out the roles of bug and drug may be all but impossible. About the best you can do is to make sure that careful medical attention is paid to the rash so that an illness cause can be attributed when that is most likely. Labeling a child as allergic to a potentially useful antibiotic if it had no causal relationship to the rash or any other allegedly allergic symptom is potentially harmful.

The only other useful treatment of middle ear infections is symptomatic. The attendant discomfort can be severe, and ordinary analgesics like acetaminophen may not be sufficient. Codeine, usually in the easily taken form of a codeine cough syrup, is a great help. Sometimes heat is soothing. Use an electric heating pad or use mineral oil or cooking oil, gently warmed in a teaspoon over the stove (careful! not too hot! the oil should feel warm on the inner aspect of your wrist), and poured into the ear canal; then plug the ear canal with a piece of absorbent cotton. If the ear is already draining fluid, the ear drum has ruptured; tell your doctor what has happened and don't put oil in it.

Because plugging of the eustachian tube is part of the problem in ear infections, it would be great to be able to decongest it and open the drainage. As I mentioned regarding the common cold and sinusitis, we don't really have decongestants worth using. I know, most doctors still prescribe them, but the truth is that they don't help ear infections to heal. In allergic kids where the swelling is at least in part due to allergy, one may occasionally get a little help with antihistamines. Some doctors also use cortisone-type drugs, either as a nasal spray or by mouth; the evidence that this helps is not wholly convincing.

When should the child with an ear infection be rechecked by the doctor? This is yet another area of medical debate. Assuming that the child seems to be getting better in the first few days, I always want to recheck him at the conclusion of the 10 to 14-day course of antibiotic therapy. If there is still a smoldering infection present, I want to treat it vigorously and get rid of it before it becomes a chronic and hard-to-treat problem. However, some physicians argue that this leads to overtreatment because some of these kids will continue to improve without any further intervention. Oddly enough, I think either of these approaches may be reasonable. It is a matter of balancing the costs of overtreatment—excessive use of drugs and increased risk of adverse reactions to them, plus increased cost of medical care, versus undertreatment—prolonged illness and impaired hearing, and an increased risk of the eventual necessity for ear surgery with its attendant costs and hazards. Which way to go should depend on the history and needs of the individual patient.

Despite the undoubted (by me!) advantages of modern treatment of ear infections, some of them don't get better. This may be due to delay in diagnosis and therapy, resistant organisms, host factors like allergy or impaired immunity, family factors like tobacco smoking in the child's environment, or simple failure

EVERYDAY PEDIATRICS FOR PARENTS

to administer the medicine in a regular and consistent manner. Furthermore, some of the kids get better, but promptly get sick again with yet another ear infection. These cases of recurrent or chronic otitis are common and difficult. The first line of defense against recurrent ear infection is long-term, low-dose antibiotic use. We generally use about one third or one half of a full therapeutic dose and give it day in and day out for many months. This use of antibiotics was pioneered decades ago in the prevention of rheumatic fever, and has been used since to good effect for other infectious illnesses as well. Antiallergy and anti-inflammatory drugs are also sometimes used as adjuncts in the treatment of the chronic, low-grade cases. Overcoming the eustachian tube blockage by inflating the ear through the nose can be quite useful; there are a number of techniques which your child's doctor can teach you. When all else fails, you and your child will find yourselves facing an ear, nose, and throat specialist who will probably advise draining the middle ears and inserting plastic tubes to keep the middle ear space aerated and healthy. These little grommets typically stay in place for months, during which time one hopes that enough healing will occur. Unfortunately, it has commonly been the practice to reinsert ear tubes several times, and this can lead to a badly scarred and not perfectly functioning ear drum. My enthusiasm for this therapeutic approach is limited, but once in a great while ear tubes are helpful. In the not too distant past, the surgical removal of the tonsils and adenoid ("T and A") was a common treatment. The idea was that chronically infected the tonsils harbored bacteria which got into the ear, and that an enlarged adenoid blocked the eustachian tubes. There is general agreement at present that the tonsils are really innocent of responsibility. On the other hand, a huge adenoid may possibly play a role, and sometimes needs to be removed.

Any illness as common and as unpleasant as otitis media deserves a summary statement.

1. Suspect an ear infection when a child with a cold acts sicker than usual, especially if there is more than a minimal fever and discomfort. Don't be afraid to "waste the doctor's time" with what may turn out to be nothing much. That's what you pay him for.
2. Hearing loss is important; if you suspect that your child is not hearing normally, either during an illness or at any other time, have him checked.
3. Treat ear infections with care. Make sure that the medicine is given *every* time. Make sure that follow-up appointments are made and kept.
4. If your child has recurrent or chronic ear infection, look for remediable causes such as tobacco smoke in the home or at day care, or underlying

medical problems such as anemia, untreated allergy, or mild immune deficiencies. Switching a child from a large day care group to home day care with only one or a few other children may sometimes help decrease the number of colds and subsequent ear infections.

5. Hang in there. Ear infections are largely a problem in the first few years of life; even the kids with the most recalcitrant problems grow out of them.

Throat Infections (Pharyngitis, Tonsillitis). It is no great surprise that people get sore throats. Like the nose, the sinuses, and the ears, our throats are the first port of call to every errant virus or bacterium that wanders into the stream of air we breath. Many of these organisms, especially the viruses, cause diffuse infections that involve our entire upper airway system, and some progress down to the middle reaches of our larynx and bronchi, or even further, all the way into our lungs. Our throats participate fully in many of these infections; a red, swollen, sore throat is often part of a bad cold, a viral laryngitis, bronchitis, or influenza. In addition to these unpleasantries, the throat has its own special problems which include a variety of germs whose major areas of attack focus on the throat. These include one bacterium, the beta-hemolytic streptococcus, and several viruses.

Strep Throat and Other Bacterial Throat Infections. The discussion of **scarlet fever** in Chapter 29 covers much of this subject from a slightly different point of view. Scarlet fever is basically an infection caused by one of the strep organisms (group A Streptococcus pyogenes) which happens to make a rash-producing toxin; some group A strep germs have this ability, some don't. Except for the rash, there is no difference for the patient. It should be noted that a strep infection in the throat is the same whether or not the tonsils are present. If the child has not had his tonsils removed, the infection may be most obvious in the tonsil area, and we tend to refer to the disease as **tonsillitis.** If the tonsils have been removed for whatever reason, strep throats can continue to occur.

For reasons which are not understood, strep throat is a rarity in the first three years of life, although an occasional baby or toddler will get a strep infection manifesting itself as a persistent bad cold. Most strep throats are accompanied by swollen glands under the angles of the jaw, headache or bellyache, fever, and a considerable degree of malaise. Cold symptoms and cough are unusual. If you can get a good look into your child's mouth you will probably see diffuse redness in the back and sides of the throat; the tonsils will become swollen and streaked with white pus. This combination of signs and symptoms is well worth a doctor visit. (To examine a child's throat, use the handle of a tablespoon as a tongue blade; to avoid gagging the patient, be careful not to insert it past the outer ⅓ of the tongue. Ask him to open as wide as he can and pant fast and hard through his mouth; saying "Ah-h-h" does not help at all. A bright flashlight is a necessity.) The doctor will nearly always need to obtain a throat culture or a fast strep-antigen test to confirm the diagnosis; various viral infections can look just the same, and it is a mistake to treat viruses with antibiotics. If the child's illness is not too severe, there may actually be some merit in waiting overnight for the result of a throat culture. The 1 day delay in starting treatment gives the body a chance to elaborate some antistrep antibodies which may help the next time a strep wanders down your child's throat.

Strep is a highly contagious organism. It is found in generous quantities in the nose and throat secretions of patients when they are acutely ill, and then gradually diminishes as the illness runs its course. Within about 1 day of the start of antibiotic treatment, a patient is no longer contagious. Many people are strep carriers; they harbor a modest number of strep in their throats for months at a time without ill effect and generally do not serve as a source of infection to others. After exposure to an adequate dose of strep germs, the new host may become ill in 2 to 5 days, or have a mild and inapparent infection, or become a carrier for a while without any symptoms, or simply not pick up the germs at all.

Treatment is the same as for scarlet fever: 10 days of penicillin or another appropriate antibiotic. This shortens the illness and the period of contagiousness and limits the risk of complications such as rheumatic fever. Recurrences of throat infections after antibiotic treatment can occur; these usually respond well to another course of antibiotic. The tonsils and the adenoid, like the various other groups of lymph glands in and around the neck, are protective structures which normally play an important role in helping to fight microbial infections. What appears to be the problem in these chronic cases is the establishment of nests of infected material deep inside the tonsils or adenoid. Sometimes the only measures which can control these recurrences are long-term antibiotic administration, or, as a last resort, tonsillectomy and adenoidectomy (T and A.)

Two rare and serious types of throat infection due usually, but not always to beta strep are **peritonsillar abscess** and **retropharyngeal abscess.** These infections are deep in the tissues of the throat, behind the tonsils or behind the back wall of the throat. They require intensive antibiotic treatment, typically in the hospital, and may need surgical drainage as well.

In addition to the beta strep infections we've been discussing, there are some other bacteria that can sometimes cause sore throats. These include certain other varieties of streptococcus, **Haemophilus influenzae** (a misnamed bacterium once thought to cause influenza, which we now know is caused by a virus), and **Arcanobacterium haemolyticum,** which can cause an illness with sore throat, rash, and cough. In the days before immunization became widespread, **diphtheria** caused epidemics of terrible infections which extended from the throat down into the deeper air passages of the chest. Even today, diphtheria still kills people in the United States who are not immunized.

Throat Infections Caused by Viruses. The majority of viral throat infections are relatively unimportant illnesses in which the throat infection is part of an upper respiratory infection with cold symptoms, perhaps a low fever, and some cough. Dozens of different viruses cause these illnesses, which can be expected to come and go within a few days or at most about 2 weeks. They are contagious and annoying, but they don't amount to much. However, there are also some specific virus infections which are decidedly more impressive. First among these is **infectious mononucleosis** which can be a difficult and debilitating disease. Because of its complexity and importance "mono" and its causative agent, the Epstein-Barr virus, are discussed at length in Chapter 36.

Another viral infection involving the throat is **herpangina,** caused by coxsackieviruses. This nasty little disease is marked by severe mouth and throat discomfort, fever, and sometimes vomiting. The back of the throat, the tonsil area, the back of the palate, and the back half of the mouth are speckled with tiny blisters or ulcers each surrounded by rings of redness. During the height of the infection mouth and throat pain can make eating and drinking painful. Herpangina spreads from child to child through fecal contamination and probably through mouth secretions as well. The incubation period is about 3 to 6 days. Treatment is not at all satisfactory. Analgesics like acetaminophen are not usually effective, but local anesthetics can be used. Benzocaine is available as a nonprescription troche or lozenge which is meant to be allowed to dissolve in the mouth. This is fine for older kids but young children often do not understand the concept. Lidocaine is a more powerful prescription anesthetic available in a syrup; it tastes absolutely awful and most kids will not leave it in their mouths long enough for it to help. About the only other thing you can do is give your child cold, sweet foods and drinks. Ice cream and milkshakes will keep them hydrated and nourished. Avoid acid beverages like orange juice or carbonated drinks like soda pop; they sting.

The **adenoviruses** cause several distinct illnesses including various types of sore throat. One of these syndromes is termed an exudative pharyngitis because the back of the throat is streaked with thick, white, pus-like secretions which look about the same as a bad strep throat. Another adenovirus causes **pharyngoconjunctival fever:** a sore throat plus red, sore eyes, and swollen glands in the neck. The adenoviruses spread in the same way as the coxsackieviruses described above.

Ear Canal Infections (Swimmer's Ear; Otitis Externa). The ear canal is a curving, skin-lined passageway, surrounded by ear cartilage in its outer part and by bone in its inner part. It is often partly filled with ear wax (cerumen) an unusual material in that it is a wax which can be dissolved in water. The main functions of cerumen are to keep the ear canal skin lubricated, and to make the lives of pediatricians and ear doctors miserable. There are racial differences in ear wax chemistry. East Asians have hard, dry, pebbly, or flaky wax. South Asians tend to have copious, soft wax. In general, people with oily skin have softer ear wax; northern Europeans who tend to have dry skins are likely to have scant and dry cerumen. There is no single, best method for dealing with normal accumulations of ear wax. Most people with dry and scant ear wax can leave it alone; it tends to fall out in small flakes. Some ear canals manufacture such vast quantities of wax that it collects in plugs which impair hearing. This can sometimes be prevented by washing the outside of the ear canal with shampoo or soap and water and letting the soapy solution run inside the ear. Reaming out ear canals with cotton-tipped applicators often has the unintended effect of shoving the wax deeper into the ear canal. If you feel the need to swab your children's ears, do it gently and only in the outer half of the canal.

All this detail about ear wax is by way of introduction to the subject of ear canal infections. These are popularly and accurately known as **swimmer's ear** infections. Repeated and prolonged immersion in water moistens and softens the wax which remains plastered wetly against the skin lining the ear canal. Skin is not well suited to this kind of chronic soaking and the normal resident bacteria are able to initiate a superficial infection in the saturated skin. Because the ear canal skin is tightly applied to the underlying cartilage and bone, there is no room for the swelling that is part of any infectious process, so the ear becomes surprisingly painful. When the doctor examines the infected ear, any movement of the outer ear will cause more pain. The pain is even worse when she attempts to remove enough ear wax to see what is going on. Unfortunately, the ear wax removal is also a necessary part of the treatment, because therapeutic ear drops can't get to the infected skin if it remains buried in cerumen. Once a good part of the wax has been gently cleaned away, treatment begins with ear drops, which combine an antibiotic agent to fight the infection and a cortisone-type drug; this decreases the swelling. Use these therapeutic drops generously; you need to saturate the entire ear canal and let the drops soak in. The patient should remain lying down with the affected ear up for several minutes each time; 3 or 4 applications a day are usual. An analgesic agent by mouth may be needed for 1 or 2 days.

Most people never get swimmer's ear infections, presumably because their ears drain dry enough. But for those who have had one episode and wish to avoid another, a simple routine of rinsing the canal with ordinary rubbing alcohol before bedtime on days when you have been swimming will usually suffice. Fill a teaspoon or the cap of the alcohol bottle with the alcohol, bend over the sink with one ear up and pour the alcohol into the ear. Turn your head and the alcohol will drain out, carrying some of the trapped water with it. Repeat the procedure with your other ear. You can also use a combination of alcohol mixed half-and-half with glycerin, used in exactly the same fashion. This is somewhat more drying in its effect than alcohol alone, but it is a great deal gooier. Various proprietary ear drops are available without prescription. These are typically alcohol plus some acetic acid (vinegar). They are often effective as preventatives but are not strong enough to cure an established ear canal infection, despite the claims on the package.

Using ear plugs to keep water out of the ears during swimming is sometimes advocated. Even if the ear plugs could keep the ear canal dry, which I doubt, they would have the disadvantage of impairing the swimmer's hearing which does not seem like a good idea.

Chapter 31

Infections of The Mouth

Infections of The Mucous Membranes of The Mouth (Stomatitis). The mucous membranes that line our mouths must cope with an astounding variety of intruders in the course of an average day: hot and cold foods and drinks, vast quantities of air containing all sorts of gaseous and particulate pollutants, and all manner of germs. Considering the amount and diversity of traffic in and out, it is impressive how healthy mouths remain. Naturally, the tissues of the mouth are sometimes involved in infections like chicken pox or measles which have widespread effects all over the body. However, what concerns us here are the several diseases whose main symptoms are eruptions in the mouth.

A variety of viruses can cause sores in the mouth, and it is not always easy to tell one from another. **Herpes simplex type 1** infects just about everyone sometime in life. The first episode of herpes infection may be completely asymptomatic or it may be an illness with small, red-bordered blisters or shallow ulcers on and around the lips and inside the mouth. The back of the mouth and the throat have few if any of these sores. Accompanying the mouth eruption are fever and swollen glands in the neck. The illness lasts a few days during which the main problem is getting the child to eat and drink enough. **Herpes simplex type 2,** which is better known as a sexually transmitted infection of the genitals, can also cause a mouth and lip infection identical to type 1. The vast majority of herpes infections are easily handled by our bodies, but both types of herpesvirus can sometimes cause dangerous infections, especially in newborns and in people who have impaired immunity. Once either type of herpes infection has taken place, the virus settles down to live permanently in our tissues. This may be a quiet and uneventful residency, or it may be marked by recurrent bouts of activity. In the case of mouth herpes, these are usually limited eruptions of "cold sores" or "canker sores" in or around the mouth. The recurrences can be triggered by other illnesses, by exposure to bright sunlight, and possibly by other sources of stress, including psychological tension.

Herpes simplex virus spreads easily in body fluids; the mouth sores are good sources of infection for many days. Both primary and recurrent episodes are contagious. The period of incubation is from 2 days to 2 weeks.

Medicines are not much help for oral herpes. Acyclovir ointment is somewhat effective in patients who have compromised immunity, but there is no evidence that it helps others. For children old enough to suck on them, local anesthetic lozenges (benzocaine, Cepacol, Chloraseptic Lozenges) can numb the inside of the mouth. Cold and sweet liquids and foods are usually the best tolerated. Some people who have recurrent cold sores learn to sense an oncoming flare-up because of tingling discomfort in the affected area. There is some evidence that prompt chilling with an ice cube can head off the development of a cold sore. Rubbing the area with a Q-tip soaked in adrenaline may have a similar effect. I have to say that neither of these remedies has been subjected to convincing, double-blinded studies, but they are worth a try.

Other viruses can cause illnesses marked by mouth blisters and ulcers. The **coxsackievirus** infection that causes **hand, foot, and mouth disease** is discussed in Chapter 29. The A4 strain of coxsackievirus can cause **herpang–ina,** an infection with tiny blisters and ulcers in the back half of the mouth. There is often fever with this uncomfortable illness, but the children are not seriously ill; recovery takes 3 to 5 days. Treatment is limited to the use of analgesics like acetaminophen, local anesthetic lozenges of benzocaine, and lots of cold, sweet liquids and foods. These viruses spread through fecal contamination. The period of contagiousness is varies greatly, sometimes lasting for weeks. The incubation period is also variable, but 3 to 6 days is typical.

The other common germ which causes mouth infections is **Candida albicans,** a yeast-like fungus about which more nonsense has been written than any other organism on God's green earth. Candida, which is also sometimes called **monilia,** is a normal inhabitant of all of our body surfaces including skin, mouth, intestinal tract, and vagina. We live in peaceful harmony with Candida albicans most of the time, as we do with thousands of other microorganisms; they don't bother us and we provide them with a convenient place to live. But the balance of nature is sometimes thrown awry, and an excess of one or another of these microscopic fellow travelers causes trouble. If an antibiotic is administered, killing vast numbers of the bacteria which normally live side by side with Candida, that fungus may find itself with extra food and lots of room for unchecked growth. The result is a superficial infection of the mucous membranes of the mouth called **thrush.** This overgrowth of Candida can also occur for no apparent reason in healthy and thriving newborns, and it is a common problem in people with defective or suppressed immunity. Thrush is marked by patches of white crud adhering to the tongue and the mucous membranes lining the mouth. These masses of fungal growth look like milk stuck to the tongue or cottage cheese adhering to the inside of the cheeks or the roof of the mouth. Attempts to remove the stuff prove that it is rather firmly attached. Oddly enough, most babies with thrush are completely uncomplaining, although a few act as if their mouths are sore. Thrush in newborns will often occur simultaneously with a Candida diaper rash (see pages 235–36), and nursing mothers may get a Candida rash of the nipples and breasts. As every woman knows, the same kind of yeast infection can occur in the vagina and vulva at any age.

Treatment of Candida mouth infections is slow, probably because saliva efficiently removes whatever medicine we apply. For years the best treatment was gentian violet, a bright purple dye which permanently stained the clothes of anyone who got too near the patient. Later, nystatin, a drug with weak anti-fungal properties, became available. It is expensive, it tastes bad, and it does not adhere well to the surfaces of the mouth, but it will eventually cure thrush most of the time and despite its drawbacks, it remains in use. Much more effective is the modern antifungal drug clotrimazole. It is available without prescription as a topical cream which can be rubbed all over the inside of the mouth several times a day. The package information does not mention the treatment of thrush because it was designed for use in the vagina and on the skin and no drug company has gone to the trouble and expense of getting FDA approval for intraoral use of the cream. As it turns out, these preparations cure thrush nicely, even without the official sanction of the federal government. There are also lozenges or troches of clotrimazole designed for older children or adults with thrush; these are FDA approved and available by prescription.

Bacterial infections of the lining membranes of the mouth are quite rare. When they do occur, there is likely to be invasion of deeper tissues of the mouth, and the patient can be expected to be seriously sick.

Infections of The Gums and Teeth. The gums are remarkably tough. It takes years of studious neglect to set up the conditions for infections of the margins of the gums, **gingivitis.** If the teeth are allowed to become deeply encrusted with bacterial plaque, irritation and eventual infection of the adjacent gum tissue will occur. Even the most limited program of casual tooth brushing is likely to keep this from happening for years. If plaque is controlled by regular use of a tooth brush, plus dental floss when teeth begin to be crowded together in later childhood, gingival infection will be a great rarity.

Dental Caries (Tooth Cavities, Tooth Decay). This is a complex process in which masses of bacteria become stuck to the surface of the teeth and secrete acids which damage the surface of the tooth enamel. This initiates destruction of the enamel and the underlying dentin, producing **tooth cavities.** The factors controlling this disease include the mineral structure of the tooth itself. If sufficient fluoride is built into the complex mineral framework of the enamel, it is resistant to this acid attack. Diet is another factor because sweets, especially sticky foods like raisins, jam, and sticky candies, provide an excellent diet for the bacteria in plaque. Even nonsticky sweet foods like milk and juices can nourish the decay producing bacteria when they are allowed prolonged contact with the teeth. This is seen frequently in babies who are put to bed with a bottle of milk or juice which they may suck intermittently all night. The resultant destruction of the front teeth is impressive to behold. Dental hygiene is another factor; the more frequently and effectively teeth are cleaned by brushing and flossing, the less plaque will be present to destroy the teeth. When infection develops deep within a decayed tooth, a **dental abscess** may form causing a red, painful swelling of the overlying gum tissue. Treatment by a dentist will usually involve removal of the affected tooth. For details concerning the use of fluoride see pages 63, and 194–95.

Chapter 32

Infections of The Middle and Lower Respiratory Tract

Laryngitis and Croup. Just below the base of the tongue, between the back of the throat and the top of the trachea lies the larynx, a complicated structure which includes the vocal cords. Infection in the vocal cords and the lining membranes of the larynx is termed **laryngitis.** In older children or adults, the illness generally does not amount to much. It is most often a viral infection, usually part of an upper respiratory bug with cold symptoms and a sore throat. The tissues become swollen, speech may become muffled and painful, but that is about all. Laryngitis in babies and small children is a different matter because the size of the larynx is so small that even a modest amount of swelling may make breathing noisy and difficult, a condition which is called **croup.** This is a generic term used to describe any acute obstruction to the flow of air through the larynx, whether it is caused by laryngitis (bacterial or viral), allergy, or even a foreign object. Common to all kinds of croup are hoarseness, a harsh cough, typically described as barking or metallic, and difficulty in breathing, especially with inspiration.

It is unusual for the larynx to be infected all by itself without adjacent parts of the airway sharing the problem. As I mentioned above, laryngitis is often part of an upper respiratory infection, usually due to one or another virus. It can also be part of an infection that extends down to the middle airways. This common form of croup is termed **laryngotracheobronchitis.** It can be caused by at least ten different viruses, and, rarely, by bacteria. For practical purposes, most pediatricians term this **viral croup.** This is a disease of babies and small children. It starts with cold symptoms and then progresses to fever, a hoarse, barking cough, and increased difficulty in breathing, especially during inspiration. Often the child will be awakened from her sleep by a coughing spell, and as she attempts to catch her breath after coughing, finds that she can not breathe in easily. This triggers crying, more coughing, and still more trouble breathing. It is terrifying to child and parents alike. These illnesses often improve in the morning and afternoon and then worsen at night. The infection generally runs its course within 1 week or less. Treatment depends on the severity of symptoms. A mild case will be manageable at home with nothing more than a mild cough suppressant and the use of a humidifier or a vaporizer in the child's room. When she awakens crying, the episode can often be brought under control by taking her into the bathroom, turning on the hot shower to make a lot of steam in a hurry, closing the bathroom doors and windows, and sitting down with the child on your lap until the croup begins to lessen. This is the only respiratory illness I know in which making the room air moist makes any difference at all. Another maneuver that can help is to bundle the child up and take her outside into the cold night air. Why this helps is a mystery, but it does. **When the illness is so severe that the child is in real respiratory distress, hospital care is mandatory.** Extra oxygen, respiratory support, and sometimes cortisone-type drugs are used. As I mentioned earlier, there are rare cases of laryngotracheobronchitis caused by bacteria. When a child seems to be sicker than she should be with what has looked like viral croup, her doctor will consider these bacterial possibilities as well.

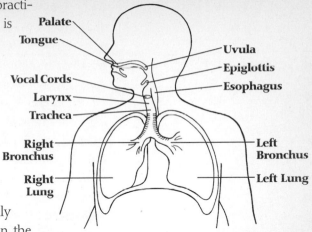

The most serious form of croup is **epiglottitis,** an infection of the larynx involving the epiglottis, the top flap that keeps food out of the lower airway during the act of swallowing. This infection is sometimes called **supraglottitis.** It is caused by the dangerous, invasive type b form of the bacterium **Haemophilus influenzae, (Hib** or **H. flu,** for short). The other members of this species, nontypable H. flu, are common inhabitants of the nose and throat which cause a large number of ordinary ear and sinus infections, but do not tend to cause serious or dangerous disease. H. flu type b germs are spread in the respiratory secretions of infected patients or of carriers who have no symptoms. Close contact within families or in day care groups increases the risk of becoming infected. The incubation period is unknown but variable. Children from 2 to 4 years of age are most vulnerable, although some cases of epiglottitis occur in older kids and even adults. The illness may be heralded by ordinary cold symptoms, but the infection of the larynx tends to appear explosively. The child has severe throat pain, trouble swallowing which may cause drooling, hoarseness, and fever. The croupy cough is not always impressive; the rapid increase in difficulty breathing is the most notable and important symptom. ***This is a medical emergency which absolutely requires immediate hospitalization for the placement of a breathing tube to keep the airway open, plus antibiotic treatment for the infection, and other supportive measures.*** The good news about epiglottitis is that is has become rare in developed countries during the last decade because of immunization of babies and small children with the excellent Hib vaccine. Unimmunized young children exposed to epiglottitis or other infections caused by Hib should be given a short course of antibiotics to prevent the disease.

Spasmodic croup is a recurrent condition which acts a lot like viral croup. The child has usually been perfectly healthy prior to the onset of symptoms, although sometimes there may have been a mild cold for a day or so. Then he awakens in the middle of the night, frightened, crying, and coughing with a hoarse bark and little or no fever. He settles down pretty well with cuddling and steaming, and then awakens again later in the night with the same symptoms. In the morning, he seems nearly all better, but the scenario repeats itself on subsequent nights. After 3 or 4 days of diminishing croup, he is back to his old self. This is a condition of small and middle-aged children. Although it seems to be an allergic response, it is not clear what the offending allergen might be. It is most common in children who are known to have other allergic problems. If your child has had it once, expect it to recur and keep your humidifier handy. I think that decongestants (specifically pseudoephedrine), antihistamines (like chlorpheniramine, diphenhydramine, or any of a dozen others), and cough suppressants (codeine or dextromethorphan) really help spasmodic croup. Give them at least at bedtime and during the night if needed.

Foreign bodies in the larynx or trachea can certainly cause croupy sounding coughs. If the cough begins abruptly without any preceding illness, or the croup fails to follow any of the usual patterns of the diseases described above, or if there is a suggestion that the child may have inhaled a small object, your child's doctor will need to look for an aspirated foreign body.

Bronchitis. Have a look at the illustration of the respiratory tract on page 319. It is obviously all one continuous set of structures, and any number of germs treat it as such, causing symptoms from the nose down to the air sacs in the lungs. I've already mentioned laryngotracheobronchitis, which reaches from the back of the throat down into the main air passages (the bronchi). However, there are also illnesses in which the bronchi themselves take the brunt of the attack. In acute bronchitis the child's main symptoms are a wet, rattling cough, some fever, and general malaise. This may occur as a primary, probably viral infection, or it can be a secondary bacterial complication during or after a virus, for example influenza. It may be quite difficult to decide if the symptoms are truly due to infection, or whether a state of hyper-reactivity of the air passages has been triggered by the preceding disease. Ordinary asthma can also sound a lot like an infectious bronchitis. X-rays and other lab studies are unlikely to clarify the picture, so your child's doctor will have to decide about treatment without complete assurance that he knows what he is doing. The therapy the doctor suggests will depend on his judgment concerning the cause of the illness. A viral bronchitis will run its course untreated except for an occasional dose of a cough suppressant. A bacterial bronchitis will respond to a properly chosen antibiotic. Asthma can be managed with bronchodilators or anti-inflammatory drugs. There are numerous medical situations where diagnosis and therapy are based only tenuously on sturdy, scientific fact. That's how it is with bronchitis today.

Bronchiolitis. The bronchi divide into finer and finer branchlets as they penetrate more deeply into the lung itself. Just before the air sacs of the lung tissue begin, at the very end of the bronchi are the tiny air passages called bronchioles. Bronchiolitis is an infection in these small structures and actually extends up into the middle-sized bronchial passages as well. It can also extend down into the lung tissue and cause a pneumonia, but most of the trouble is in these terminal divisions, so the disease is honored by their name. The usual but not sole culprit is the **respiratory syncytial virus (RSV)** which is an exceptionally successful microbe, indeed. Everyone gets RSV infection in early childhood, and most of us get reinfected off and on all our lives. In older people it causes colds or bronchitis, rather than bronchiolitis. RSV spreads through the air and also on objects, including the hands of playmates or caretakers. The contagious period lasts at least several days and in infants may last for up to 1 month. The incubation period is 2 to 8 days.

The baby or small child with bronchiolitis comes down with what seems like an ordinary cold, and then gets sicker, with increasing cough, and faster, more labored breathing. There is often fever early in the illness, but it tends to disappear. Most kids with this disease are only moderately ill and can be taken care of at home without any special treatment. But the sickest kids will need to be hospitalized and their care can become demanding. Some of them improve a bit faster if they are given ribavirin, an antiviral agent. After an episode of bronchiolitis, many children prove to have increased airway sensitivity; they may get repeated episodes of wheezing with every little cold, or actually develop chronic asthma which can last for years. It is these long-term effects of RSV infection that have spurred efforts to develop an effective vaccine; considerable progress has been made and a vaccine will probably be available in the near future. Children under age 2 years who have had a chronic lung problem called bronchopulmonary dysplasia or who were born prematurely are particularly susceptible to serious RSV infection. They may be given a specially prepared RSV immune globulin to provide temporary protection.

Whooping Cough (Pertussis). I get angry just writing about this disease. Whooping cough is a serious and dangerous infection which had nearly disappeared from the United States and many other developed nations because of the widespread use of an effective vaccine. Then, a couple of decades ago, the claim was advanced that the vaccine was more dangerous than the disease. Despite excellent evidence to the contrary, this became a media sensation and millions of alarmed parents refused to have their children immunized. In several countries, including Great Britain, Germany, Japan, Sweden, and the United States, epidemics of whooping cough returned, and the death rate from the disease climbed. When the use of the vaccine began to increase again, the incidence of the disease promptly decreased. Whooping cough is no joke. The WHO estimates that 600,000 children die every year from it. It seems to me that the publicists and physicians who promulgated the distorted and misleading scare stories about the vaccine bear a grim responsibility for the results of their efforts.

Whooping cough is caused by **Bordetella pertussis**, a bacterium that infects the lining tissues of the entire respiratory tract from nose to lungs. The illness starts with what seems like an ordinary cold that drags on for about 2 weeks; then, as the germ moves down to the bronchi, an increasingly severe, racking cough appears. The character of the cough is caused by the effort of the child to clear the sticky, heavy secretions from her air passages. After a series of repeated, hard, painful coughs, she finally brings up some phlegm and then takes in a huge breath to refill her lungs. This inspiratory effort is the "whoop" of whooping cough. During or after an exhausting series of coughs, she will vomit as well. The pattern of cough in infants may vary; they may fail to clear their airways and whoop, and, most dangerously, they may have periods without breathing which can cause brain damage or death. The severe coughing stage of pertussis lasts for about 2 weeks, and then the child begins to heal. The acute illness lasts for about 6 weeks, and the exhausted and debilitated child may have recurrent bouts of severe cough and be more prone to respiratory infection for many months thereafter. In the United States today, when babies under the age of 6 months get whooping cough, 20% get pneumonia, over 2% have convulsions during the illness, nearly 1% have brain damage, and 1% die. Adults infected with this bacterium rarely get full-blown whooping cough, but commonly develop a milder but prolonged bronchitis which is rarely recognized as such.

The whooping cough germ is spread from person to person by coughing and sneezing, the patient being most contagious during the first few weeks of the disease. The incubation period is 7 to 14 days. The attack rate is nearly 90% in nonimmune individuals.

Treatment for whooping cough is only partially satisfactory. Antibiotics shorten the course of infectivity and somewhat lessen the severity of the illness. A variety of drugs have been used with only modest success to ameliorate the cough. Babies nearly always need prolonged hospital care because of the dangers of impaired breathing and consequent brain damage.

Vaccination against whooping cough prevents the disease in most and moderates it in nearly all the rest. The old vaccine we have used since the late 1930s typically causes fever, fussiness, and local soreness where the shots are given. On rare occasions it can cause severe and frightening allergic reactions. The question of whether the old vaccine itself can cause permanent brain damage has been studied exhaustively. A massive British study and several American studies have concluded that such vaccine-caused damage is either exceedingly rare or nonexistent. From a public health point of view, the debate about vaccine safety ignores the facts: 5,000 to 10,000 American children died from the disease every year in the decade before whooping cough vaccine came into use, and only 5 to 10 American children died from whooping cough in the early 1980s, when vaccine use was at its peak. Happily, a new whooping cough vaccine has been developed which is much better tolerated. It is already in use for booster shots and probably will be approved for use for the primary vaccination series. Presumably, this will allow the controversy over whooping cough vaccination to disappear, and we will once again be able to consign this nasty disease to the dustbin of history for American children.

Influenza or "The Flu." Every fall, as regular as clockwork, our annual visitation of influenza reaches the United States. The first cases are usually reported in the eastern part of the country, and the tide slowly sweeps west until midwinter when influenza can be expected to reach California. About two years out of three, the tide is in the nature of a flood when a true epidemic of influenza occurs, and every 10 or 20 years, the flood is torrential when we suffer a worldwide pandemic of influenza. These variations in the intensity of influenza outbreaks are due to continuing changes in the virus itself. An attack of influenza confers immunity only to one specific strain of influenza because our immune systems learn to recognize the virus by the characteristics of its outer coat. When the coat changes, our immune systems may fail to recognize the invading organism early enough to prevent the disease. When a major change in the virus occurs, everyone's immune systems will be fooled, and we will all be susceptible.

Influenza is largely an infection of the respiratory tract, but the patient hurts all over. It begins suddenly with chills and fever, headache, muscle pain, and general malaise. Respiratory symptoms of runny nose, sore throat, and harsh cough soon appear. Nausea, vomiting, and abdominal pain can occur, especially with influenza type B, but this is not a major aspect of the disease. When people speak of "stomach flu," an illness whose major symptoms are in the gastrointestinal tract, they are not referring to true influenza. After about 3 days of total misery, the fever generally diminishes and by about 1 week most victims are well on the road to recovery. But not everyone is so fortunate. A substantial portion will have a continuing bronchitis, either viral or bacterial or both, or a pneumonia. Healthy children usually handle influenza infections quite well, but children with chronic diseases or impaired immunity are at increased risk from complications. Deaths from influenza are mostly among the aged.

This virus spreads via respiratory tract secretions, from person to person, or person to object to person. The incubation period is 1 to 3 days, and the period of contagiousness is about 1 week.

In general, treatment is directed at relief of symptoms, but in truth, medicines do not do a great deal of good. Bed rest will be desired by the patient at the height of the illness. Acetaminophen may help the headache and muscle pain. Children should not take aspirin or nonsteroidal anti-inflammatory drugs like ibuprofen (Advil, Nuprin) or naproxen (Aleve) because of the possible risk of Reye syndrome. Cough suppressants are welcomed. Bacterial bronchitis or pneumonia require antibiotics. Two antiviral agents, amantadine and rimantadine, can sometimes be used against influenza type A. If either is given before exposure to the virus the incidence of infection is sharply reduced. If given within 2 days after the onset of the infection, the severity and length of influenza is lessened. Amantadine has a number of unpleasant side effects which have created limited enthusiasm for its use; it may cause insomnia, depression, and other nervous system problems. Rimantadine seems to be somewhat less toxic. Neither of these drugs has any effect against influenza type B. Once an outbreak of influenza is underway, public health labs can identify the responsible viruses, so that doctors will know whether one of these antiviral drugs is likely to be useful.

Vaccination against influenza has had a checkered career. The early flu vaccines tended to cause, or at least were blamed for, fevers and other unpleasant reactions. The currently available flu vaccines cause fewer and milder side effects. The "swine flu" vaccine used in 1976-77 caused some cases of a neurologic disorder called Guillain-Barré syndrome in adults; subsequent vaccines seem to have been free of this risk. Furthermore, the viruses that cause influenza are in constant flux. If the wrong mixture of virus types are included in a given year's vaccine, it may fail to protect adequately against an unexpected new strain of influenza. Virologists have to decide many months ahead what next season's likely flu viruses will look like; their track record is generally excellent but they have been known to be mistaken. Despite these difficulties, the vaccine confers a very useful amount of protection from influenza, in the range of 70 to 80% fewer cases in vaccinated populations. This can be difficult to discern for a given individual because so many other viral infections can mimic influenza that a true protective effect may not be recognized. You may get through the winter unscathed by influenza, but a terrible cold in January and a nasty viral bronchitis in February may lead you to the erroneous conclusion that the flu shot didn't help. Because influenza viruses change so fast, and because the immunity induced by the vaccine weakens rather quickly, yearly "flu" shots are needed to keep up immunity. Most healthy kids can weather an episode of influenza nicely, so routine immunization against this disease is not recommended for all children. Those with chronic illnesses such as cystic fibrosis, chronic asthma, and certain heart diseases, children who are taking aspirin for arthritis, or who are immune-suppressed are all candidates for yearly influenza immunization. Members of families in which there are people at increased risk from influenza should also receive the vaccine.

Pneumonia. Pneumonia means infection in the alveoli or air sacs, the gas exchanging tissues of the lungs. The term pneumonitis is often used interchangeably with pneumonia, although technically pneumonitis means inflammation, rather than infection. If you have read the preceding pages about infection of the respiratory tract, you'll remember that any number of germs can cause infection from the nose to the lungs, from top to bottom in this continuous set of structures. In addition, there are some microbes whose main effect is deep within the lungs themselves. For every age of childhood, there are specific groups of agents that are likely to cause pneumonias. In early infancy the usual culprits are germs that the baby acquires from his mother during birth; prominent among these are the **group B streptococcus** and **Chlamydia trachomatis,** a sexually transmitted bacterium. In later infancy and early childhood a variety of viruses commonly cause pneumonia. These include **respiratory syncytial virus (RSV)** which is discussed in the preceding section on bronchiolitis, and the **influenza viruses,** plus lots more. Among middle-aged children over 5 years of age, a peculiar bacterium called **Mycoplasma pneumoniae** is probably the most common agent. However, at any age the common invasive bacteria **Haemophilus influenzae type b,** the **pneumococcus (Streptococcus pneumoniae)** and a handful of other ordinary denizens of the nose and throat can cause serious and even life-threatening infections.

It is not possible to outline a general clinical picture of a case of pneumonia since the disease varies so widely depending on the age of the patient and the germs involved. For example, Chlamydial pneumonia is likely to be a mild illness of infants in the first months of life, characterized by cough and rapid breathing and not much else. In contrast, pneumococcal pneumonia in an older child is a dramatic and dangerous infection with an abrupt onset of high fever, severe cough, painful breathing, and the appearance of extreme toxicity. In the middle-aged child with Mycoplasma pneumoniae infection, there is a nasty cough which just drags on and on, but not much fever. This disease is often termed "walking pneumonia" because the patients are rarely sick enough to stay in bed. Because of the variety of germs which may be involved, it is impossible to specify mode of spread of infection, period of contagiousness, or incubation period. A fairly safe assumption is that a patient is contagious at least as long as the fever continues, but there are exceptions to even this simple guideline.

Pneumonias are not easy to assess because it is difficult to be sure which germ is causing the trouble. Most tests for virus infection take too long to be of any assistance, and there is no simple way of discovering what bacterium may be causing infection deep inside the lungs. For that matter, it can be hard to know if the lungs are actually involved at all, or whether the infection is limited to the upper and middle respiratory tract. X-rays are a big help, but we really don't want to use any more radiation on our patients than is absolutely necessary. Certain infections cause characteristic changes in the white blood count, and there are a few other lab tests that can give helpful hints. But when push comes to shove, the pediatrician depends on her clinical judgment and her prior knowledge of the patient in deciding how a particular child and his pneumonia should be treated. For the bacterial pneumonias, antibiotics are great. For the viral pneumonias, treating the symptoms to keep the child comfortable is about the best we can do. Cough suppressants, perhaps something for fever, tempting drinks and ice cream to provide fluid and calories for the sick child who has lost his appetite, and lots of tender, loving care—that is the complete list.

Cystic Fibrosis: See Chapter 40 — Gastrointestinal Problems, page 382.

Tuberculosis. Writing about tuberculosis is a sad task because this is the story of a partial public health success which has become a public health failure. Tuberculosis is an infection caused by **Mycobacterium tuberculosis** and less often by related organisms. It can affect any part of the body but the main sites of infection are the lungs and lymph nodes. This is an ancient disease which has been recognized for many centuries, all over the world. During the time of the rise of great cities in the nineteenth century, the combination of crowding and poverty seems to have led to an increased prevalence of the disease. It became known as the "white plague," and was one of the leading causes of death. During our own century, the gradual improvement in the lives of city people began to limit the depredations of tuberculosis. Pasteurization of milk plus the control of tuberculosis in herds of milk cows led to the decline of milk-borne TB. Public health measures including case finding and the provision of treatment in sanitariums removed some contagious cases from the community. After the World War II, the development of antituberculous antibiotics made a cure possible. The rates of infection and death from TB dropped dramatically in every developed country. Then, in the 1980s, public health funds for TB control were cut, health services for the poor became less available, and the conditions of life in our decaying inner cities worsened. People with AIDS are particularly susceptible to TB and exceedingly hard to diagnose when they have it. As AIDS spread, especially among drug abusers, TB spread as well. Even worse, many cases are now resistant to the inexpensive and easily administered antiTB agents which once worked so well. Costly and complicated multiple antibiotic regimes are now often required. Increased public health efforts instituted in the past few years seem to have brought the rate of new infections down, but TB remains a substantial problem in our country. In the developing world, TB has never been well controlled; worldwide, it continues to infect 8 to 10 million and kill 3 to 5 million people every year.

When a child inhales TB-infected droplets, the organisms make an initial infection in the lung tissue and the lymph nodes of the chest. Most of the time there is no sign of illness, and after a period of 6 months to several years, the body successfully walls off the infected areas with fibrous tissue. TB organisms may persist for decades in these scarred areas, and they may become reactivated and cause disease at any time later in life. Teenagers are particularly vulnerable to the development of adult-type, chronic TB from these previously quiescent spots on the lung. Sometimes the child's body fails to control the initial TB infection and a variety of serious consequences can follow, depending on where the expanding infection goes. The most dangerous TB infections are spread through the blood stream, causing disease in the brain, liver, bone marrow, and nearly everywhere else in the body.

Adult-type, reactivation tuberculosis can occur at any time of life. Symptoms are typically those of a chronic lung infection including cough, low fever, weight loss, and malaise. Sometimes the disease is so mild in its manifestations that Grandpa's chronic cough will go undiagnosed and untreated for many months, until a grandchild's brand new tuberculous infection leads to examination of the rest of the family in the search for the source.

TB can be diagnosed with the help of the tuberculin skin test. A minute amount of noninfectious protein material derived from TB organisms is injected into the skin of the forearm. If you have been exposed to TB and developed sensitivity to the organism, a swollen red area will usually appear in 2 to 3 days. Once you have developed skin test positivity as a result of infection, future skin tests throughout your life will nearly always be positive. Therefore, the test simply indicates that you have been exposed to the germ at some time in the past. TB organisms can also be grown directly from sputum coughed up by the patient; children swallow any sputum they produce so we examine stomach contents instead. Chest x-rays are also invaluable.

In the days before antibiotics, the quite unsatisfactory therapy of tuberculosis was limited to bed rest, partial collapse of the lung in an effort to rest it, and a good diet. Lots of patients died. Today, most are cured within a year or less by strict adherence to a regimen of antiTB drug treatment. A crucial part of treatment is case finding. Primary childhood TB is rarely contagious; each new case is due to an adult contact with active TB, and that contact must be sought.

Prevention of this disease is a public health issue. Poverty, crowding, undernourishment, drug abuse, and AIDS fueled the comeback of tuberculosis, and will continue to keep TB a major American problem until we develop the social will to attack these issues in more effective ways. A live vaccine against TB **(BCG; Bacillus Calmette–Guerin)** has been available for many years, and has proven to be of some limited use. In many European countries every child is routinely vaccinated with one or another strain of this weakened, live, cow tuberculosis organism. In the United States, BCG has had its largest use among Native Americans whose children are particularly prone to TB. In general, BCG has not been considered to be worthwhile in our country, in part because it induces a positive tuberculin response which can make diagnosis of active TB more difficult.

Because adult-type TB may remain a mild illness for considerable periods of time, and because it is so effectively spread by coughing, it is crucial to make sure that adults involved with the care of children do not have active tuberculosis. In many parts of the United States today, our childcare workers are disproportionately likely to be blacks, Hispanics, and recent immigrants from Latin America or Asia, all groups with high rates of the disease. *Yearly TB testing of adults employed in child care and education is a necessity.* At the risk of making you paranoid, I must remind you that this includes all the adults who are in close and frequent contact with your children—babysitters, house cleaners, day care providers, and your in-laws. If they have negative TB tests today, the tests should be repeated every year. If they have positive TB tests, they need to see their doctors to find out whether or not they are contagious and if they require treatment.

Chapter 33

Infections of
The Gastrointestinal Tract

Acute infections of the gastrointestinal tract are among the most common diseases of childhood. A variety of microorganisms, most of them viral, can be involved. The stomach and the duodenum (the uppermost portion of the small intestine) may be affected, along with the rest of the small intestine and sometimes the large intestine as well. These vary from mild cases of "stomach flu" to dangerous episodes of vomiting and diarrhea that can cause severe or fatal dehydration. These illnesses, are distinct from the less common and often longer lasting conditions called **gastritis, duodenitis,** and **peptic ulcer** in which the stomach lining or the duodenal lining are inflamed and sometimes ulcerated, without any involvement of the rest of the gastrointestinal tract. Some cases of gastritis or duodenitis are caused by irritants like aspirin or alcohol, or develop in response to extreme physical stresses like major surgery or a bad burn. But most cases are puzzlers.

These children have chronic or recurrent abdominal pain, often in the night, sometimes with vomiting, sometimes relieved by eating. Like adults with similar complaints, they are often unusually tense and rather driven people. For a long time, we thought these kids were suffering from a psychosomatic disease, and our treatment was a combination of medicine to relieve the symptoms plus psychotherapy to deal with the underlying patterns of behavior. This approach was successful in the short term, but quite a few children had relapses in later childhood or in adult life. Then, a little over ten years ago, two Australian doctors proved that **Helicobacter pylori,** a previously ignored bacterium that lives in the stomach and duodenum, can cause gastritis. Since then, the world of gastroenterology has been in an uproar, largely because no one wanted to admit that we had ignored this little bug for so long. The consensus that has recently emerged is that H. pylori does play an important role in this group of diseases, and therapy for ulcer-type symptoms now includes antibiotics as well as ordinary antiulcer drugs. It remains to be seen whether the long-term results will be any better than in the old, preHelicobacter days, but so far, it appears that the addition of antibiotic treatment results in more real cures, with far fewer relapses. The question of a psychological component to this illness seems to have been put aside for the moment while gastroenterologists try to incorporate the infectious component into their understanding.

Gastroenteritis (Stomach Flu; Turista). Acute infection of the gastrointestinal tract may be caused by viruses, bacteria, or parasites like giardia and various amoebae. Worldwide, there are billions of these illnesses and they kill about 4,000,000 children every year, mostly in developing countries. In the United States 400 children die annually from these infections. ***Take this disease seriously; gastroenteritis kills children.***

These are acute illnesses, often, but not always, starting with vomiting and abdominal pain, and progressing to diarrhea. The big problem with gastroenteritis is the loss of body fluids, leading to the risk of dehydration. If the child is vomiting as well as having diarrhea, replenishing fluids by mouth becomes difficult, and dehydration is worsened. In mild cases, the child may not act terribly unwell, the volume and frequency of watery stools is not great, and the illness comes and goes in a few days. With increasing severity of the infection, all the symptoms are worse, fever is likely to be higher, appetite declines, and the child begins to look dry; the lips and mouth become dry, tears are scant, the area around the eyes may look dark and lined. When dehydration is severe, the eyes look sunken and in infants the fontanel (soft spot) on top of the head is depressed. Children who are dehydrated to this extent are dangerously ill. They require prompt and careful replenishment of their body fluids which, in this country, is usually accomplished with intravenous fluids. It can sometimes be done with fluids administered by mouth under expert supervision.

Because there are so many different microbes that cause these illnesses periods of contagiousness or incubation vary depending on each type of germ. In general, these illnesses are likely to be spread through fecal contamination of water, food, or objects such as shared toys or the hands of adult caretakers. There are also some viral agents which are spread via nasal and mouth secretions. To cause even more confusion, seemingly identical illnesses are caused by food poisoning which is not an actual infection with a germ, but is due to toxins produced by germs which have had the opportunity to grow in unrefrigerated foods.

Treatment is aimed primarily at the replacement of lost body fluids. In most instances the body eventually rids itself of the causative organism, so that antibiotic treatment is not usually indicated. Antidiarrheal drugs have only a tiny place in the management of these diseases. The commonly used antidiarrheals like diphenoxylate (Lomotil) and loperamide (Imodium, etc.) are narcotic derivatives which work by partially paralyzing the gut. They certainly decrease the number of stools, but they have a variety of dangers which limits their usefulness and safety with children. One concern is that the paralyzed gut is less able to rid itself of the invading organism, giving it that much more opportunity to do damage. Another class of alleged antidiarrheals are the absorbents like kaolin and pectin (Kaopectate). These thicken the stool but don't do anything useful for the disease process; they are a waste of time and money. Bismuth subsalicylate (Pepto-Bismol) is a mild intestinal antiseptic as well as an absorbent; it may sometimes be worth using although there is concern because it is a salicylate and may therefore be linked to Reye syndrome. Another absorbent is cholestryamine, a gritty powder which is so unpalatable that it is nearly impossible for small children to use. Antivomiting agents are needed on rare occasions.

Fluid therapy has two parts: The replacement of lost mineral salts and water, and the provision of salts and water to provide for ongoing requirements. Water alone is not enough; the fluids lost in vomit and diarrhea carry away a considerable amount of the mineral salts the body needs for its functioning. If the illness is mild and brief, it is possible to manage the salts and water requirements with a wide range of liquids. Even if an optimal balance of mineral substances is not provided, the clever kidneys of a healthy child can make do nicely. But when vomiting or diarrhea are severe, it becomes imperative to provide the right stuff—sodium, potassium, and water in the correct amounts, plus sugar as a source of calories and because it helps the intestine to absorb water and sodium. During diarrhea there is impairment of the intestine's ability to absorb sugars, and this has led to the suggestion that milk sugar (lactose) in particular should be avoided. In practice, lactose-free solutions don't seem significantly better than any others so this advice is now less widely offered. Solutions with a high concentration of any sugar will overwhelm the ability of the injured gut to deal with the sugar, and the diarrhea may actually worsen. For that reason it important to avoid very sweet liquids like apple juice or grape juice, unless they are diluted about one half. Sweet solids like Jell-O are also too concentrated, but liquid Jell-O made with twice as much water as usual may be well tolerated.

For mild and brief episodes of vomiting and diarrhea:
1. Stop all solid foods until the vomiting has stopped.
2. Offer very small amounts of liquid every few minutes for the first hour or two; the volume can be as small as 1 teaspoon at a time for an infant, 1 or 2 ounces for a middle-aged child. Breast fed babies should be nursed briefly

and frequently, or they may be given one of the fluids listed below. If the vomiting stops, slowly increase the volume of each liquid feeding and decrease the frequency, The goal is to maintain the child's normal fluid intake and to replace the fluids lost in vomitus and stools. This is difficult to estimate with any accuracy, but figure on ½ to 1 cup of solution for every average-sized stool. Be aware that super-absorbent diapers can hide a lot of stool volume. ***If the vomiting does not stop, your child needs to be seen by a doctor.***

3.   Most illnesses with vomiting and diarrhea are accompanied by loss of appetite. Since providing fluids is most important during the acute illness, there is no need to insist on solid foods. As soon as his appetite allows, resume offering his usual foods. Those likely to be accepted and best tolerated are starchy and bland foods like bread, crackers, pasta, white rice, dry or cooked cereals, plain cookies (like animal crackers), potatoes, bananas, apples, yogurt, and soft vegetables. Meats, eggs, and cottage cheese can be added later. Wait before adding sweetened fruit juices, solid Jell-O, heavily sweetened cereals, dried fruits like raisins, or undiluted soft drinks because they may provide more sugar than the gut can handle early in the illness. Fatty foods can slow digestion, so take your time before reintroducing them. Do not give high fiber foods like whole grain or bran cereals and raw vegetables which can be intestinal irritants.

4.   The body needs water, sugar (which can be supplied as either simple sugar or as easily digested starches), and two crucial minerals—sodium and potassium. An ideal solution to maintain the body's functioning and to replace losses from vomiting and diarrhea must contain all these elements. WHO/UNICEF Oral Rehydration Solution, Infalyte, Pedialyte, and generic Pediatric Electrolyte solutions are properly balanced solutions which can be used by themselves. Flavored electrolyte solutions can be made into frozen "juice" bars.

Several substitutes can be used for mild illnesses if balanced electrolyte solutions are not quickly available; note that *none* of these solutions by itself provides an ideal mixture of water, sodium, potassium, and sugar. Simple combinations of solutions can be chosen which are satisfactory for the treatment of mild dehydration.

•   Gatorade has inadequate amounts of sodium, a little potassium, and excess sugar.

•   Apple juice has little sodium, adequate potassium, but excess sugar.

- Chicken broth has excess sodium, little potassium, and no sugar.
- Soda pop has hardly any sodium or potassium, and excess sugar.
- Tea (real tea, not herb tea) with a rounded teaspoon of sugar for every 8-ounce cup provides very little sodium, a small amount of potassium, and adequate sugar.
- Rice water is the liquid in which rice has been boiled. Its composition varies but it generally provides little sodium, adequate potassium, and adequate sugar.
- Rice gruel made from infant rice cereal is a fairly well balanced solution. Use ½ to 1 cup powdered infant rice cereal, 2 cups water, and ¼ teaspoon table salt.

Depending on the age and preferences of the child, it is possible to supply reasonably adequate amounts of the essential nutrients with various combinations of these liquids. Either **tea with sugar, plus a little chicken broth,** or **rice water, plus a little chicken broth,** is good. **Diluted apple juice, plus a little chicken broth** is also well tolerated. If solid foods are also being taken, variable but probably adequate amounts of sodium, potassium, and sugars are likely to be present. Bananas are a good potassium source and are usually happily accepted.

Avoiding Turista. Safe water supplies, and properly produced and carefully inspected meats, fish, and poultry are among the foundation stones of basic public health. Increased public investment in these services certainly decreases the incidence of these illnesses. Cholera epidemics in our country stopped when we chlorinated our water; food-borne illnesses like trichinosis and cow tuberculosis are now vanishingly rare, thanks to government supervision of agriculture and food production. Of course, problems still exist, such as the 1994 outbreak of a devastating disease, hemolytic-uremic syndrome, caused by a germ spread through fast-food hamburgers. But as soon as we travel to areas where public health is ignored, we are subject to a myriad of food and water-borne illnesses. The standard rules are a help: Drink only boiled or treated water; eat uncooked fruits and vegetables only if they can be peeled; avoid soft drinks and frozen desserts because they may be made with contaminated water; avoid foods most prone to spoilage like unrefrigerated meats and sauces. Prevention by the use of prophylactic anti-infection drugs is partially successful, but there are difficulties. The multiplicity of infectious organisms makes it impossible to protect against them all. Furthermore, the use of these drugs will inevitably increase the prevalence of organisms resistant to their effects. Lastly, each of the prophylactic agents has side effects, some of which are worse than gastroenteritis. In short, travel in the developing world is a hazardous business; think twice before exposing babies and young children to these illnesses.

Intestinal Parasites: Giardia, Worms, Amoebae. The most popular intestinal parasite of the decade is **Giardia lamblia.** In countries with unsafe water supplies, giardia has been and remains a major problem; St. Petersburg, Russia, for example, is famous for the permanent population of giardia in its drinking water. Until recently, giardiasis was something of a rarity for American children. The little organism lived a quiet life in the small intestines of various animals, was excreted in their stools, and contaminated streams and lakes. Unwary hikers drank the water and after a week or more developed nasty infections with bellyache and diarrhea. Sometimes pet owners managed to get the disease from their infected dogs or cats. Then a major change in the ecology of giardia occurred—the advent of mass day care. What had been an oddity became an everyday disease as the germ spread on stool-contaminated hands and objects in the warehouses for babies we call day care centers. Baby A excretes giardia cysts in her stool; Caretaker B changes her diaper; then, without washing her hands, Caretaker B prepares Baby C's bottle and transfers a few cysts to the unfortunate recipient. In a week or two, Baby C gets good and sick. After recovery from the acute illness, she continues to excrete giardia cysts for weeks or months, and shares them with Baby D and Baby E, etc. Even more effective than the day care method of spread is the practice of swimming lessons for the very young. Both the neophyte swimmers and their adult teachers can confidently be expected to acquire the organism.

The diagnosis of giardiasis used to be difficult and expensive, but a new stool test can quickly and accurately detect giardia antigen. Treatment with one of several drugs eventually cures the disorder, but repeated courses of medicine may be required.

Worms. Of the many worms that can cause infections within the human intestines, **pinworms (Enterobius vermicularis)** are the most common in American children. The female pinworms, tiny white things about ½ inch long, live in the intestines until they are ready to lay their abundant eggs. They migrate down through the anus onto the surrounding skin or up to the vulva and vagina, trailing eggs as they go. This process typically takes place at about 11o'clock at night, and the unhappy child who has been host to the pinworms is awakened by intense anal or vulvo-vaginal itching. If the child is too young to report with any accuracy what is troubling her, parents may be confronted by an exceedingly upset and miserable kid who knows that she is miserable but doesn't quite know why. Examination of the area around the anus and of the genital area may reveal one or more worms, sometimes dead, sometimes alive and wriggling. If pinworms are not seen but the symptoms suggest their presence, sticky cellophane tape can be pressed against the perianal skin and then attached to a glass slide; examination under a microscope will show the pinworm eggs. These sticky tapes may need to be collected every morning for several days to find the culprits.

First aid can be given by sitting the child in a cool bath; the itching stops quite promptly. Next morning, call your doctor for a prescription for one of the excellent pinworm-killing drugs. The eggs are light as feathers and will float all over the house, settling on every surface, to await ingestion via someone's fingers. Luckily, most of the eggs die a natural death within a few days, but a few may persist for 2 or even 3 weeks. During this period it is easy to get reinfected, so a follow-up dose of medicine is always a good idea. It is a complete waste of time to try to rid the environment of pinworm eggs; there are just too many of them. If repeated infections occur, just treat the whole family every 2 weeks for about 3 cycles of medication. Many families react to pinworm infestations as they do to lice with annoyance, disgust, and embarrassment. None of these responses is much use; playing host to these little fellow travelers is not a sign of moral turpitude or social failure. Just kill them, and get on with living.

Another intestinal parasite worth mentioning is the **roundworm (Ascaris lumbroides).** These earthworm-sized organisms have a complex life cycle requiring human fecal contamination of soil, incubation of the roundworm larvae in the soil, and then contamination by the larvae of water or food. Depending on the number of worms living in the intestine, and also on the presence of larva or adult worms in several body tissues, the host may have no symptoms at all or he may have a wide variety of troubles ranging from pneumonia to an itchy rash to intestinal obstruction. But more often than not, the infestation is light, and the first and only sign of roundworms is the surprising and rather revolting appearance of one or more of them in the diaper or the toilet. Treatment with any of several drugs is usually simple and effective.

Amebiasis is an infection with one of the single celled protozoan organisms called **amoeba** or **ameba.** Many amoebae live harmlessly in our intestinal tracts, but some can cause disease. The most important of these is **Entamoeba histolytica** which is common in tropical countries, and fairly common in the American South and Southwest. It spreads by way of fecal contamination from person to person or through food and water. Amoebic infections can cause a wide variety of intestinal complaints, the most dramatic of which is a bloody diarrhea. Treatment with antiamoebic drugs is somewhat complex but effective.

Hepatitis means inflammation of the liver, a process which can be caused by a considerable number of infectious agents. Some of these are viruses which do most or all of their damage to the liver itself, and these are the causes of what is generally termed hepatitis. But there are also viruses and some other germs which cause liver inflammation as one part of their attack on the human body; **infectious mononucleosis** caused by the Epstein-Barr virus is an example. When we talk about hepatitis per se, we are not referring to any of these other agents. So far, five different and quite unrelated viruses have been discovered which cause five somewhat different types of hepatitis. The important types in our country are **hepatitis A, B, and C; D** or **delta,** and **E** are uncommon. **C** and **E** were previously termed **non–A** and **non–B.**

Hepatitis A is a very common liver infection that usually causes a fairly mild disease marked by fever, loss of appetite, nausea and vomiting, dark-colored urine, light-colored stools and the development of jaundice, a yellow discoloration of the skin and the whites of the eyes. Most of the time, the infection is so mild that few if any symptoms are ever noticed; 30% of adult Americans have evidence in their blood of having had hepatitis A in the past, but most of them never knew it. The virus spreads through fecal contamination from person to person, or through fecal contamination of food and water. The period of contagiousness is 1 to 3 weeks, mostly before the acute illness symptoms appear; the incubation period is about 1 month.

Treatment of hepatitis used to be strict bed rest, presumably on the theory that one should not exercise a sick liver. But livers are not muscles, and there is really no way to rest a liver. So, treatment at the moment is limited to as much rest as the patient seems to want, plus avoidance of alcoholic beverages, since they are known to be toxic to the liver. Recovery may take a month or more.

A vaccine against hepatitis A has recently been approved. It is not yet clear how this agent will be used, but it may prove to be helpful in the immunization of day care and other child care workers, to avoid unnecessary illness in group care settings where hepatitis A tends to spread. It can also be used by travelers to areas of high hepatitis A incidence, by health care workers, and others with an increased risk of the disease. Temporary protection against hepatitis A is afforded by immune globulin (gamma globulin). This is commonly used for travelers and also to protect family and other contacts of newly diagnosed patients.

Hepatitis B is a quite different and decidedly more serious disease. The hepatitis B virus spreads through body fluids, including blood, saliva, semen, and vaginal secretions. Current blood screening programs have nearly stopped the spread of this disease through blood transfusions. Abuse of injected drugs, heterosexual and homosexual intercourse, and exposure of newborns during the birth process account for most cases in the United States. Nonsexual family contact with a patient or a carrier also occurs.

The acute phase of hepatitis B infection may be asymptomatic, as it is in hepatitis A, or the child may have an overt disease, very much like that of hepatitis A. The incubation period is 1½ to 5 months, the course of the illness tends to be less acute and dramatic, but recovery is slower. The big problem with this disease is that 5 to 10% of patients become chronically infected; they continue to excrete the virus in their body fluids, so they are permanently contagious, and they have an increased risk of developing destructive liver inflammation, cirrhosis, and liver cancer. Newborns infected with the virus have an 80% risk of becoming chronically infected. Worldwide, hepatitis B is a major problem. Some population groups have very high incidences of infection. These include people from Asia, eastern Europe, much of the Middle East, Africa, the Pacific islands, the Amazon basin, and Native Americans from Alaska.

Treatment, so far, is unsatisfactory; experimental drugs have some effect but not much. This is a disease we need to prevent, and fortunately we can. Hepatitis B vaccine is a synthetic material derived from recombinant DNA technology which uses ordinary baker's yeast to produce a hepatitis antigen. The body learns to recognize it and then produces an effective antibody against the disease. This vaccine is a triumph of high technology; with it we have a real chance to rid humanity of a disease which kills untold thousands of children and adults year after year. In the case of infants born to hepatitis B infected mothers, the risk of infection is so acute that the baby also needs temporary protection. This is provided by giving the infant an injection of antihepatitis B immune globulin (HBIG) as soon as possible after birth. The combination of HBIG and the recombinant vaccine prevents the vast majority of newborn infections. Obviously, this strategy will only work if the mothers with chronic hepatitis B infection are recognized before the baby is exposed to the virus at birth. This is why universal screening is needed during pregnancy.

Hepatitis C is also spread through the blood. It was an important cause of blood-transfusion associated hepatitis until screening tests allowed infected donors to be excluded. Hepatitis C remains a risk for the users of illicit drugs and it can be spread by sexual (especially homosexual) intercourse. Like Hepatitis B, it often leads to chronic liver disease including cirrhosis and liver cancer. Treatment so far is unsatisfactory, and there is no preventive vaccine.

Chapter 34

Infections of The Genitourinary Tract

Kidney Infections (Pyelonephritis). Not only are the acute episodes of kidney infection miserable for all concerned, there is the small but real possibility of chronic infection which can lead to serious impairment of kidney function in later years.

If an older child's kidneys become infected, she is likely to have a fever, possibly some chills, often pain at one side of her mid to low back, and perhaps belly pain and vomiting. Her urine may be foul smelling, and urination may be frequent and painful if the infection involves her bladder as well as her kidneys, as it often does. In contrast, a baby with a kidney infection will be feverish and miserable, but he is unable to let his parents know where he hurts. At any age, kidney infections are sometimes low grade, smoldering affairs, with no specific symptoms whatsoever.

Kidneys can become infected in two different ways. Bacteria gain access to the bloodstream from time to time, and if enough of them land up in the kidneys, an infection may develop. This is the usual source of kidney infections in babies. For reasons that are not even slightly clear, boy babies are much more likely to develop kidney infections than girls. And they are most often babies who have not been circumcised. We don't understand this, either. In any case, kidney infections in infancy are rather rare. After infancy, kidney infections become increasingly common among girls and less frequent among boys, a pattern that persists thereafter. The other route for germs to reach the kidneys is by spreading upstream from the bladder. Bladder infections are quite common, especially in girls and women. This seems to be the result of the shortness of the female urethra; it is no great distance from the outside world to the inside of the female bladder, and it is easy for a variety of bacteria to find their way in. Once established in the bladder, bacteria may be able to reach the kidneys. The ureters, which are the tubes that connect the kidneys to the bladder, are fitted with a muscular, one-way valve which is supposed to let urine into the bladder from the ureters, but keep urine from refluxing up the ureters back to the kidneys. During urination the bladder contracts to express the urine out; if the ureters' valves are incompetent, some of the urine is flushed upstream to the kidneys, and kidney infection can result.

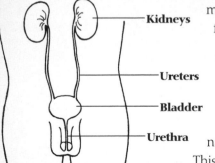

Determining the presence of a kidney infection requires a clean urine specimen, as freshly voided as can be obtained, and uncontaminated by its passage through the urethra to the waiting sterile container. This is a good trick. When the donor of the urine specimen is an older child or an adult, careful explanations, meticulous cleaning, and some manual dexterity may make this possible. In males, the foreskin must be retracted or the urine specimen will reflect the washing out of the tightly apposed inner surfaces of foreskin; examination of such a specimen is nearly useless. In females, the vulva must be cleaned and the flow of urine must come directly from the opening of the urethra, without washing over the labial surfaces. In both sexes, the only reliable part of the specimen is what is called the "midstream," which is a sample of the midportion of a single, uninterrupted act of urination. In younger children we often settle for a "bagged" specimen, collected in a plastic bag which has been attached with adhesive to the skin around the genitals. Thorough cleaning of the area before attaching the bag, removing the bag promptly when the child has voided, and refrigerating the specimen immediately will increase the value of bagged urine specimens. Alternatively, a truly accurate specimen can be collected by catheterizing the bladder (inserting a slender plastic or glass tube through the urethra and up into the bladder) or "tapping" it with a long needle inserted through the skin of the lower abdomen, just above the pubic bone. Neither of these are particularly nice things to do to small children, although skillful catheterization is not so bad.

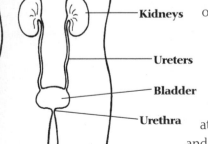

Further diagnostic study is often needed as it can be difficult to tell whether a urinary tract infection is confined to the bladder alone or whether it involves the kidneys as well. X-rays, ultra-sounds, and radioactive tracers may be necessary to clarify the situation.

EVERYDAY PEDIATRICS FOR PARENTS

Treatment of kidney infections with antibiotics generally works nicely. If there is some sort of obstruction to the flow of urine, surgical treatment may be required, but this is relatively unusual. Because recurrent and chronic kidney infections are potentially so destructive, follow-up urine studies are important. In some instances, kidney infections recur so often that a low dose of a sulfa drug or some other effective antibacterial is used for a period of months or even years.

Bladder Infections (Cystitis). A goodly number of older girls and women are plagued by bladder infections throughout their lives. As mentioned earlier, the direct and short route from the great outdoors to the inside of the female bladder is a major reason for this. Other reasons include the existence of certain bacteria which adhere to genital tissues with great persistence, and the proximity of the urethra to the anus, allowing bacteria from the gut easy access to the urinary tract. A considerable fuss is always made about teaching girls to wipe themselves with toilet paper from front to back, rather than back to front. This sounds like a reasonable idea but I don't know any studies that confirm its usefulness. After the age of puberty, sexual intercourse is a major trigger of bladder infection. Vigorous or repeated intercourse provides ample opportunity for any bacteria in the vicinity to be pushed into the urethra. So-called "honeymoon cystitis" is by no means restricted to honeymoons. Bladder infections in males are most unusual; the occurrence of even one certainly provides ample reason to search for a specific cause.

The symptoms of cystitis may be due to causes other than infection. Anything that irritates the bladder or the urethra causes an increased frequency of the urge to void, and discomfort during or after the act. This can include external chemical irritants such as bubble bath. Once in a while symptoms can be caused by an allergic reaction to something in the diet. When a bladder infection is the cause there may be fever and malaise as well. The diagnostic dilemma outlined in the discussion of kidney infections applies equally here, but most children with bladder infections are old enough to cooperate with the collection of a specimen.

Treating bladder infections is easy because the kidneys do a good job of excreting antibiotics into the urine in concentrated form; the antibiotic-rich urine bathes the bladder walls and the germs don't stand a chance. Increasing fluid intake is usually advised; the effect of this is to wash infected urine out of the bladder as rapidly as possible to prevent the bacteria from reproducing at their leisure. Several home remedies have been popular, especially drinking large amounts of cranberry juice. The theory is that the juice changes the acidity of the urine and helps kill the offending bacteria. Personally, I would rather depend on a properly chosen antibiotic, but cranberry juice is at least a good source of extra liquid. The other aspect of treatment that is often forgotten by doctors is pain relief ; the patient may not look all that sick but she really hurts. An old fashioned but effective drug is phenazopyridine (Pyridium), which has an analgesic effect on the lining membranes of the bladder and urethra. It is a dye which turns the urine an amazing orange-red color while it is being used.

When bladder infections are triggered by sexual intercourse, a simple ritual is often enough to prevent further episodes. Instructions for the patient: Before love-making, drink a glass of water and empty your bladder. After love-making, empty your bladder again. If this fails to prevent cystitis, ask your doctor for a prescription for a urinary tract antiseptic like nitrofurantoin (the macrocrystal form Macrodantoin, and other brands, is the best tolerated form of this drug); one capsule is taken before intercourse or soon afterwards. See the preceding section on kidney infections regarding other preventive measures.

Urethritis. The lining membranes of the male urethra connect with the bladder on the inside and the skin covering the head of the penis on the outside. The outside connection of the female urethra is continuous with the delicate mucous membranes of the vulva and the vagina. These differences in neighboring structures have a lot to do with the differing propensities of male and female urethras to get into trouble.

The skin covering the head of the penis, like skin everywhere, is resistant stuff, and rarely infected or irritated. Sometimes uncircumcised boys and men get an infection due to trapping of secretions from the inside of the foreskin. This is especially likely to happen if the foreskin is tight and cannot be retracted and washed. About the only time male urethas get infected is with sexually transmitted diseases where the mucous membranes of the urethra are directly exposed to infected secretions. Bladder infections in males are rare, so the combination of cystitis and urethritis, common in females, is almost never seen.

The female urethra can also be involved in any infection or irritation of the adjacent vulvar and vaginal mucous membranes. This can be a sexually transmitted disease like chlamydia or gonorrhea, or a yeast infection. Chemical irritants like bubble bath, detergent, or even shampoo in the bath water are potent causes of irritative urethritis.

In any of these circumstances, treatment will obviously depend on the particular cause. Prevention is also a matter of specifics, varying from avoiding the use of bubble bath to choosing sexual partners with care and using condoms.

Sexually Transmitted Diseases. What an uncomfortable subject for both pediatricians and parents. Thinking about the possibility of these infections in infancy and childhood automatically raises the question of sexual abuse. Thinking about them in adolescence involves facing the reality that our children become sexually active at an early age. Add to that the current nationwide hysteria about the alleged repression of child abuse memories, and parents and child care workers and teachers and pediatricians begin to look at each other with suspicion and anxiety. Who can be trusted? Who can be believed? What a scenario for paranoia.

Sexually transmitted diseases (STDs) in preadolescent children are not common, despite what is known or suspected about the ubiquity of sexual abuse of children. However, the incidence of these infections in childhood has increased in recent decades. Part of the increase may be due to more accurate diagnosis as physicians have begun to face the necessity of looking for STDs in young children. Unhappily, part of the apparent increase is surely a symptom of the fraying of the social fabric in America. In the context of family dysfunction, absent parents, inadequate and unsupervised child care outside of the home, and the continuing epidemic of drug abuse, it is hardly surprising that children become the victims of adult sexual impulses.

The list of microbial agents of STDs is long, and the list of possible symptoms even longer. Many of these diseases cause genital or urinary symptoms such as painful urination or urethral discharges, some cause skin rashes, sore throats, swollen joints, or weight loss and failure to thrive in early childhood. The symptoms are so varied that it is pointless to say to parents "Watch out for symptoms such as these; they may signal STDs."

On the other hand, it may be worthwhile for parents to be aware that unexplained behavioral changes in a child or an adolescent *may* be signs of sexual abuse. These include depression, school avoidance or failure, eating disorders, and fearful responses to previously accepted adults, for example. The trouble with a list like this is that a myriad of other causes may be involved instead. Leaping to the conclusion that sexual abuse is happening can easily be both mistaken and damaging. Focusing on sexual abuse when that is *not* the problem can deflect attention away from an accurate understanding, and raising the issue of sexual abuse within a family, a classroom, or a school can have devastating effects on innocent people. Physical signs suggesting sexual abuse include any signs of vulvar or vaginal trauma, hymeneal scars, and any sort of genital or anal bruising. It has turned out to be quite difficult to separate innocent injuries from inflicted trauma. A straddle bruise from a playground fall can look just the same as a sexually inflicted injury. The hymen can be injured by rape but it can also be torn by masturbation. A rush to judgment in these situations can be a costly, even tragic mistake.

So, what can you do to keep your kids safe? **1) Hold on to a sense of proportion.** Automobile accidents are a bigger threat to our kids than babysitters; cigarette smoking kills more people than syphilis. **2) Don't inadvertently put your child in harm's way.** Make sure that adequate supervision is available at day care, at summer camp, and in school. Big, impersonal institutions may not screen their employees as well as they should. Small group settings where the adult workers are few and know each other well may minimize risks. **3) Listen carefully when a still, small voice inside tells you that something is not well with your child's behavior. 4) Don't expect kids to protect themselves.** The recent fad of trying to teach young children to fend off unwanted and inappropriate adult advances assumes a degree of maturity and power that children are not likely to have. It is our job to protect them, not theirs.

Chapter 35

Infections of The Nervous System

This brief chapter is a joy to write. Two major infections of the nervous system, poliomyelitis and bacterial meningitis, were once among the worst health concerns of American parents and pediatricians. Today, because of the development of safe and effective immunization, polio is conquered in our country and we are well on the way to controlling it all over the world. The leading cause of bacterial meningitis has also met its match in a vaccine, and the incidence of that terrible disease has fallen rapidly in countries where the Hib vaccine is in use.

Poliomyelitis (Polio; Infantile Paralysis). The year before the first poliomyelitis vaccine was introduced 18,000 Americans developed paralytic polio. Some of them recovered completely, but many were left with crippling disabilities and some required assistance in breathing for the rest of their lives. When Jonas Salk's inactivated polio vaccine became available in 1956, the whole world celebrated. Within a few years we were presented with Albert Sabin's live vaccine. The ease and economy of administration of this oral vaccine made it the standard in the United States, and polio due to wild poliovirus has disappeared here except for rare cases contracted overseas. However, the live, oral vaccine is responsible for a handful of cases of paralysis, about 1 case for every 700,000 first doses of vaccine. Subsequent doses are nearly devoid of risk, about 1 case for 6,900,000 doses. There are also a few cases in family contacts of vaccinated children; the risk is increased for people who have immune deficiencies. The total number of vaccine related cases in the United States averages 9 per year. There is increased interest in using a combination of killed Salk vaccine plus follow-up doses of live Sabin vaccine; this should decrease the risk of vaccine related polio even further. Debate among the experts continues but I expect that this will become the new routine.

In many parts of the developing world, polio vaccine campaigns have already controlled the disease, but polio is still present in Africa and much of Asia. In the developed world, polio continues to flare up where groups of people have remained unprotected, usually for reasons of religious belief. Polio has also returned to the former Soviet Union and Yugoslavia where public health practices have collapsed. No matter where you live or travel, it is important to be fully immunized against this disease.

Bacterial Meningitis. During all my years as a pediatrician, there was nothing I dreaded more than the telephone call from a parent telling me that a child had a fever and a stiff neck. Maybe it was just stiff from an inflamed gland, maybe it was just a muscle strain, but perhaps it was bacterial meningitis.

Meningitis is an infection of the membranes that surround the brain. Many microbes can cause meningitis, among them a wide variety of viruses and several bacteria. Viral meningitis may be a mild, nearly trivial disease, with headache and fever for a few days, or it can be a severe illness capable of causing permanent brain damage. Even the ordinary viral illnesses of childhood like measles, mumps, and chickenpox sometimes cause meningitis, but bacterial meningitis is the biggest concern. Before the advent of the antibiotic age, bacterial meningitis was nearly always fatal. Even with antibiotics, these infections remain dangerous, hard to treat, and capable of causing permanent disability or death.

Bacterial meningitis usually makes the child act dramatically sick; high fever, obvious discomfort, loss of appetite, increasing immobility—all the signs that an important illness is underway. There are, of course, exceptions. Some cases start slowly and progress bit by bit: a sick child who just does not seem to be improving, a fever that hangs on, an undefined misery. When the doctor discovers that the child cannot comfortably flex his neck, a spinal tap will be done, the sample of spinal fluid will be examined for pus cells and bacteria, and the diagnosis made. Treatment consists of intravenous antibiotics in the hospital. In addition, a cortisone-like drug is often given to reduce brain inflammation; this is thought to decrease the risk of nerve damage and subsequent deafness. In all children who have recovered from meningitis it is crucial to obtain follow-up studies of hearing.

Of the several bacteria that can cause meningitis in childhood, **Haemophilus influenzae type b** has been the most common. Hib vaccine has been available for several years and it has nearly eliminated the disease in countries like ours, wealthy enough to afford widespread use. In the rare instances where the disease still occurs, it is important to protect susceptible children by prophylactic use of an antibiotic for family contacts. There are as yet no effective vaccines against the other common bacterial causes of meningitis.

Chapter 36

Miscellaneous Diseases

Cat Scratch Disease. Families who decide to keep pets should realize that, like nearly everything else in life, pets are a package deal. If you keep turtles, you can expect to be harboring Salmonella germs in the terrarium; dogs carry fleas and canine tapeworms; ferrets spread Camplyobacter diarrhea and also have a nasty tendency to chew off various human body parts; and cats? Well, cats cause a wonderful variety of human allergic reactions, they also carry fleas which they willingly share with their human housemates, and kittens, those darling, fuzzy, playful, little things, carry cat scratch fever.

The microbe that causes this disease eluded investigators for years, but it has recently been identified as a **rickettsia, Bartonella henselea.** The rickettsia are miniature bacteria which live as parasites within animal cells, and usually spread to their human hosts via ticks, lice, or fleas. This particular rickettsia is different in that it seems to be spread directly by a scratch or, less commonly, a bite. A week or so later, when the scratch has probably already healed and been forgotten, a small pimple develops; days or weeks later, a neighborhood lymph gland becomes swollen and sore, and the patient may become sick and feverish.

Most of the time, the whole process simmers down slowly all by itself without the necessity for treatment. Sometimes the sore lymph gland requires draining; there are also rare complications, especially in immune-deficient persons. Severe infections seem to respond fairly well to antibiotic therapy.

Prevention is simple: Avoid cats, especially young cats. If this is not possible, don't give it a lot of thought; it is a rare disease of no great importance.

Chronic Fatigue Syndrome (Epidemic Neuromyasthenia; "Yuppie Flu"). This alleged disease is such a can of worms that it is tempting to pretend it doesn't exist and ignore it altogether. A substantial body of opinion in the medical community holds that there is actually no such disease; a fair number of doctors are not so sure; and a small number are noisily convinced that chronic fatigue syndrome is both real and important.

Whatever the cause or causes, there are older children, adolescents, and adults who become ill with a variety of hard to describe "virusy" bugs, the sort of illness with a little fever and some respiratory or intestinal symptoms that can be expected to disappear in a few days. Instead of recovering, these people stay sick. They are headachy, depressed, feel weak, are easily fatigued, have muscle discomfort, cannot concentrate on anything, and, in general, give a convincing imitation of someone with a nasty, chronic, infectious disease. However, thorough medical investigation is nearly always negative. Some patients show evidence in their blood of past infection with any of several viruses, but actually no more than can be found in the blood samples of healthy persons who are symptom-free. Several aspects of this illness have suggested a psychological cause. It has frequently been described as occurring in outbreaks among young people in schools or other living groups. The element of suggestibility in these circumstances appears to be a factor, as it is in a number of well-studied outbreaks of hysterical symptoms. Furthermore, psychological evaluation reveals that many of these patients had significant depression and anxiety *before* becoming ill. My own suspicion is that this is a wastebasket diagnosis which includes a quite small number of people with a specific post-viral neurological disorder, plus a decidedly larger number of people whose symptoms are actually psychological. However, given the present state of our knowledge, I fail to understand how anyone can speak about the causes of this condition with much assurance. For further discussion of the problem of adolescent fatigue in general see the section on the Hypochondria of Change on page 166.

When chronic fatigue syndrome is a possibility both patient and doctor are left with a dilemma. The doctor does not want to miss the diagnosis of an illness for which effective treatment might be instituted. The patient does not want to be left with the statement that "It's all in your head." It is rarely clear how anyone should proceed. In this situation, the predictable happens: The patient hears that wonderful cures of the disease are available through chiropracty, aromatherapy, yeast-free diets, or with the help of herbs or acupuncture. Whether the eventual improvement of patients with chronic fatigue syndrome is due to these or any other therapies is unknown and unknowable by either practitioners or patients. It is worth remembering that the human body has wonderful recuperative powers *all by itself.*

Infectious Mononucleosis (Mono; Epstein–Barr Virus Infection). The virus called Epstein-Barr is one of the most faithful fellow travelers of the human race. One way or another, nearly all of us manage to become infected with this member of the herpesvirus family. Most of these infections are so mild that we are wholly unaware that we have been colonized; the virus takes up residence in our noses and throats, and stays there for months or forever. During at least the early part of this process, the saliva is contagious, and the virus spreads by kissing or on saliva-contaminated objects. We still do not know how long people remain capable of sharing their infection.

A minority of people infected by this virus develop the syndrome called infectious mononucleosis, "mono" for short. The incubation period from exposure to illness is a month or even longer. The clinical picture is that of a slowly worsening illness with fatigue, headache, a little fever, and increasing malaise. These symptoms are often ignored until the sore throat begins; it is usually so severe that it must be attended to. By the time he sees his doctor, the typical patient feels truly terrible. The physician's examination reveals a red throat partly covered with thick, gray secretions, swollen lymph glands below and behind the ears, and a swollen, tender liver and spleen. If the liver is badly involved, there may be jaundice as well. Because the virus can spread widely throughout the body, a shopping basket of other, less common symptoms may also be found. The usual case worsens during its second week and then improvement gradually begins. By the end of the third week, the patient is feeling fairly human although his energy and stamina may not return completely for weeks to come.

In babies and very young children the symptoms are often less well-defined. The child may have a sore throat, or just the swollen liver and spleen, or just seem generally unwell with no localizing signs. When people with immune deficiencies become infected, they may suffer quite severe illnesses from E-B virus; AIDS patients may get a pneumonia from it.

Treatment is symptomatic: aspirin or acetaminophen or ibuprofen for the sore throat; sometimes one has to add codeine as well. Don't let anyone give the patient amoxicillin or ampicillin because it can trigger a dramatic rash. Cortisone-like drugs are sometimes used for certain severe complications but should be avoided when possible. Recovery is slow, and it is difficult for the teenaged patient to believe that it will ever arrive, but it does.

The relationship between the E-B virus and the so-called chronic fatigue syndrome was the subject of much interest in the recent past. There is no doubt that a few patients with mono experience a very slow recovery, with periods of apparent relapse alternating with periods of improvement. These eventually resolve, but it can take many months. It was therefore natural to search for evidence of a preceding E-B virus infection in patients with chronic fatigue syndrome who had no obvious acute mono infection. Expert opinion now generally holds that there is no evidence of a causal relationship, but, as is often the case in medical matters, there is still some controversy on this issue.

Since we all acquire an E-B virus infection at some time in our lives, it is clear that no preventive measures are known. In the developing world, E-B virus infection is typical within the first year of life, presumably because of increased ease of spread of the virus in crowded quarters. These infections are more likely to be mild than full-fledged mono acquired at a later age, an interesting unintended disadvantage of economic progress.

Kawasaki Disease. Here is an example of that peculiar and puzzling category, newly discovered diseases. In 1967 a Japanese pediatrician, Tomisaku Kawasaki, recognized what appears to be a brand new illness. It is characterized by redness of the eyes, throat, mouth, and lips; a generalized rash; a firm swelling of the hands and feet; and a swollen lymph node in the neck. During the course of the illness other areas of the body can become involved including the joints, heart, and blood vessels. The patients generally get better after a few weeks, but some develop serious heart problems, and a few die. Most of the patients are under the age of 5; more boys than girls are affected. It soon became clear that the disease is seen worldwide, although the incidence is much higher in Asians. Despite nearly three decades of study, a cause has yet to be found. Kawasaki disease looks like an infectious process, but it does not seem to spread from person to person. It is not a particularly common illness; in the United States about 2000 to 4000 cases are found every year.

Happily, treatments have been devised which effectively shorten the course of the illness and appear to minimize the long term problems. A combination of immune globulin (gamma globulin) given intravenously plus aspirin by mouth is administered as early in the illness as possible.

Kawasaki disease remains the focus of intense investigative interest. Obviously, preventive measures cannot be devised until the cause and the mode of spread are discovered.

Lyme Disease is as good an instance as one could wish of the importance of ecology in human illness. Human disease due to the **spirochete Borrelia burgdorferi** was a rarity until several ecological changes occurred sequentially: Large numbers of humans began encroaching on the habitats of deer; because humans had destroyed the predators which had once kept the deer population under control, the deer population exploded; the deer carried ticks and the ticks in turn carried the germ that causes Lyme disease. The deer invaded our gardens, we invaded their woods, and, one way or another, we began to share their ticks. Result: an epidemic of Lyme disease.

This illness starts when a minute tick attaches to a human host to obtain a meal of blood. After many hours of attachment, Borrelia organisms migrate from the tick into the skin of the new, host-to-be. A small red pimple then develops at the site of the bite, and surrounding it a ring-like rash begins to spread. Other similar areas of rash may pop up elsewhere on the body, and a variety of constitutional symptoms appear, including fever, malaise, aches and pains everywhere, and stiff neck. This stage of the illness subsides spontaneously, and then, during the following weeks and months, the nervous system, heart, eyes, and joints may come under attack. The joint involvement can look exactly like juvenile rheumatoid arthritis. That was the diagnosis made on 12 children in the town of Old Lyme, Connecticut in 1975. Two local mothers became aware of this bizarre cluster of cases and reported it to the state department of public health. Their report stimulated medical detection which eventually elucidated the entire story, from bacterial cause to ecological trigger, of what has become a common and important disease, now known to occur all over the world. In the United States, cases are clustered on the Eastern seaboard, the upper Midwest, and California, all areas of increasingly close contacts between lots of people and lots of deer.

When antibiotic treatment is begun in the early stage of the illness, rapid cures can be expected, but later treatment is both more difficult and less effective. Once it is well established in a human host, Borrelia burgdorferi is hard to dislodge.

Prevention is best accomplished by avoiding deer ticks, but this is not so easy if you live near deer. The ticks can be found in brush, grass, and trees. Clothing which has been sprayed with permethrin insecticide will kill ticks. The best tick repellent for use on the skin is DEET; this should be used sparingly, and should not be used on children's faces, hands, or abraded skin. After possible tick exposure, careful head to toe inspection will allow the early detection of these tiny ticks. If they are removed before 24 hours of attachment, the risk of becoming infected with Borrelia is very small. To remove a tick, grasp it gently with a fine tweezers or with a facial tissue held between your fingers. Pull it slowly, gently, and firmly; the tick will eventually relax its hold on the skin and, if you haven't pulled it too vigorously, will come off intact and alive. If you have pulled too hard, the head parts will remain in the skin; your doctor can decide whether to leave it alone or remove it. Wash your hands after handling the tick. It is not usually necessary to give a prophylactic antibiotic after a deer tick bite, but circumstances vary; ask your doctor.

Mumps. Here is a viral disease, previously a standard part of growing up, which has become something of a rarity since the widespread use of the mumps vaccine. Mumps is systemic, which means that it affects the whole body. It is known by its most obvious manifestation, the painful swelling of the parotid salivary glands inside the cheeks below and in front of the ears. Mumps also causes an inflammation of the lining membranes of the brain—a viral meningitis—which is typically mild. The most serious problems with mumps are inflammation of the testes (orchitis) and deafness. Testicular inflammation occurs most often in teenagers and adults; it is not only painful but can lead to destruction of one or both testes. The precise incidence of permanent deafness from mumps is unknown but probably small.

Mumps is spread through respiratory secretions. The patient is contagious for a few days before parotid swelling makes the diagnosis obvious, and he remains contagious for over a week. The incubation period is 12 to 22 days.

Treatment of the uncomplicated case is limited to the easing of discomfort. Mild pain killers are used, and sometimes cold packs held against the swollen cheeks give temporary relief.

The good news is prevention by the use of mumps vaccine. Before its introduction in 1968, we had about 150,000 cases a year in the U.S.; now we have only about 5,000. Mumps vaccine is usually given in the combined measles, mumps, and rubella (MMR) vaccine; two shots provide a high degree of protection.

Chapter 37

Immunizations

There seem to me to be so many confusions and misapprehensions concerning the subject of immunizations that some general comments may be in order.

The theory of immunization is straightforward and simple; expose a person to a weakened or modified agent of disease and the person's immune system will learn to recognize it. If later exposed to the living, virulent organism or the toxic material, the immune system will be able to overcome it before any significant damage is done. Some immunizing agents are living, whole organisms of disease which have been weakened to eliminate their ability to cause illness; oral polio vaccine is an example. Some are killed organisms, either whole or some significant and recognizable part. Salk polio vaccine is an example of killed, whole virus; the new acellular pertussis vaccine is an example of a vaccine made from an extract of killed organisms. Some modern vaccines are small, noninfectious parts of organisms produced by yeast cells modified through recombinant DNA technology; the hepatitis B vaccine we use is made in this way. A few vaccines, like diphtheria and tetanus, are toxoids, substances similar to the toxins produced by disease germs, but altered enough to be harmless. In all these cases, the modification is designed to avoid any harm to the recipient of the vaccine, but close enough to the real thing to allow the body to recognize it when necessary.

It is a tribute to human intelligence that the first and quite successful immunizing agents were devised before anyone had proven that there were any such things as germs. Since ancient times in Africa and Asia and since at least the sixteenth century in Europe, it was a folk custom to inoculate healthy people with material from the scabs of a patient with smallpox. They then developed a mild infection which conferred immunity. A similar and safer custom came to be termed vaccination, after the bovine disease vaccinia or cowpox. Farmers had noted that a person who had contracted cowpox was thereafter protected against smallpox. A small amount of cowpox scab was scratched into the skin of the healthy person, causing the production of a local infection and a generalized state of immunity. The practice of vaccination led to the first complete victory of the human race over a deadly disease. The WHO's campaign has eliminated smallpox for the entire planet; since 1980, the disease has been wiped out.

The end of the nineteenth century and the early decades of the twentieth saw an enormous flowering of information about the microbes that cause disease, and consequent excitement about the possibility of devising immunizing agents. Vaccines against rabies, tetanus, diphtheria, pertussis (whooping cough), typhoid, tuberculosis, and other diseases were developed. For a period after World War II the promise of the newly discovered antibiotics caused a shift in attention away from vaccines, but in recent decades research has once again accelerated. In addition to the older vaccines, we now have immunizing agents against poliomyelitis, measles, mumps, rubella, chickenpox, hepatitis A and hepatitis B, Haemophilus influenzae type b, influenza, pneumococcus infections, and a host of less well known infectious illnesses. Vaccine development continues with malaria and HIV as major targets.

The perfecting of immunizing agents has been a difficult undertaking, and there have been many fatal mishaps along the way. Early rabies vaccines contained nerve tissue, and recipients ran the risk of serious allergic reactions. The first commercial batches of polio vaccine were incorrectly manufactured and cases of polio resulted. An early killed-type measles vaccine caused peculiar allergic illnesses. The swine flu vaccine caused some cases of Guillain–Barré disease, a nervous system disorder. Furthermore, not all vaccines work very well. BCG vaccine against tuberculosis is useful but far from perfect; typhoid vaccines have never been completely reliable; a number of vaccines require follow-up doses to boost waning immunity. Nor do any vaccines result in immunity for 100% of the recipients. For reasons largely unknown, small numbers of people fail to benefit from properly prepared and administered vaccines. Lastly, many vaccines induce fevers, malaise, soreness at the site of inoculation, and other adverse reactions.

Given these problems, it is no surprise that both physicians and patients have sometimes approached the introduction of a new vaccine rather warily. This seems to me not a bad idea. Before I start administering a vaccine to my patients, I need to be convinced that the risks are very small and the benefits very great. Happily, that is the situation with the great majority of the vaccines being offered to American children today. The vaccination of our children offers them excellent protection against an array of very nasty and sometimes deadly diseases. It enables them to travel to parts of the world where these diseases are still rampant. Their immunity will also add to the sum total of protection of the whole American population; not only is there less risk to them but they will be less likely to be a risk to others who may not yet have been immunized.

In some of the preceding chapters I've mentioned the controversies surrounding the use of certain vaccines, and, lest I have failed to make my point with sufficient clarity, I'll underline it now. There is now and has always been a certain amount of opposition to the use of vaccines. Some of this is based on religious belief, and is therefore not really accessible to argument. Some opposition comes from nonmedical practitioners who seem not to accept the germ theory of disease. Some of the opponents of immunization are homeopaths whose theories of disease seem to be compatible with immunization, but who oppose it anyway. And with embarrassment and fury, I must admit that a few, vocal, honest-to-God doctors still think immunization is a terrible mistake. I wish I could understand how anyone could receive a medical education and fail to appreciate the gift of immunity granted to us by the use of vaccines. Do these physicians want to return to epidemics of smallpox, diphtheria, whooping cough, and polio? Do they look forward to the day when more babies are born with congenital rubella? Have they never seen a child whose mind has been twisted by measles encephalitis? Is liver cancer from hepatitis B such a great idea? I simply do not understand what they can be thinking. In my decades of pediatric practice I met a small number of parents who had embraced these anti-immunization notions. Trying to provide adequate medical care to their children while knowing that they were vulnerable to quite awful illnesses was a harrowing experience. This may explain why the tenor of this paragraph is so different from nearly everything else in this book. In the first chapter I said that this book was designed to help you understand your choices and make the ones that were right for you. But when it comes to protecting your children by having them immunized, I don't think your range of choices amounts to much. **Immunizations save lives.** It is as simple as that.

End of sermon. What follows below is a summary of available, everyday vaccines, their mode of employment, effects, and problems.

Vaccine	Efficacy	Side Effects and Problems
Diphtheria Toxoid (injection)	Superb vaccine, usually given with tetanus (DT) or tetanus and pertussis (DTP) excellent protection, lasts 10 years or more.	Soreness at site of injection is common; occasional fever; very rare severe allergic (anaphylactic) reaction.
Haemophilus Influenzae, Type B; "Hib" (injection)	4 similar vaccines; all produce good but not 100% protection.	Side effects are mild.
Hepatitis A (injection)	Brand new vaccine, long-term efficacy not yet known.	Not yet known, but seems well tolerated so far.
Hepatitis B (injection)	90–95% efficacy, good persistence of protection.	Occasional pain at site of injection; occasional fever.
Influenza (injection)	70–80% protective; vaccine must be altered every few years to match influenza viruses in current circulation. Recommended for children whose health status would be seriously affected by influenza.	Yearly boosters required; current vaccines cause many fewer adverse reactions than old products.
Measles (injection)	95% protection record; usually given as part of MMR (measles, mumps, rubella).	Same kids develop a mild fever and rash; allergic reactions are rare; encephalitis caused by measles may also, very rarely, be caused by the vaccine, but this is unproven.

Vaccine	Efficacy	Side Effects and Problems
Mumps (injection)	95% efficacy and long persistence; usually given as part of MMR.	Very well tolerated; rarely reactions of any kind.
Pneumococcal, Polyvalent (injection)	Gives only limited protection against 23 common types of this bacteria; most useful in people with a high risk of these infections.	Generally well tolerated; boosters probably necessary; very poor efficacy in the first two years of life; not recommended for general use in children.
Poliovirus, Inactivated; IPV or EIPV (injection)	E (enhanced) IPV is an improved Salk-type killed vaccine; gives nearly 100% protection and long-lasting immunity.	No serious side effects; because it cannot spread from person to person, this vaccine lacks the ability of live vaccine (OPV) to infect and thus protect unvaccinated contacts. IPV and EIPV are safe for people with problems of immunity.
Poliovirus, Live; OPV (oral)	Sabin vaccine has gives long-lasting immunity in nearly 100% of vaccinees.	Can cause polio in immune-deficient people; risk of polio in immune-competent people is 1 per 700,000 first doses of vaccine, 1 per 6,900,000 subsequent doses; risk is *lower* in children than in adults.
Pertussis (Whooping Cough), Whole-Cell (injection)	Imperfect but useful vaccine that has made a common illness rare; long-term protection may diminish; usually given with tetanus and diphtheria; will probably be replaced by new acellular vaccine.	Causes soreness and swelling at injection site, fever, and fussiness; very rare severe reactions include anaphylaxis, fever convulsions, prolonged crying, transient but frightening collapse; permanent neurological impairment has been alleged but this has not been confirmed by large scale studies.

EVERYDAY PEDIATRICS FOR PARENTS

Vaccine	Efficacy	Side Effects and Problems
Pertussis, (Whooping Cough), Acellular (injection)	Newer vaccine, used for years in Japan. It has none of the bacterial cellular components that cause many of the side effects of the older, whole-cell vaccine, appears to be equally effective; approved for booster shots for toddlers and older children, and will probably be approved for the initial series.	Fewer adverse effects than the whole-cell vaccine.
Rubella (injection)	This vaccine has reduced the incidence of rubella in the US by 99% ; congenital rubella from pregnancy has practically disappeared; well tolerated in babyhood and early childhood, with long lasting immunity; generally given as part of MMR.	Mild fever and rash occasional; rare incidence of prolonged joint inflammation in teenagers and adults; risk of this is less than risk of arthritis after naturally occurring rubella.
Varicella (Chickenpox) (injection)	Introduced for general use in 1995; it is well tolerated; immunity appears to be sustained for at least 10 years, but boosters may be needed.	The major questions regarding this vaccine are 1) whether immunity will wane in adulthood, leaving people susceptible to chickenpox at an age when it may be more serious, and 2) whether the live virus will cause an increased incidence of zoster (shingles) at later ages.

As I've mentioned in the chart above, many immunizing agents cause fussiness or fever or a sore arm or leg in the lucky recipient. If your baby is miserable for hours after his first DTP, make sure he gets a dose of acetaminophen before the next shot in the series. It may make his response less uncomfortable. A less common problem is the formation of a firm pea-to-jelly bean-sized lump under the skin where the shot was given. This is an area of irritation which will disappear in a few months.

Noninfectious Disorders

Chapter 38

Allergy

Allergy is a messy and unsatisfactory subject. Until the last few decades, studies of allergic phenomena were handicapped by a lack of precise laboratory measures; medical opinion considered the field of allergy to be excessively subjective and vague. This caused many physicians to develop a dismissive and uninformed approach to allergic disease. Into this relative vacuum have swooped a colorful and zany batch of medical and nonmedical quacks, and self-anointed adepts in allergy. I suspect that the real allergists, sober and well-grounded in their field, must find these pretenders an embarrassment and a trial. What all this means for the itching, sniffling, and congested public, actually suffering from allergic disease and seeking surcease, is that much of what is printed or spoken on the subject is suspect; let the wheezer beware.

Allergy Defined

Allergy is a state of abnormal, increased sensitivity (hypersensitivity) to any substance (an allergen) or physical state (such as cold) resulting in an undesirable tissue response because of an alteration in immunologic functioning. This long and technical definition is necessary to differentiate allergic responses from a variety of other situations in which the body reacts in an abnormal way to a usually innocuous substance or state. Ordinary milk is an excellent example. Allergy to milk protein can result in all sorts of symptoms, including abdominal cramps. But absence from the small intestine of the enzyme (lactase) needed to digest milk sugar (lactose) can also cause cramps, and this is in no sense an allergy. In both cases, there is intolerance of milk, but the allergic intolerance is based on an abnormality in the functioning of the immune system, and the lactose intolerance is not.

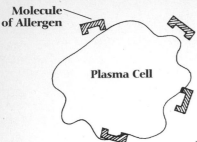

fig. 1

Molecule of Allergen

Plasma Cell

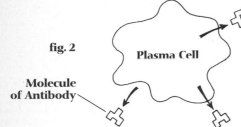

fig. 2

Plasma Cell

Molecule of Antibody

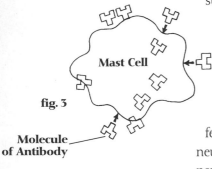

Mast Cell

fig. 3

Molecule of Antibody

The great advance in our understanding of allergic disease occurred three decades ago with the discovery of immunoglobulin E (IgE), the particular substance that is required for a typical allergic reaction. A substance (an allergen) enters the body and is recognized as foreign and unwelcome by plasma cells (fig. 1). The plasma cells respond by producing a specific form of IgE called an antibody (fig. 2). An antibody can identify and attach to a particular allergen if it shows up again. Many thousands of copies of a given antibody are produced. The IgE antibodies then moor themselves to the surfaces of certain cells called mast cells and basophils (fig. 3). These cells are loaded with chemicals known as mediators which play an important role is initiating allergic reactions. If a molecule of a specific allergen attaches to adjacent molecules of the matching IgE antibody on the surface of these cells (fig. 4), the cells rupture and pour out a stew of biologically active chemicals into the tissues and bloodstream (fig. 5). One of these chemicals is histamine, which sets off an immediate allergic reaction. Depending on where this occurs, it may include a runny nose, wheezing, a hivey rash on the skin, or abdominal cramps. Other chemicals initiate a slower developing allergic response, called a late phase reaction. An immensely complex sequence of biochemical and tissue changes can ensue which explain the wide variety of allergic disorders from which we can suffer. In addition to this classic allergen-plus-IgE interaction, other mechanisms exist which can disrupt these chemical mediator-laden cells. These include the presence of various drugs, all sorts of normal body constituents, and physical stimuli such as cold. (Sometimes you will see the term **antigen** used nearly synonymously with the term **allergen.** An antigen is a substance capable of inducing an immunological response; if the response it induces is an allergic response, the antigen is serving as an allergen. Many immunologic responses are nonallergic, for example immunity to a disease germ.)

People who are prone to allergic disease tend to have abnormally high levels of IgE in their blood and more than usual amounts of IgE attached to their mast cells and basophils. They also may have subtle differences in the functioning of their nervous systems and the chemicals called neurotransmitters. In addition to our central nervous system and its attached nerves that traverse our bodies, we have what is termed an autonomic nervous system which regulates all sorts of body functions. There is good reason to believe that this system is likely to be out of balance in people with allergies. As

EVERYDAY PEDIATRICS FOR PARENTS

if that was not enough, there also seem to be abnormalities in the concentration of some of the many chemicals that regulate the transmission of information along the autonomic system.

Allergic disease is a family affair. The vast majority of people with allergy have relatives with allergy. If both parents are allergic, the chance of their child being allergic is about 80%; if one parent is allergic, the chance of an allergy developing is about 60%. Allergy is also common; about 1 American out of 6 has an allergic disorder.

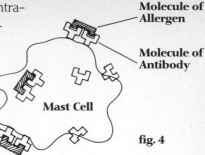

Molecule of Allergen

Molecule of Antibody

Mast Cell

fig. 4

What Constitutes An Allergen. A wide range of substances can serve as allergens: foods, pollens, various other plant materials (poison ivy and poison oak oil, for example), bacteria, fungi, insects (most notably house dust mites), animal hair and danders (bits of skin or feathers), medicines, metals (most often nickel), and a batch of assorted chemicals. There is agreement among allergists about most of these materials. Clinical studies have clearly demonstrated causal relationships, laboratory tests can confirm specific immune substances directed against particular antigens, and removal or hyposensitization can elicit improvement. In addition, there is a long list of what one might call candidate allergens, substances suspected of allergenic potential but without sufficient data to convince careful observers. It is here that allergy tends to slide into the realm of the true-believers, zealots of various persuasions, practitioners of "clinical ecology," inventors of devices to ward off "environmental allergy," and snake oil salesmen. When I am confronted with the startling and wondrous claims of these folks, what bothers me the most is that there may actually be something true hidden in all the nonsense. Because they refuse to apply the methods of science to their notions, it remains impossible for anyone to determine what is true (possibly a little) and what is fantasy (probably a lot). When I complained about one of these fringe-dwellers to a fellow physician, he responded "Well, Elmer, you have to understand that he really is more a poet than a pediatrician." I guess that is a fair assessment, but I wish they would all go away.

fig. 5

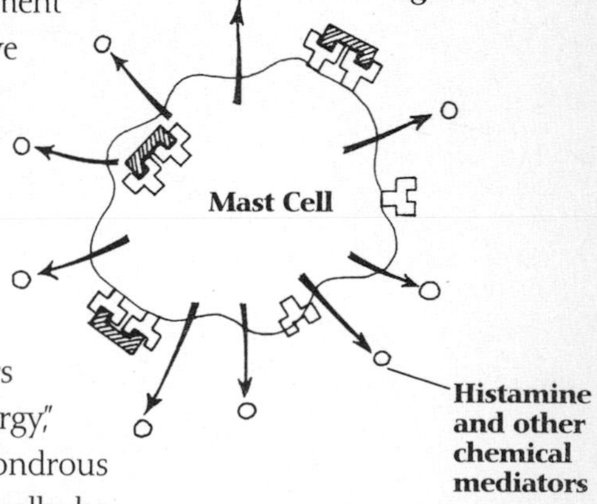

Mast Cell

Histamine and other chemical mediators

How is allergy diagnosed? Not easily. As I noted above, nonallergic causes can cause the same symptoms as allergic causes, and the task of the diagnostician is to sort these out and then to discover the specific triggers of allergic disease. Far and away the most powerful tool in the medical investigation is an old fashioned, time consuming, low-tech combination: A thorough history is taken to determine what is happening to the patient, and when, where, and why it's happening—plus a careful and complete physical examination. By the time this is accomplished, the physician is likely to have a pretty good idea about the nature and even the causes of the illness. Some simple laboratory tests may be needed, commonly a blood count to look for the typical increase in the numbers of the eosinophil blood cells often found in people with allergies. If the patient has nasal symptoms, a smear taken from the mucous membranes will be examined for the same cells.

If the physician has done a meticulous examination and elicited an accurate history, and the allergic problem is not too complicated, the diagnostic process may be completed. Usually, further investigation will be needed. The amount of IgE antibodies in the blood can be measured; it is very likely to be elevated, but that information is of little use. Specific IgE antibodies directed at particular allergens can be measured in the blood using any of several excellent tests. These studies are expensive and certainly not devoid of error, but they will often direct attention to the proper area for allergy management. Allergists have generally been disinclined to use these studies of specific IgE, preferring instead to do skin testing, which they consider to be more informative. A skin test is done with a dilute solution of an allergen injected or scratched into the surface of the skin. The development of a reddened and swollen area indicates allergy. This method is uncomfortable, time consuming, and requires a high degree of patient cooperation—a good trick for a 3-year old!—and properly prepared, freshly manufactured, and accurately administered extracts of large numbers of potential allergens be on hand for testing. It is often an expensive ordeal. Call me cynical, but I think the main reason allergists prefer skin testing is that it is practically a monopoly of their specialty. Other doctors are unlikely to have the scores of test antigens at hand, nor the trained personnel in the office to do these tests, but any doctor can order a RAST or MAST, the blood tests that look for the same answers.

The next diagnostic tool is continued observation. This may be observation without intervention, for example, carefully noting the circumstances under which an allergic symptom appears. Does the child cough and wheeze only when she visits Grandma who has a cat? It can also include observation during a period of changed circumstances. Does she still cough and wheeze at Grandma's a few months after the cat has died? The most fruitful diagnostic intervention is likely to be an elimination diet. The best elimination diet is one limited rigidly and exclusively to a small group of foods with very little potential for inducing allergic responses. If the symptom disappears during a 2 or 3 week period on the diet, other foods are then reintroduced very slowly, one at a time. If the symptom flares, the offending item can be identified. This is one of those great ideas which are very tough to carry out with success. It requires that the child live in a household where mistakes are never made, where no one ever unthinkingly slips the kid a bite of graham cracker, and where the child has absolutely no independent access to food. It also requires a family willing to ingest the same awful diet as the patient, or be heartless enough to eat a normal diet in the presence of a toddler screaming for a bite of whatever is on the plates of everyone else. It should be clear from this description that elimination diets of this type are a snap until the age of about 8 months. At later ages, these diets are a major family ordeal. A simpler elimination diet removes only those foods most likely to be allergens. This is not so easy either. The list of likely allergens includes so many basic foods that constructing an acceptable diet is difficult. A further obstacle is the complexity of the foods we all habitually eat. A glance at the list of ingredients in prepared foods will illustrate my point. And to make matters worse, ingredients in foods may be incompletely described, or their identities not fully understood. A diet excluding corn may run afoul of a soft drink sweetened with corn syrup which was listed simply as "natural sweetener" or "sugar syrup." Milk may masquerade as "whey" or "caseinate." I have known parents who gave their child wheat bread as part of a supposedly wheat-free diet, because the label said it contained "white" flour and the parents had not realized that white flour is made from wheat. A third type of elimination diet omits just one food that is suspected of being an allergen. The problem is that your chances of picking the right food to avoid are not very high. Also, multiple allergens are common, so eliminating just one may not make any perceptible difference. I suppose I should mention a fourth elimination diet which eliminates absolutely everything except a nonallergenic, predigested formula. It is close to impossible to coerce any child past early infancy to accept and subsist on this stuff for weeks at a time. If you still want to try an elimination diet despite all these difficulties, here are two ways to proceed.

The Go–For–Broke Eliminate Nearly Everything Diet. Limit the diet to the following foods, plus salt, pepper, and herbs for seasoning if desired:

Lamb, white potato, sweet potato, spinach, carrot, pear, peach, apricot, plum, rice plain rice crackers, baby rice cereal, safflower oil.

If life on this diet is insupportable, the following foods may be added:

Chicken, turkey, lettuce, squash, asparagus, broccoli, cauliflower, apples, grapes, raisins, barley.

If the allergic symptoms do not begin to subside after 3 weeks on this diet, the likelihood of food allergy is remote.

If symptoms do subside, start adding 1 new food every 3 to 5 days, and watch carefully for the reappearance of symptoms. When deciding which foods to add, it makes sense to choose those which have been missed the most; these are usually milk and wheat. If you ordinarily give your child a vitamin preparation, reintroduce it as if it were a possibly allergenic food.

A More Modest Elimination Diet. Remove from the diet the following foods:

Milk cream, sour cream, cheese, cottage cheese, yogurt, kefir, ice cream, sherbet (unless specifically milk-free), products containing casein, caseinate, and whey; eggs; wheat and all products made with wheat including pasta (even vegetable-flavored pasta), white flour, cereals with wheat, farina, semolina; corn, corn starch, corn syrup, corn oil; oranges and orange juice; soy, soy sauce, tofu, soy milks; peanuts, peanut butter; fish; shellfish; chocolate.

If the allergic symptoms fail to improve after 3 weeks, give up for the moment. At a later date, after everyone has recovered from this initial effort, consider trying the Go-For-Broke Diet.

If the symptoms do subside, begin to add back 1 forbidden food every 3 to 5 days and observe closely for the reappearance of symptoms.

A last word concerning elimination diets: Allergies come and go, especially in childhood where kids really do "out-grow" them. So, even if you can demonstrate beyond a shadow of a doubt that your child is allergic to tuna fish today, he may not have any allergic reaction to tuna fish next year. It is a mistake to limit a child's diet forever on the basis of a past allergy. Cautious reintroduction of suspect foods makes good sense unless the child has had a severe allergic reaction like hives all over the body, difficult breathing, or anaphylactic shock. Foods like nuts, peanuts, and shellfish have the worst records of that sort of allergic reaction, and reintroducing them is a matter for serious consultation with a skilled allergist.

Allergy Treatments. Without any question, the best allergy treatment is **avoidance of the allergen,** but this is not always possible. Cats, peanuts, pollen grains, stinging insects, and any number of other potent sources of allergic reactions can appear unbidden at our doors, nostrils, or mouths. If your

EVERYDAY PEDIATRICS FOR PARENTS

child's allergy can be mitigated by avoidance, you will need to work closely and patiently with your doctor. Devising an environment with a reduced burden of allergens is not always easy.

For children with a food allergy, the first step is **accurate recognition of all the foods which cause symptoms.** Every effort should be made to minimize the number of forbidden foods. Improvement in symptoms when the food is withheld and worsening when it is given provide the initial evidence to justify putting it on the list of foods to be avoided. Occasional retrials are important so that a food is not excluded unnecessarily. Otherwise, it is too easy to end up with a diet with so many exclusions that it cannot be followed. If important, basic foods are excluded it is worthwhile to consult a pediatric nutritionist to insure that the diet actually eaten meets all the child's nutritional needs.

The tactics for **avoiding inhalant allergens** may include air filtration systems in the home, finding new homes for the family's birds, cats, hamsters, pet rats, and dogs, and attempting to provide a environment which is inhospitable to dust mites. House dust mites thrive in mattresses, blankets, pillows, rugs, upholstered furniture, and stuffed animal toys. Encasing mattresses and pillows in special allergen-proof and dust mite-proof materials, banishing rugs and upholstered furniture, especially from the child's bedroom, and occasional hot water laundering of stuffed animals and blankets can reduce the exposure to the mites. There are also two chemical treatments which seem to decrease house dust mite exposure. Benzoyl benzoate in the form of a damp powder can be applied to rugs to kill the mites. A benzyltannate spray is also available; it is supposed to render the mites less allergenic. Unfortunately, there is, as yet, little real evidence that these chemical measures are useful.

If you can't avoid an allergen, the next best thing is to minimize your allergic reaction to it. One way is with **hyposensitization treatment.** This is a very long course of injections of the offending substances, starting with exceedingly minute concentrations and gradually increasing the amount as the body becomes accustomed to it. The method works best for people allergic to pollen and insect stings. The disadvantages are cost, the prolonged nature of the treatment, some discomfort from the shots, and a risk of adverse reactions. If too strong a dose is administered, the patient may experience a temporary worsening of symptoms. There is a tiny but real risk of severe and even life threatening allergic reactions. For this reason, most doctors who do hyposensitization treatment insist that the patient come to the office for the shots and remain there under observation for up to half an hour. It can be a time consuming undertaking. In an attempt to avoid these problems, a method of oral hyposensitization with drops given into the mouth or under the tongue has been proposed, especially by the "clinical ecologists." It is a wonderfully simple and painless approach, and there does not seem to be any evidence that it works.

If neither avoidance nor hyposensitization is the answer, there are medicines that can be an immense help. The **antihistamines** have been available for over half a century. Without any doubt, they can block the effects of histamine release, at least to a degree. For some allergic states like mild hay fever or allergic conjunctivitis (an allergic reaction of the lining membrane of the eyes) antihistamines may be sufficient. The main adverse effect of this group of drugs has been sleepiness, and the newer antihistamines are much better in this regard. The deficiency of antihistamines is that they target only histamine, which is just one of the many chemical mediators of allergic reactions. A second group of antiallergy drugs, cromolyn and nedocromil, work differently. They act by stabilizing the mast cells and basophils that contain the chemical mediators so that they are less apt to rupture when an allergen appears. These are excellent drugs, nearly devoid of side effects. However, they generally require frequent administration, work best if taken before exposure to allergens, and must be used as locally applied drops or sprays, since they are not absorbed if taken by mouth. The most powerful antiallergy medications are the cortisone-like drugs. This family of drugs are called **corticosteroids,** or **steroids,** for short. This leads to confusion since the anabolic steroids, male hormone–like drugs used by some athletes, are also called steroids. The two groups of drugs are quite different in their effects on the body although they share chemical similarities which accounts for their confusing nomenclature. Corticosteroids block many allergic manifestations as part of their general anti–inflammatory action. Depending on the allergic disease, they can be used locally as ointments or sprays, or systemically by injection or by mouth. They have become the mainstay of treatment for illnesses as diverse as eczema, asthma, and hay fever. But there is no free lunch; the list of their side effects is pages long. The hazards attendant to their use are sufficient that no cortisone preparation can be purchased without a prescription excepting only the mildest hydrocortisone creams. I am not suggesting that these drugs should be avoided; they are life and health savers. But they are serious and powerful agents with the capacity for producing some nasty problems. Approach them with caution.

Nasal Allergy (Allergic Rhinitis). We all lead with our noses; the nose is right up there in front of us, meeting the world, and naturally, meeting all the neighborhood allergens. Small wonder that nasal allergy is so common. Some nasal allergies are seasonal. Pollen allergy (hay fever) requires pollen in large amounts, and this depends on the time of year when one's least favorite pollinator is in bloom. Grass and weed allergies tend to be spring and summer events. Fungal spore allergy is a major cause of allergic rhinitis in certain areas during the fall when there is a bloom of fungus in fields after the harvest of certain crops. Other nasal allergies are perennial, because the cat lives in the house all year long, or because house dust mites are always part of the family. And some perennial nasal allergy has nothing to do with what we inhale into our noses because it is caused by the milk we drink or the bread we eat every day.

Nasal allergy is unusual in infancy; it tends to appear later in childhood or adolescence. The stuffy, itchy, drippy nose makes diagnosis apparent. The allergic child may also have dark-circled eyes (allergic shiners), a horizontal crease across the middle of the nose from all the nose rubbing, and a chronic cough from the post-nasal drip. The mucous membranes inside the nose are wet, swollen, and usually pale. If the allergic state is sufficiently severe, the child may act quite unwell. It is clear that much more than a few square inches of nasal tissue are involved.

Treatment of **seasonal allergic rhinitis** is nearly always satisfactory with appropriate use of antihistamines, topical cromolyn, or topical corticosteroids. (The term "topical" means locally applied, in this instance as nose drops or sprays, in contrast to "systemic" which means that the drug is given to the whole body in the form of tablets or shots.) Very severe cases may require a brief oral course of systemic steroids, but this is the exception. Environmental control of the patient's bedroom or even the entire house can be attempted. Expensive but fairly effective filtration systems can decrease the amount of pollen to manageable amounts, at least during the hours spent indoors. For the most troublesome cases of pollen allergy, hyposensitization is the last resort.

The control of **perennial allergic rhinitis** requires precise delineation of the offending allergens. Getting rid of house dust mites is not going to help the child who is allergic to corn or chocolate. Avoidance of the allergen is high on the agenda. Otherwise, one ends up with the necessity of staying on medication year in and year out, which is expensive, time consuming, and burdensome. Furthermore, if antihistamines and cromolyn-type drugs fail to provide sufficient relief, all that is left is the use of corticosteroids. The chronic systemic use of these drugs is out of the question because of their adverse effects on growth, the risk of cataract formation, changes in appetite and mood, and other unwanted results. The topical use of cortisone-type sprays directly into the nose is safe for the short term, but there are measurable amounts of medication absorbed into the body, and the long-term effects are not completely understood. Clearly, it is worthwhile making every effort to keep clear of the allergens and therefore be spared the chronic use of cortisone.

Eye Allergy (Allergic Conjunctivitis). The typical case of allergic conjunctivitis is an acutely red, watery, itchy eye which flares up when the child walks over a newly mown lawn or plays with a neighbor's cat. Sometimes the conjunctiva—the membrane covering the white of the eye—is so irritated that it swells up like a layer of egg white. Allergic conjunctivitis can be part of a larger allergic reaction like nasal allergy or asthma, or it can be quite limited with no other part of the body involved. The diagnostic approach to allergic conjunctivitis is similar to that for nasal allergy, except that food allergies play no discernible part. The causes are usually pollens and animal danders.

Seasonal, pollen-triggered allergic eye symptoms are nicely handled by eye drops. Antihistamine drops work pretty well, although they tend to cause some stinging. Cromolyn eye drops work better and hardly sting at all. At this writing, they are not on the market because of production problems, but they will doubtless reappear. Prednisolone and other cortisone derivatives are available as eye drops and they work beautifully. Because they can have serious adverse effects on the eye, their use must be monitored by your child's physician.

Eye allergies caused by animal danders can sometimes be forestalled by pretreatment. If you give your child an antihistamine by mouth before an expected exposure to an animal known to cause allergic trouble, the visit may be rendered harmless. In the long run, avoidance of known animal allergens is the best approach. Convincing your spouse, that a beloved family pet must go...well, that can be pretty tough.

Asthma will be included in this section even though asthma is by no means only an allergic illness. It could just as well be described in the section on chest infections since infections play a significant role in setting the stage for asthma in many children.

Asthma is a disorder in which the bronchi (the tubes that carry air to the lungs) become hypersensitive to a variety of irritants. The small muscle fibers surrounding the bronchi tighten, constricting the airway and making it especially difficult to exhale, the mucous glands lining the bronchi secrete excessive amounts of fluid, and the lining membrane swells, further interfering with the flow of air. All this causes coughing, wheezing (which means wet, squeaky noise especially during exhalation), and shortness of breath. As you might expect, the sensation of being choked causes immense anxiety. When doctors talk about asthma these days they often use the terms **reactive airway disease** or **hyperactive airways** more or less synonomously. Sometimes the term **asthmatic bronchitis** is used, especially if an infectious component is suspected. Some asthma is straightforward, obvious allergy, with a clearly identified set of known allergens. Sometimes asthma is a hypersensitivity state triggered by a previous viral infection; this is most likely to have been bronchiolitis caused by the respiratory syncytial virus (RSV) in infancy. For months or years thereafter, the child may react with asthma to new respiratory infections or other irritants. This kind of asthma seems to be most common in the first several years of life. (See pages 321–22 for details.) Some asthma is triggered by exercise, particularly in cold air. Tobacco smoke, either first or second hand, causes asthma; children in households where an adult is a smoker have a far greater incidence of asthma. To confuse matters further, many asthmatics can be shown to have multiple causes for their disease. For example, a child who wheezes after drinking milk may also worsen after a bad cold or a visit to a tobacco smoke-filled house.

From the 1930s to the 1950s, it was suspected that asthma was a response to psychologically inept parenting. It does seem to be true that asthma becomes a focus of parent-child friction and struggle in certain families. And asthma does apparently flare up in response to psychological stress in some children. But this is a far cry from the notion that the parents are, in some sense, the cause of the asthma. My late partner, Percy Jennings, who was both a pediatrician and an allergist, organized a long-term study of families with asthmatic kids, and his findings laid this idea to rest. He demonstrated that families with asthmatic kids are neither better nor worse than any other families. Of course a chronic illness like asthma can become a focus for family fights, but families never have any trouble finding something to fight about. We have learned to quit blaming parents for their children's wheezes (unless they are smokers.)

The main contribution of families to asthma is genetic. Since asthma is in large measure an allergic disorder, and since the tendency to develop allergies is, to a considerable degree, inherited, this comes as no surprise. What one inherits is an increased *general* susceptibility to having an allergic disease; Dad may have eczema, Mom may have hay fever, and Junior may get asthma. One does not inherit Dad's specific inability to tolerate shellfish or house dust mites.

Asthma Treatment. The medical management of asthma can proceed in one of two ways. Because the antiasthma drugs available today are powerful and effective, it is possible to treat asthma as a series of unconnected acute illnesses, treating each episode when it comes along, and paying very little attention to the underlying causes. This kind of approach is nearly inevitable for patients who get their medical care in urgent care clinics or emergency rooms, and it may be one of the reasons why an increasing number of people die every year of acute asthma. Obviously, the best way to treat asthma is to invest as much time and effort as needed to elucidate the causes for each person's individual, particular case. This will include a thorough allergy study, and a careful investigation of the environment to discover possible asthma triggers. It should lead to the development of a treatment plan which takes into account the family realities of the patient's life.

The center of asthma therapy should be **prevention.** This may take the form of house dust mite control, a diet free of foods known to cause asthma, getting rid of the family cat, or reforming the family cigarette smoker. For exercise-induced asthma, it may mean providing a prophylactic medication to be inhaled before sports. For asthma triggered by respiratory infection, it may involve starting antiasthma medicine at the first sign of a cold. Very rarely, it may mean hyposensitization shots.

Some people with asthma live in a state of incipient wheezing, not quite asthmatic at all times, but easily nudged over the line into a full-fledged attack. For these quite numerous folks, long-term, daily use of antiasthmatic medications makes sense. For the last several decades, the medical profession has been debating how best to do this. Although authoritative directives are issued from time to time by various expert groups, I think the jury is still out on the subject. Without doubt, your child's doctor will have strong views on how to proceed.

Antiasthma drugs commonly used today fall into 5 groups:

Beta–adrenergic bronchodilators are drugs chemically related to adrenalin which relax the smooth muscles that surround the bronchi. Adrenalin, metaproterenol, albuterol, salmeterol, and terbutaline are drugs of this class. They are most often used by inhalation, although oral, subcutaneous, and even intravenous forms are available. Generally, they work quickly but they have no effect on the other parts of the asthmatic condition—the swelling and wetness of the mucous membranes inside the bronchi. For decades, they have been used in vast quantities both for acute asthma and for long-term control of symptoms. Currently, their everyday, long-term use is somewhat in disfavor, in part because certain bronchodilators may be linked to an increased risk of asthma death.

When bronchodilators of this type are used for children, inhalation from a hand-held metered dose inhaler or from an electric pump-driven nebulizer is possible. If a bronchodilator is prescribed for your child, it is absolutely imperative that precise instructions be given regarding proper and effective use. The printed information that accompanies the medicine is all very well, but you really need an experienced professional to show you what to do.

Anticholinergic bronchodilators (ipratropium and atropine) are fairly new but not very important drugs for asthma. They are designed to have the same effect as the other, so-called adrenergic bronchodilators, but mediated through a different set of nerves and chemical substances. The fact that these drugs are used at all should serve as a reminder to physicians about the tenuousness of our knowledge. Until a decade or so ago, the wisdom among pulmonary specialists was that no drug of this kind should ever be used in patients with asthma. Some over-the-counter cough remedies which have weak atropine-like effects still carry a warning against their use by patients with asthma. In any event, these drugs have not proved useful for children with asthma.

Theophylline and its chemical cousin **aminophylline** are antiasthma preparations which have been used for most of this century. Like other bronchodilators, they act by relaxing the smooth muscles that surround the bronchi. For decades, theophylline preparations plus adrenalin were the mainstays of asthma therapy, but they have become less widely prescribed since the advent of the newer bronchodilators and the corticosteroids. The main problem with theophylline is that adverse side effects appear often and easily; there is not much room between a desirable therapeutic dose and a potentially hazardous overdose. Even at appropriate dose levels, many patients complain of jitteriness or sleeplessness. This is not surprising since these drugs are closely related to caffeine. With a careful choice of preparation and adjustment of dose, it is often possible to take advantage of theophylline for asthma. The long-acting tablets or granules make infrequent doses feasible. This is particularly appreciated by children who would otherwise awaken wheezing in the middle of the night.

Cromolyn and **nedocromil** are described in the previous discussion of antiallergy medicines. Unlike the bronchodilator drugs just mentioned, these agents do not reverse any of the symptoms of asthma. They are pure and simple prophylactic drugs which block the release of the chemical mediators that cause asthma attacks. When they are inhaled several times a day they slowly alter the tendency of the mast cells and basophils to rupture. When they work well, it takes a greater allergic insult to result in asthma, and the asthma may be less severe. Because it often requires weeks of therapy before any effect is noted, both patients and doctors tend to become impatient, and the drugs are often abandoned long before they might have done some real good. This is a pity because they are exceptionally safe agents, practically devoid of any side effects; I regret that they are not more widely and effectively used.

Corticosteroids by inhalation or systemically by mouth or injection are powerful antiasthma drugs which work through their anti-inflammatory effects. Because the whole-body or systemic use of these drugs is attended by such profound and often damaging effects, every effort must be made to minimize their use in a chronic disease like asthma. It is often tempting for patient, family, and doctor to have recourse to short courses of prednisone or similar preparations; a few days of treatment often leads to a prompt recovery. The problem is that these short courses tend to be repeated more often than is wise, and a cumulative effect may be taking place which may elude discovery for a long time. The local use of corticosteroid inhalations is now standard treatment for thousands of asthmatics. The main effect of these agents is preventative, warding off asthmatic reactions. In the presence of an acute asthma episode, they have a modest antiasthma effect but not enough to count on. They have no bronchodilator effect. All this means that these drugs must be used in conjunction with either inhaled or injected bronchodilators like albuterol or adrenalin, or oral agents like theophylline. Systemic effects are much less of a problem with inhaled corticosteroids compared to systemic steroids. However, studies have shown that enough inhaled steroid is absorbed to have measurable effects on pituitary and adrenal function, and perhaps on body growth. For this reason, I consider inhaled steroids to be appropriate only if comprehensive antiallergy management plus drug therapy with cromolyn, beta-adrenergic bronchodilators, and theophylline have failed to control the child's asthma. Inhaled steroids are a seductive shortcut, but, like other seductions, the results may not be what one had in mind.

Skin Allergies. The most common skin allergies are **eczema** and **contact dermatitis** which are discussed at length in Chapter 26. Regarding eczema, see pages 233–35 and 236–37on infant and toddler skin; regarding contact dermatitis, see pages 245–47 on middle-aged children's skin.

EVERYDAY PEDIATRICS FOR PARENTS

The other major skin allergy is **hives,** or **urticaria,** an eruption characterized by raised, red, itchy patches. Some of these are round, some have a pale center, some are irregular in shape, and some blend into each other and cover large areas of skin. Rarely, hives can occur in the mouth or the throat and interfere dangerously with breathing.

The problem with hives is finding out the cause. It can be due to a drug allergy, a food allergy, or even an allergic reaction to a germ or to insect bites. A few cases are due to odd reactions to chilling and some are due to overheating! There are hives associated with a variety of systemic diseases, and there is a rare, hereditary form of hives. I have to admit that, most of the time, we never do figure out the cause. This is of little importance for a single episode of hives, but once in a while hives recurs and then finding the cause becomes quite a challenge. Fortunately, the treatment of hives is generally simple; antihistamines nearly always work well.

Gastrointestinal Allergy. When the stomach and intestines suffer an allergic reaction it is, naturally enough, to food. Foods are, for practical purposes, the only allergens to which our gastrointestinal tracts are exposed. But interestingly, most food allergies are not expressed in the GI tract. Our stomachs and intestines process allergenic foods which are then absorbed into the blood stream. They then have the opportunity to react with tissues all over the body. Depending on the target organ, this can lead to allergic rashes or sniffles or wheezes or temper tantrums. Our guts are most often innocent bystanders to all this action.

On those occasions when the GI tract itself is the site of allergic disease, it has only a limited number of ways to manifest its distress. Stomach cramps, vomiting, diarrhea, and bleeding are the usual allergic responses.

Babies with colic act as if they are suffering from stomach or gut cramps, and perhaps they are; we really do not know. For that reason, and because there is so little that controls colic, there has been much interest in the investigation of possible allergic causes. It appears that a few formula fed babies improve on hypoallergenic formulas, and perhaps 1 out of 4 colicky breast fed babies improve when cows' milk is excluded from the mother's diet. But for most colicky babies, food allergy seems not to be the problem. In later childhood, cramps or vomiting are rare but possible reactions to food allergy. Infant colic is discussed at length in Chapter 7.

Among the many causes of diarrhea, allergy surely ranks low; at least, that is the opinion of most doctors. I think the reason so many parents suspect allergy as a cause of diarrhea is that they are misled by an apparent cause and effect relationship: I gave him canned salmon for dinner and he was up all night with a tummyache and diarrhea. If you act on that observation and omit salmon from his diet thereafter, you are likely to remain convinced that you have identified an allergy. Well, probably not; it was most likely a viral infection. So, why didn't the rest of the family get it? Well, probably because they are older, and they are already immune to that particular germ. Be brave, wait a few days, and try a little canned salmon once again. If he gets diarrhea, I'll be convinced. If he does not get diarrhea, you will have returned a valuable and delicious food to his diet, and you will have avoided labeling him inaccurately as an allergic person.

This is not to say that GI allergy to foods is nonexistent. When it occurs, there may be either hidden, chronic blood loss leading to a significant anemia, or actual, visible blood in the stool, or a quite persistent chronic diarrhea. None of these patterns of illness is at all common. Constipation as a sign of allergy is even rarer.

Central Nervous System Allergy. Many of my pediatric colleagues would have put a question mark at the end of the phrase "central nervous system allergy." It is not a widely recognized entity, but I think it exists, and it can be a bear when it does.

This is the field of allergy at its messiest. The alleged allergic effect is **behavior,** an utterly subjective symptom nearly impossible to measure. There are no reliable laboratory correlates that would enable us to study behavioral allergy in a reproducible and objective fashion. The net effect is that central nervous system allergy has attracted the attention of whole squadrons of half-baked pseudo-experts. The few careful investigators in the field can hardly be heard for the purveyors of noisy nonsense.

Two somewhat different patterns have been ascribed to central nervous system allergy. Many years ago, the **allergic tension–fatigue syndrome** was described by several careful investigators. They reported that many allergic children acted tired or tense and grumpy. Needless to say, these are not exactly rare forms of childhood behavior. The difference was that these behavioral symptoms diminished or disappeared when the offending allergens (usually milk and chocolate) were removed form the child's diet. When the foods were returned, the symptoms followed. Does this prove that the nervous system itself is reacting in an allergic fashion? Perhaps all this means is that some kids with

EVERYDAY PEDIATRICS FOR PARENTS

untreated food allergies feel rotten and act miserable because of their itchy skin or stuffy noses until the foods are removed from their diets. However, there are a few children whose behavioral response to certain allergenic foods seems to be much more intense than could be explained on the basis of the malaise associated with a stuffy nose or itchy skin. They certainly act as though their brains were having a terrible time. As I mentioned, the children who manifest these behavioral symptoms have other allergic problems as well. Over the years I have searched assiduously for children whose only allergic problem was tension-fatigue syndrome, but I have never been able to convince myself that I found one.

The other pattern which has been blamed on nervous system allergy is attention deficit hyperactivity disorder (ADHD), a term which describes children who have trouble focusing their attention, are easily distracted, and consequently have great difficulty with studying and learning. It is alleged that these are symptoms of nervous system intolerance to food additives, coloring agents, and naturally occurring salicylates in foods. The only way to determine this scientifically is to give the children the supposed allergenic material hidden in capsules, and compare their behavior when they are given identical appearing capsules with nothing allergenic inside. This experiment has been done and it has shown that intolerance to these substances is not a factor for the vast majority of children with hyperactivity and attention problems. It appears likely that a very few children do react adversely to some food coloring agents. If you suspect that your local wild man is one of them, try a food coloring-free diet for a few weeks; it probably will not help but the test is certainly harmless.

This is a good place to comment (once again!) on the notion that sugar can cause hyperactivity, presumably through some sort of effect on the nervous system. I don't expect you to believe me, but it simply is not true. Not one large and carefully done study has ever indicated any such effect. If high blood sugar caused excitement, people with diabetes (who quite often have elevated levels of blood sugar) should be running around screaming half the time—and they don't. You can try a simple experiment: Add some extra sugar to your child's fruit juice and watch for any change in behavior. I'll bet you don't see any at all.

Chapter 39
Eye Problems

Vision and Its Development

Newborn babies have some definite problems in gaining useful information from the world by looking at it. At birth, a full-term infant has a visual acuity of 20/200 to 20/400. That means they sees as much detail at 20 feet as they will eventually be able to see at 200 to 400 feet. Their color vision is equally faulty; babies see intense, saturated, primary colors best and they tend to pay the most attention to red. Surrounding babies with pastels is a matter of parental or grandparental preference, not a response to infant choices. Furthermore, the coordination of the eye muscles takes a while to be perfected, and it is not unusual for babies' eyes to cross or wander off to the side. It may take several months until perfect and reliable binocular vision is always present. Despite this somewhat primitive ocular equipment, alert, unsedated newborns seem quite interested in what they can see. They focus best on objects somewhat less than a foot away from their eyes, a handy distance from which to examine Mom's face during a feeding. Even during the first days of life, babies stare with obvious interest at the faces that surround them.

As the months pass, visual acuity rapidly improves. Late in the first year, babies focus accurately on small objects like flies or raisins. One can even test infant vision by placing such interesting but minute materials within a baby's reach and observing the reaction. By the end of the first year, vision is in the range of 20/40 to 20/60, nearly approaching adult levels of precision, although it may take until age 5 for 20/20 vision to be attained. Like nearly everything else in human development, this process is essentially automatic. Provide a baby with normal eyes and something to look at, and nature takes care of the rest. Babies do not need fancy visual targets to study, nor "learning toys" to hone their visual skills. They will not harm their eyes by using them in dim light, nor will they get cross-eyed by examining objects held a few inches from their noses. It is a great system, tested over the millenia, and requiring no assistance from the early learning industry.

Testing Vision. One area in which routine medical examinations are most useful is in detecting abnormalities of vision at an early age. Accurate vision is the key to so much learning during infancy; the correction of deficient vision can make a major contribution. Even more important is discovering the child who is not using both eyes equally. If undetected and untreated, this can lead to a permanent decrease in vision in one eye. For these reasons, your child's pediatrician will look into her eyes for congenital cataracts, test her eye muscles for proper coordination, and observe her ability to use her eyes for depth perception (as a test of binocular vision). As she grows, her visual acuity will be tested with increasingly precise techniques; it is important that these tests be repeated throughout childhood and adolescence since abnormalities of vision can develop quite unexpectedly at any age.

Myopia (Nearsightedness) is a condition in which the eyes are too long from front (the cornea) to back (the retina). This causes the lens of the eye to focus images in front of the retina instead of directly upon it. The retina gets a blurry picture, especially of objects far away. It gets a fairly good image of near objects, thus the term "nearsightedness." The eyes of infants tend normally to be just the opposite of this, that is, farsighted. As they grow, the farsightedness diminishes and nearsightedness may appear sometime in middle childhood or later. We know that many instances of nearsightedness are inherited. Nearsighted parents have more than their share of nearsighted kids. There is also the theory that nearsightedness results because human eyes are not well designed for the amount of close-up work we require of them these days, but, even if true, there is not much we can do about that.

Children who are becoming nearsighted rarely complain about their increasingly blurred vision; they just seem to accept that the world is a rather fuzzy place. If your child complains that the blackboard at school is hard to see, if he looks puzzled when you point out a particular star or a distant airplane, or if he holds his books increasingly close to his nose, have his vision tested. None of those clues is diagnostic of myopia, but they are surely worthy of your attention. You will notice that I did not include headache in the list of symptoms suggestive of nearsightedness; there is rarely, if ever, any connection.

Hyperopia (Farsightedness) is a condition in which the eyeball is too short from front to back. It is the opposite of nearsightedness. A small degree of hyperopia is the norm in infancy and early childhood, but it isn't a problem unless it is quite extreme. The child's eyes can accommodate to a somewhat farsighted shape because of the flexibility of the lens. (As the lens becomes less flexible in later adult years, farsightedness becomes more troublesome, and bifocals or granny glasses become necessary for near vision.) Farsightedness is sometimes blamed for "eyestrain" or headaches; the idea is that the little internal muscles of the eye become tired from the work of changing the lens' curvature to improve focusing at nearby objects. I must say that I have never seen a case of headache due to farsightedness and cured by glasses, so I am a bit dubious about this idea.

Astigmatism is a third type of refractive error which is considerably harder to define and explain. The eye has surfaces (the cornea and the lens) which bend or refract incoming rays of light and focus them as an image on the retina in the back of the eye. These refractive surfaces should be spherical, like a portion of a large ball. If instead they are shaped more like the curve of a tablespoon (longer in one direction than in others) they focus a smeared image rather than cleanly defined points of light. That condition is astigmatism. It may accompany either near- or farsightedness, and, like them, is corrected with suitable lenses.

Amblyopia is not one of the refractive errors, although it may be caused by them. Amblyopia is reduced vision in one or both eyes due to some sort of interference with normal visual development during the early years of life. This can occur if the retinas are presented with images so different that they cannot be made to fuse into a single binocular, stereoscopic image. When this happens, the brain learns to ignore or suppress the image arising in one of the eyes, usually the one which presents the least sharp, least useful image. If this situation remains uncorrected for long, it is exceedingly difficult and often impossible to restore adequate vision in that eye, even though one may be able to correct the image by supplying a corrective lens, removing a cataract, or correcting a muscle imbalance. After the brain has decided that the information coming from that eye is useless, it may be unaffected by the receipt of new and better information.

Strabismus is a condition where one eye turns too far in (a crossed eye) or too far out (a walleye). In either case, the images projected on the two retinas will be too dissimilar for fusion to be achieved. The straighter eye wins, and its image is used by the brain; the image from the other eye is gradually suppressed and vision in that eye becomes less and less useful. Amblyopia can also occur if the two eyes have differing refractive characteristics. For example, if one eye has normal refraction and a clear retinal image while the other eye is nearsighted with a blurred image, the nearsighted eye becomes amblyopic. The same situation occurs if one eye has a congenital cataract or any other impediment to the formation of a clear pattern projected on its retina.

EVERYDAY PEDIATRICS FOR PARENTS

Amblyopia is one of those problems in which time is of the essence. The eyes and the visual cortex of the brain develop rapidly after the child is born. It is crucial to diagnose and treat problems such as congenital cataract within the first several months of life. Treatment of strabismus and of unequal refraction can usually be done satisfactorily if instituted within the first years. Patching the good eye (to force the unused eye to function), eye drops (to blur vision in the good eye), glasses, and eye muscle surgery all have a place, depending on the particular situation.

As noted above, strabismus is the failure of the two eyes to line up properly, with one eye turning in or out or even up or down. The risk of amblyopia is the most important reason for attending to strabismus, but it is also makes depth perception impossible, and it is a major cosmetic problem. Most instances of crossed eyes or walleyes have no known cause. However, some crossed eyes are due to excessive farsightedness. Farsighted eyes require their owners to make a constant effort of accomodation, which involves altering the shape of the lens. The nerve impulses controlling lens shape seem to spill over to the muscles which turn the eyes toward the midline, and one or both eyes begin to cross. This is most likely to occur with prolonged use of the eyes for close work, or when the child is thoroughly fatigued. Strabismus of this type is usually effectively treated with glasses to correct the farsightedness. Other kinds of strabismus may require a variety of therapies. The rule that applies to strabismus, amblyopia, and refractive errors is **Grossman's Law of Eye Problems: *Pay attention!*** Vision is important; eye problems cannot be ignored.

Pseudostrabismus, a nonproblem, deserves mention as well. This is the condition in which the eyes appear crossed when in fact they are quite straight. The nasal bridges of many infants are quite flat and wide. The effect of this is an relative excess of skin which partially covers the inside edges of the eyes, next to the nose. There is then less white of the eye visible on the inside corner of the eye than on the outside corner. The illusion produced is that the eye is turned in. Pseudostrabismus can be quite confusing, even if one recognizes the lack of symmetry of the skin folds around the eyes. The easy way to differentiate it from true strabismus is by taking a full-face flash picture of the baby. If the eyes are actually straight, the flash reflections in the baby's eyes will be symmetrical. You may be able to see the same thing by using a small flashlight held a few feet away from the baby's face.

During the early weeks and months of life, it is common to see some tearing from one or both eyes, accompanied by a collection of mucusy or pus-like goo at the inner corner of the eye. This is caused by an **obstruction of the nasolacrimal duct.** This tiny tube is designed to carry tears from the eye down into the nose. When the duct forms in fetal life, it is sometimes left partly blocked at the nasal end. Tears back up, germs start to grow in the stagnant puddle at the top of the duct, a wide spot called the lacrimal sac which is right next to the inner corner of the eye, and a low-grade infection gets underway. The large majority of these cases resolve all by themselves, but parents tend to get disturbed by the combination of tears and pus. The simplest treatment is to instill antibiotic eye drops or ointment 2 or 3 times a day until the pus clears up. It may be necessary to continue at least once daily for several months to control the tendency to frequent relapses. A second treatment that is often suggested is to massage the area of the lacrimal sac, the idea being that one can increase pressure in the plugged-up duct and eventually force the duct to open. It sounds like a reasonable idea, but I doubt that there is any evidence that it works. Furthermore, both infants and parents eventually tire of the exercise. For the small minority of children who reach the age of 1 year or thereabouts without any sign that the duct has opened, the solution is surgical probing by an ophthalmologist. This works very well indeed. We used to advise probing at much earlier ages, but careful observation made clear that spontaneous resolution often took place if we were patient.

Teary eyes in early infancy are not always due to plugged tear ducts. A rare condition, **congenital glaucoma,** can also cause tearing and requires prompt treatment by an ophthalmologist. This is one more reason to have your baby's doctor check any case of eye discharge.

Foreign Bodies. Considering the frequency of exposure of children's eyes to dirt, sand, wood chips on the playground, and miscellaneous debris everywhere, it is amazing how little trouble they have from foreign objects lodged on the surfaces of their eyes. Part of that happy state is due to active blink reflexes; eyes close with striking rapidity when a visible threat approaches. It is also due to the cleansing action of the tears. However, a certain number of bits of flying junk get stuck under an eyelid or imbedded in the cornea (the clear area of the front of the eye), and when they do, it hurts.

Examination of a screaming child who is telling you that he has something in his eye is not one of parenthood's brighter moments. If you can calm him down, take a careful look in three areas. Even the smallest object stuck to the **surface of the cornea** or imbedded in it causes an impressive amount of pain. Hold the eyelids open and use a bright light. Sometimes you will be able to see the object best with the light held to one side. To get better traction on the eyelids, put a bit of facial or toilet tissue under each fingertip. It helps to have about six or eight hands in this situation. Sometimes corneal foreign bodies can be washed off by having the child open and close his eyes with his face held partly in a bowl of water. Kids who know how to swim can usually manage this quite nicely. Nonswimmers are likely to assume that you are trying to drown them, and they react predictably. If washing fails to dislodge the object, have the child keep his eye closed until you can get him to a doctor. If this is absolutely impossible, you can try to remove it with a wisp of wet cotton from a cotton ball or Q-tip or the corner of a wet handkerchief.

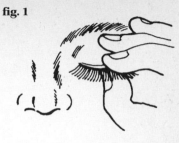

fig. 1

    The next area to examine is the **underside of the lower lid.** Be sure to pull the lid down enough to allow a good look in the area next to the eyeball, and in each corner as well. Eye washing or the use of a wet Q-tip, wisp of cotton, or handkerchief will serve to remove most debris. The tough place to examine is **under the upper lid.** Just pulling up on the lid may not suffice. You will need to "flip" the lid, a weird but necessary maneuver. The upper lid contains a piece of firm connective tissue called the tarsal plate. This structure allows the lid to be turned up and the underside seen. To accomplish this, have the child look down. Grasp the eyelashes next to the lid margin (fig. 1), pull the lid down and away from the eyeball and then fold the lid back (fig. 2), holding a finger against the upper part of the eyelid to act as the fulcrum around which the eyelid can fold (fig. 3).

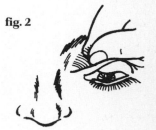

fig. 2

    Removing a foreign body will instantly cure the discomfort unless the object has caused a **corneal scratch** or **abrasion.** These hurt, although the pain is much less when the eye is closed. There is really no way for you to tell whether you are dealing with such a scratch or with the continued presence of an imbedded object. Get you child to a doctor who can relieve the pain with a drop of local anesthetic and do a complete examination.

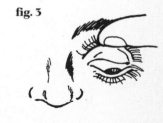

fig. 3

Chapter 40

Gastrointestinal Problems

The Esophagus Is A Two-Way Street

The upper end of the gastrointestinal tract is the esophagus, a tube connecting the back of the throat to top of the stomach. Although its main function is to get food down to the stomach, there needs to be a way for ingested material to be rejected if, for example, the stomach decides that the stuff wasn't food after all. At the lower end of the esophagus there are circular muscle fibers which tend to keep the esophagus partly closed except during the act of swallowing. Furthermore, the angle of attachment to the stomach is such that the fuller the stomach, the more the lower end of the esophagus is compressed. The combination of these anatomical factors help keep stomach contents down where they belong most of the time. An actual act of forceful vomiting is usually needed to overcome the impediments to reverse flow.

Spitting Up. Early in life, however, neither the valve-like function of the muscles of the esophagus, nor the pinching off of the esophagus by the top part of the stomach works perfectly. When the stomach is full of milk or bloated with swallowed air, stomach contents can easily flow back up the esophagus, and out it comes through the mouth and nose. When this happens without actual vomiting, which is to say without an effortful contraction of the stomach, the event is described as spitting up. This is messy but usually without importance. Some babies spit up so much and so often you may begin to wonder if anything is staying down at all. If the infant is growing and gaining normally, the answer is yes. Babies like this may just be getting more milk at a feeding than they can handle. Often, babies spit up if they are handled too enthusiastically right after a feeding, or if they are put to sleep belly down before they have had a chance to burp up the swallowed air. With increasing age, the esophageal sphincter mechanism matures, and spitting up gradually diminishes somewhere around the first birthday.

Gastroesophageal Reflux. Technically, spitting up is an example of gastroesophageal reflux, the medical term for stomach contents going backwards into the esophagus. A certain amount of GE reflux is a perfectly normal part of human life; everybody does it from time to time. When the stomach contents erupt high into the esophagus and the back of the throat,

EVERYDAY PEDIATRICS FOR PARENTS

we have the unpleasant symptom called **heartburn.** In early infancy when the stomach manufactures relatively small amounts of gastric acid, the refluxed material can flow up into the esophagus and result either in some spitting up or simply return back into the stomach, and no harm done. Later, as stomach contents become increasingly acidic, the refluxing material can be quite irritating. It can cause inflammation of the esophagus itself, or it can even spill over into the lungs if some of it is inhaled through the larynx into the trachea. This is a rare but real cause of chronic cough in infancy and early childhood.

The tricky business here is to differentiate reflux which can cause real trouble, from ordinary reflux occurring harmlessly in a child who has other unrelated symptoms. The physician may be misled by tests which show that reflux does indeed occur but which do not actually prove that the reflux is making the child sick. This is a good example of how wonderful technology can lead to lousy medical care. When methods were first devised to measure the presence of acid reflux into the esophagus, enthusiasm for using the tests outran good sense in judging what they meant. Medical journals began to fill up with articles blaming GE reflux for everything except the Cold War and inflation. Fortunately, we have finally figured out that demonstrating reflux *alone* does not prove anything. In the relatively unusual instances when GE reflux actually causes problems, we have a variety of treatments, none of them much good. These include thickened feedings, holding the child in peculiar positions with the help of special chairs or saddles, medicines, and even surgery. Satisfactory solutions have proved elusive.

Vomiting

The functions of the stomach are straightforward: Receive food and drink, add appropriate enzymes and some gastric acid, mash everything up, and propel the resultant puree to the small intestine for further processing and absorption. When the stomach is left in peace to do its job, it is a remarkably efficient and trustworthy organ; it demands little attention and we notice it rarely, if at all. However, it is also a vulnerable organ at the mercy of its owners who may throw all sorts of indigestible foods into it. It is also required to cope with all sorts of medicines, bits of dirt, coins, chalk, eraser heads, and whatever else comes down through the esophagus. Furthermore, it is under the influence of the nervous system, which may send it confusing and upsetting messages. It is responsive to blood-borne hormones and, despite its protective barriers of mucus and acid, it can be infected by bacteria. Understandably, there are circumstances when the stomach, so to speak, throws up its hands.

Viral Gastroenteritis. When a child vomits, our immediate thought is likely to be that something of an infectious nature is happening in or around the stomach or intestines. This surmise is frequently correct; viral gastroenteritis is certainly a common culprit. This is an acute illness marked by vomiting followed by diarrhea, and accompanied by malaise and a little fever. It is one of the illnesses that people call "stomach flu," a misleading label because it implies a relationship with the real "flu," which is influenza, a respiratory illness. Details concerning the diagnosis and treatment of gastroenteritis are in Chapter 33.

Food Poisoning. When we speak of food poisoning we are really talking about two quite different types of illness, each of which can be caused by a wide variety of agents. Ordinary food poisoning is exactly that: The food that causes the illness has a poison in it. The toxin is usually a staphylococcal enterotoxin, a substance excreted by staphylococcus bacteria which have had a few hours to grow in unrefrigerated foods. Staph grows with special enthusiasm on mixed up, starchy-proteiny foods like egg and potato salads, cream sauces, and cream-filled cakes and pastries, as well as ham and poultry. It takes anywhere from 30 minutes to 7 hours for the victim to begin to experience the cramps and vomiting which usher in a miserable few hours of malaise and diarrhea. Another bacteria, Bacillus cereus, can cause a similar illness transmitted in cooked rice. These illnesses usually last 1 day or less. Treatment is the same as for viral gastroenteritis; please see the pertinent paragraphs in Chapter 33.

There are also some uncommon causes of food poisoning which don't happen to cause vomiting. The bacteria Clostridium botulinum can grow in improperly home-canned foods; it produces a powerful nerve poison which causes a paralytic illness called **botulism.** Shellfish contaminated with certain microorganisms can also harbor paralytic nerve poisons.

All of these are illnesses caused by foods which contain already formed poisons. In distinction are the illnesses transmitted by foods contaminated with bacteria which can grow inside our bodies and produce disease. Some of these germs create toxins which cause the damage; others are actually invasive organisms which get into our intestinal tissues and even our bloodstreams. The toxin-producers include some species of Shigela, Clostridium perfringens, some strains of Escherichia coli (E. coli), and Vibrios, including the one causing cholera.

Of these, E. coli is the most common in the United States. These infections tend to be develop more slowly than ordinary food poisoning; vomiting is much less common, and cramps, diarrhea, and fever are often worse. Like the more common staphylococcal food poisoning, these illnesses may strike whole groups of people who have had the ill fortune to eat the same batch of contaminated food.

Other Causes of Food–Associated Vomiting. The association of foods and vomiting is not limited to food poisoning or food-borne infections. **Allergy** to a food may induce vomiting, although rarely. People allergic to food are much more likely to react by breaking out into a rash or having breathing problems. Vomiting after eating a food may also have a behavioral basis. When he was a young boy, my son Mike was prone to car sickness. On one occasion, he had the misfortune to follow a fish dinner with a long and twisty car ride, with predictable results. For years afterward he would vomit if he ate fish.

Vomiting Caused by Chemicals and Medicines. Any number of materials including household chemicals and medicines may be vomited either because of a direct, irritating effect on the stomach or by other mechanisms. The vomiting center in the brain can be set off by codeine, theophylline, adrenalin, many anticancer drugs and other agents. Medicines that may bother the stomach directly include aspirin, other nonsteroidal anti-inflammatories (ibuprofen, naproxen, etc.), erythromycin and other antibiotics, and anything alcoholic.

Vomiting Triggered by Other Illnesses. Vomiting may also be a response to infections in other parts of the body. It not infrequently appears at the beginning of a strep throat, during a kidney infection, pneumonia, or hepatitis. Noninfectious illnesses, far removed from the stomach may also include vomiting. Migraine headaches or the migraine equivalent called **cyclic vomiting** are examples. (A migraine equivalent is an episode of migraine without the headache, but with the same underlying mechanisms. It can be manifested by dizziness, vomiting, or temporary loss of vision.) Various processes in the head, from a concussion to a brain tumor, can provoke vomiting.

Intestinal Obstruction. An important cause of vomiting is intestinal obstruction. In infancy, this is likely to be caused by **pyloric stenosis,** an overgrowth of muscle at the far end of the stomach where it connects to the beginning of the small intestine. Sometime after the first weeks of life, babies who develop this condition begin to vomit forcefully after feedings. The vigor of the vomiting has led to the use of the term **projectile vomiting,** a dramatic and overused phrase which simply means that the vomited milk meal can end up a couple of feet from the infant. It is worth noting that a single episode of vigorous vomiting does not necessarily mean that pyloric stenosis is present, but repeated occurrences are a convincing indication that something is up. These babies usually do not act sick at all; they will cheerfully accept another feeding immediately after having spread the preceding meal over every adult within reach. Because so little food can get through the swollen pylorus, affected infants become constipated and begin to lose weight. The diagnosis is made by physical examination or ultrasound; the treatment is a simple surgical procedure.

At any age children may develop obstruction lower down in the intestines. This condition may be signaled by the appearance of cramping, abdominal pain, and golden or green-tinged vomit. A special kind of obstruction that occurs mostly in late infancy and early childhood is **intussusception,** the telescoping of a portion of intestine into the next part of the intestine further down the line. Babies with intussusception abruptly begin to scream with pain and they often draw up their legs during the periods of discomfort. Then they tend to settle down and act quite normal until the next bout of cramps. Later, they may pass a bloody bowel movement. Intussusception and any other kind of intestinal obstruction require prompt medical attention.

Diarrhea

Although I've written about diarrhea in other chapters, diarrhea is an important symptom in its own right and merits separate attention. Diarrhea means increased frequency and wateriness of stools. This definition does not specify frequency compared to what, nor does it tell us how much water there should be in a stool. The reason for my lack of precision is that what is normal for stools depends on the age and the diet of the child. Young infants generally have stools every time they are fed; the gastrocolic reflex empties the colon as soon as the stomach is filled. Breast fed infants often continue to have frequent stools for months, and their stools may be so liquid that the diaper looks like it has been coated with yellow paint. Babies on formula have a rapidly diminishing number of stools per day, and the bowel movements are thicker, darker, and drier. With increasing age, stool frequency diminishes, no matter what the diet. In childhood and later, the indigestible fiber content of our foods becomes the major determinant of how often our colons empty themselves. High fiber diets containing whole grains, legumes, other vegetables, and fruits result in a large volume of stool. The gut responds by producing a bowel movement at least once a day, and frequently more often. In contrast, low fiber diets are characterized by refined grain products like white bread or white rice, an increased intake of fats and sweets, and lots of milk, juice, and soda pop. The gut has less to do when presented with this reduced volume of indigestible material, so it slows down and produces fewer and firmer stools, often resulting in chronic constipation.

For practical purposes, we tend to define diarrhea in terms of what is the normal pattern for a particular child. When a child who generally has a single, formed stool every day begins to have several loose stools, that's diarrhea. Diarrheal stools may also exhibit unusual colors. Our livers produce yellow-green bile which is excreted into the small intestine. During the transit down the gut, these bile pigments are gradually turned brown. During diarrhea, transit time is faster, and the unaltered bile may color the diarrhea stools green.

Acute diarrhea in childhood is most often caused by infection in the gastrointestinal tract. When the infection has passed, improvement may not be complete, and some diarrhea may continue for many days or even months. This is due to damage to the lining membranes of the intestine which repair themselves slowly. This is one of the rare instances where children heal more slowly than adults. These post-infectious diarrheas can be puzzling and difficult to manage; everyone gets pretty tired of sopping diapers and sore bottoms, but healing does happen.

The Many Causes of Diarrhea. Like vomiting, diarrhea can be a nonspecific symptom associated with all sorts of infectious processes. It is also a major symptom of food poisoning. Sometimes an excess of a particular food will cause acute diarrhea by overloading the capacity of the gastrointestinal tract to digest it. This is probably most likely to happen after overindulgence in sugary foods like soft drinks, fruit juices, and sweet fruit. Chronic diarrhea can also be caused by food overloads. I've seen a few children who simply eat so much that their intestines could not deal with the volume. The offending foods tend to be starches like cereal and grains like rice.

Toddler diarrhea is a harmless, annoying, and poorly understood condition of older infants and children in the first few years. These kids are perfectly healthy, happy, often quite strapping youngsters who eat heartily and produce more and looser stools than anyone wants to see. They are not sick but they are a mess, several times a day. This is down-to-the-shoes diarrhea. Despite the obvious good general health of these kids, we end up studying them at length for various unlikely diseases, and after spending hundreds of dollars of someone's money, we find nothing at all. Three thousand washing machine loads later, they get better. About the only treatment that may work is increasing the fat content of the diet which tends to slow down intestinal activity. Of course, everyone freaks out about this because they think the whole milk, cheese, peanut butter, and meat will clog his arteries on the spot; this concern is a trifle exaggerated.

An important instance of an imbalance between the capacity of the gut and the burden of digestion is a deficiency in one of the enzymes needed for processing food. The most common of these is **lactase deficiency** which leads to **lactose intolerance.** Lactose is the sugar normally present in the milk of humans and other mammals. It is a large molecule, a double sugar, which must be split into two simple sugars, galactose and glucose (also known as dextrose), which are then absorbed into the body. Lactase is the enzyme which does the job of splitting. During the evolution of our species, milk was available to humans only from the mother's breast and only in infancy and early childhood. After weaning, the gut had no opportunity to digest lactose, so the need for lactase disappeared. By middle childhood, lactase production gets turned off or at least turned down in most human beings. When a lactose load is presented to the lactase-deficient gut, it passes the lactose undigested down to the large bowel where it ferments, producing cramps, gas, and diarrhea. This is extremely common, especially in people of Asian, African, and Mediterranean ancestry. People from northern Europe and from cattle-herding African tribes tend to keep their ability to produce lactase throughout adult life. Apparently, continued lactase production conferred a survival advantage, since milk and milk products are such important parts of the diet in those groups. If a child develops lactase deficiency, lactase can easily be supplied as drops or tablets, to be taken before a lactose-containing meal. Alternatively, the amount of milk and milk products can be limited to whatever is tolerated without symptoms. Some children can digest cheese and yogurt, which have less lactose than milk itself. Lactose-free or reduced lactose milk is also available.

Temporary lactase deficiency often occurs when the capacity of the small intestine to produce lactase is damaged by intestinal infections. This can cause a partial lactose intolerance for weeks or months with the result that diarrhea persists. Eventually, the gut recovers and milk can be digested without difficulty.

EVERYDAY PEDIATRICS FOR PARENTS

It is an undoubted fact that a decrease in lactose production is a normal phenomenon in most human beings past early childhood. This has led some observers to question the necessity of feeding milk and other lactose-containing foods to ourselves and our children. Why, they ask, should we fly in the face of Mother Nature's wisdom, and force our poor small intestines to deal with an out-of-date nutrient for which they may no longer be equipped? Furthermore, milk and milk products include fat, which, at least in the view of some cardiologists, has replaced the love of money as the root of all evil. The answer to these objections is that milk and its products are really terrific foods. Milk protein supplies all the amino acids our bodies need; the calcium in milk is well absorbed; vitamins A, B-complex, and D are abundant in milk; human beings like the taste; and it is cheap. Take milk out of your child's diet and you will be hard-pressed to devise affordable substitutes. I can imagine what my kids would have said if I told them that they would have to make do with soybean curd, oatmeal, almonds, and cruciferous vegetables. (As Marie Antoinette might have said: "Let them eat kale.")

There may be disadvantages to consuming a high protein, high calcium diet. It seems to result in bigger, taller people, with stronger bones and less osteoporosis, but it may also lead to more and earlier heart disease if large amounts of milk fat are included. The conclusions I draw are as follows:

1. Milk and milk products are excellent foods and good value.
2. Some people are allergic to milk; they should not drink it.
3. Some people can't digest lactose; they can either avoid milk or use lactose-free milk, or take a lactase supplement.
4. A high milk fat diet may not be a great idea (except for the Tutsi cattle herders in Africa who seem to thrive on it); use fat-reduced milk, at least after the first year or two of life. Limit the intake of cream, ice cream, and butter to modest levels.
5. Try not to get panicked by the Antimilk Lobby.

Cystic fibrosis is another condition in which diarrhea may result from a lack of digestive enzymes. The problem here is an exceedingly widespread abnormality of function in many body tissues. In this inherited disease, cell membranes lack the ability to transport chloride ions in a normal fashion. This leads to abnormally thickened secretions in the lungs, liver, pancreas, nose, sweat glands, and reproductive organs. In the pancreas, the thick secretions prevent the normal flow of the enzymes needed for the digestion of food within the intestine. The result is the inability to digest and absorb food, and the production of greasy, smelly, and often loose stools. Treatment with replacement enzymes is a major help in managing this aspect of the illness. The problem in the lungs is the production of gooey, thick secretions which become infected. A chronic pneumonia develops which is partly controllable with antibiotics and other agents. Children with cystic fibrosis used to die in infancy or early childhood. Now, survival into early or midadult life is commonplace. The problems in the lungs have remained difficult, although some new approaches have begun to show real promise.

Lactase deficiency and cystic fibrosis are both examples of malabsorption due to the inadequate availability of digestive enzymes. Another kind of malabsorption occurs with an inherited intolerance to a protein called **gluten.** This disorder is called **celiac disease,** or **gluten–enduced enteropathy,** or **nontropical sprue.** Gluten is a protein present in wheat, rye, oats, and barley. Abnormalities in the small intestine lead to an inability to tolerate this protein and to the development of diarrhea and other symptoms. Children with celiac disease grow poorly and tend to be peculiarly miserable and unhappy. The symptoms persist throughout life unless the gluten-containing grains are removed from the diet. This may sound like a food allergy, but it is technically different because other, nonallergic immunologic mechanisms are involved.

Allergic reactions to foods can cause diarrhea, although this is uncommon. As I mentioned regarding vomiting, most food allergies are manifested in the skin or respiratory tract rather than in the gut. The lining membranes of the gastrointestinal tract seem to be able to protect themselves pretty well against allergenic foods. When allergic diarrhea does occur, it can result in bloody stools or in a protein-losing state with leakage of blood proteins into the stool.

Inflammatory bowel disease occurs in two forms: **Crohn's disease** and **ulcerative colitis.** I've included these uncommon conditions in this chapter because they are serious and important. These are poorly understood but seemingly related illnesses in which portions of the bowel become intensely irritated and inflamed. Bowel cramps, diarrhea, often with bleeding, weight loss, and fever may occur. The underlying cause appears to involve abnormal immune function, perhaps peculiar responses to infectious agents. Inflammatory bowel disease tends to run in families; this is at least in part due to a genetic predisposition, but environmental factors also are suspected. Crohn's disease usually occurs at the lower end of the small bowel. When it begins, the only sign may be an unexplained fever or a decrease in the child's rate of growth, but diarrhea eventually appears in most cases. Ulcerative colitis occurs anywhere in the large bowel. Most cases start with abdominal cramps and diarrhea. In both types of inflammatory bowel disease there may be disease outside of the bowel, especially in the joints. When doctors are faced with treating illnesses whose causes are unknown, we are often limited to therapies which attack particular symptoms. That is the situation with Crohn's and ulcerative colitis; a variety of treatments are in use, both medical and surgical, but control is only fair. Most patients survive for many decades, and many live out a normal life span, but we don't have any cures.

Managing illnesses like inflammatory bowel disease and cystic fibrosis is a massive strain for the patient and the family. For the child, the illness means all sorts of physical discomfort, frequent episodes requiring frightening medical attention and hospital stays, limitation of normal childhood activities, and the ever-present reality that a normal life span may be impossible. It is hard enough for mature adults to face their mortality; the burden for children and adolescents is nearly unthinkably heavy. For the brothers and sisters of a chronically sick child, family life is inevitably distorted; the sick child needs a disproportionate amount of attention and energy. The parents' lives are also subjected to endless demands and constant worry. Staying sane and keeping a family together in these circumstances is discussed in Chapter 48.

Abdominal Pain

In the preceding pages I've talked about abdominal pain in relation to vomiting and diarrhea, and noted that it can also occur as part of various nonabdominal illnesses. But how about abdominal pain as an isolated symptom? What does it mean and what should be done about it? When I was learning to write for my school newspaper, my teacher taught me that every news story required reporting WHO, WHAT, WHEN, and WHERE—a good framework for approaching the child with a bellyache.

WHO has the bellyache? The significance of abdominal pain depends, to a large degree, on the owner of the belly. Children, like adults, have their favorite ways to be sick. I am not implying that this is a matter of choice, just that it is a matter of fact. Some people get headaches, others just don't seem to. It is the same with the bellyaches. Some children will complain of abdominal pain with absolutely every illness that comes their way. They are neither lying nor exaggerating; they are simply reporting what they feel. When they are unwell anywhere, by golly, they have abdominal pain. If you are reasonably sure that this describes one of your children, you have doubtless already learned that evaluating his belly pain requires that you look further afield than the belly button to find a likely cause. By contrast, the child who never has belly pain should have your full attention when she reports abdominal discomfort. Whether it turns out to be something in the abdomen or outside it, it is likely to be significant. Experienced parents also automatically factor in the child's overall style of dealing with the problems of existence. Some kids are stoics and complain as little as possible; others employ noisy histrionics and squeeze every last bit of parental concern from each episode, no matter how trivial.

The other aspect of who has the bellyache involves the age of the child. Recurrent episodes of apparent abdominal pain in early infancy usually means colic. It is easy to assume "Oh, that's his 6 o'clock colic" when you have lived through several such evenings and you know what is going on. It is more difficult when the first attack explodes, and he is screaming at full blast. Is the baby eating well? Does he have a normal body temperature? (I mean actually measured with a thermometer; you really need to know.) Can he be comforted, at least for a while, with nursing, or a pacifier, or rocking and cuddling? If the answer to all these questions is yes, you can be reassured that colic is the likely problem, and not some exceedingly rare and awful intra-abdominal catastrophe. If you are unconvinced, you need to talk to your doctor as soon as possible.

WHAT kind of pain is it? And WHERE is the pain? Is the pain mild or severe, constant or episodic, cramping or burning or squeezing or a feeling of pressure? Older children usually provide reasonably complete responses to these questions which may help both you and your doctor to figure out what is going on. But babies and toddlers may barely be able to localize the pain at all, let alone describe it. An imprecise but useful rule of thumb was offered years ago by the English physician John Apley. Apley's Law states that the closer the pain is to the navel, the more likely it is to be "functional," that is to say without a diagnosable, organic cause. A partial exception to this rule is the early pain of acute appendicitis which often is first felt at the navel and then moves southwest to the right lower quadrant of the abdomen, over the appendix itself, as shown in the illustration. For the parent trying to evaluate her child's bellyache and decide whether or not to call the doctor, **severity** is the main criterion. Take into account the child's history of dealing with pain, as previously discussed. Other indicators are the child's appearance and activity. If he looks pale or sweaty, refuses to eat, and lies quietly in bed—don't hesitate; phone immediately.

WHEN the pain occurs may also provides important clues. Every parent will eventually be faced with a child suffering from Monday Morning Bellyache, reputedly of such severity that going to school is out of the question. (And surely you will recall having had, or faked, identical symptoms during your own childhood.) Look for the other indicators of illness, measure the child's temperature, and inquire tactfully about the problems the child is anticipating at school that day. You don't really want to send the kid to school who is incubating a strep throat or about to embark on a roaring case of gastroenteritis; on the other hand, you don't want to play into an unrewarding pattern of school avoidance. The first episode of Monday Morning Bellyache may be hard to diagnose, and may even earn the sufferer an inappropriate but welcome holiday at home. Any subsequent examples should be met with interested concern mixed with skepticism.

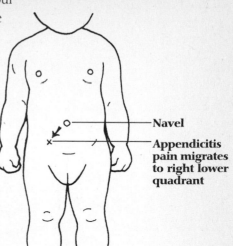

Navel

Appendicitis pain migrates to right lower quadrant

Monday mornings won't be the only challenging times ahead. My wife relates that when she was a young child she developed a bellyache and vomiting during the automobile trips down a winding road to visit her formidable and frightening grandmother. Her parents attributed this to car sickness, never noticing that their daughter never had any discomfort during the trip back home up the same winding road. In short, knowing that a child is facing a stressful situation, whenever it might be, can provide the key to understanding belly pain and any number of other stress-related complaints.

Other types of abdominal discomfort where timing is significant include **menstrual cramps** which can fool everyone, especially early in adolescent development. Most girls start their menstrual periods without any discomfort at all. After months or years, cramps may begin to appear. The first time or two, cramps occurring the day before the menstrual flow may be confusing. A rather uncommon condition called **mittelschmerz** (German for middle-pain) is lower abdominal pain caused by ovulation, occurring in the middle of the menstrual cycle, between two periods.

A few other causes of chronic abdominal pain, in the absence of other symptoms, should be noted. Lactose intolerance usually comes with diarrhea and excess gasiness, but not always. An ill-defined condition called the "irritable bowel syndrome" can cause cramps, sometimes associated with diarrhea, sometimes with constipation. Peptic ulcer in kids is not common, but can express itself as recurrent bellyache. The parasite giardia usually causes diarrhea, but occasionally only bellyache. Low-grade kidney infections are always worth looking for in kids with this complaint. Adolescent girls may have abdominal pain from a variety of pelvic problems, including sexually transmitted infections.

Noninfectious Disorders: Gastrointestinal Problems

Organic or Functional? The distinction of organic versus functional is a difficult and potentially misleading idea that has dominated medical thought for centuries. Organic implies that somewhere in the body there is a derangement causing the illness or the symptom. We hold the faith that, if we only knew enough about disease, we could find some change in a tissue, some deflection from normal in the way an organ works, some invading organism, or some peculiarity of cells that would explain what is wrong. For an impressively large number of human ills, this theoretical construction works beautifully. Unhappily, for an even larger number of the children and adults, the category "organic disease" does not work at all. The patient has appeared with his complaint, and the doctor has dutifully searched for a definable, namable, organic cause. Doctors are taught that the worst sin the physician can commit is the failure to find a disease by neglecting to think of it and look for it. There is just enough reality in this to prod the practitioner into ordering obscure lab tests or suggesting multiple consultations when she knows deep down that this little boy has a bellyache because he hates P.E. class or is upset by his parents' screaming fights. This kind of understandable but ill-advised medical meandering wastes money, involves potentially painful or dangerous tests, and often manages to convince the child and the family that something awful must or might be wrong.

Eventually, the physician calls off the wild goose chase and has to come up with some sort of a conclusion. She has several options. Number 1: "There is nothing wrong with you." The problem with this answer is that the bellyache has not gone away. Maybe the doctor has just overlooked something? Number 2: "It's all in his head." Unconvincing. "Doctor, you should see him when he is having one of his spells!" Number 3: "It is a functional pain." Well, what does that mean? As an answer, the diagnosis "functional" is incomplete, but it is actually significant. It suggests that there is indeed a derangement in some aspect of the workings of the body. We know that every part of our human machinery is affected and controlled by our hormones and our nervous systems. The balance of these regulating forces can go awry, and organs can malfunction. We may lack the ability to measure all these factors with enough precision to lead to a satisfying "organic" diagnosis, but the malfunction is none the less real. So, it turns out that organic and functional are closely related. **Organic** implies that we can find, or see, or measure a cause of disease and demonstrate its effects. **Functional** implies that a cause exists and its effects are real, but we do not yet have the diagnostic machinery to demonstrate it. The danger in this way of thinking is that we will try to reduce complex emotional phenomena to simple, physical, or chemical variables. If we someday discover that sadness is associated with a high level of a particular brain hormone, it would still be foolish of us to overlook the real life causes of the sadness, and focus solely on minimizing the concentration of the hormone.

All of which brings me to this point: Chronic bellyache in children can have many causes, but when it is present in an otherwise healthy child with no other symptoms, both pediatricians and parents need to think about emotional factors. It is impressive how often abdominal pain disappears when a child is given the opportunity to talk about, or play out, his particular fears and worries. This does not mean that every child with a psychosomatic bellyache needs 4 years of psychoanalysis. Sometimes a parent or a pediatrician can unleash a therapeutic torrent of feeling just by mentioning to the child that bellyaches can happen when people are worried about something. Could it be that something is worrying you? The first time you suggest this possibility you may be met with silence or denial. If so, try again later, perhaps rephrasing your remarks. At the very least, you will have expressed your interest and your concern, and you will, in effect, have given him permission to acknowledge and give vent to his feelings. For many children, that permission will be a gift of real value.

Chapter 41

Genital Problems

Vulvar Adhesions (Labial Adhesions). A common development in early infancy is the formation of delicate adhesions between the inner lips of the vulva. This usually occurs in plump little girls whose fat thighs press the vulvar lips (labia minora) together. These tissues are naturally moist and growing, and they begin to stick together, covering the lower part of the vaginal opening. Often the adhesions progress northward, covering the entire vaginal opening and eventually hiding most of the urethral outlet as well. You look at these babies and wonder how on earth the urine is going to find its way out. In fact, I've never seen a baby who could not manage to pee, adhesions or no adhesions, so it does not seem like a very big deal.

If you see this process starting with your daughter, increase the efficiency and vigor of bottom washing, spreading the labia more completely, and then

Clitoris

Urethral Opening

Beginning Adhesion of Inner Lips

Inner Lips (labia minora)

Outer Lips (labia majora)

Vaginal Opening

Anus

apply a little petroleum jelly (Vaseline) or some other bland, gooey cream on the inner surfaces of the labia. It's okay if some of the goo gets into the vagina. *Don't* try to undo any stuck areas; it will hurt, and the unstuck parts will just stick back together again. Don't let your doctor unstick them, either; it hurts no matter who does it. If the adhesion is so complete that you or your doctor are sure she'll never pee again, it is possible to unstick the labia by applying a dab of estrogen-containing cream over the area once or twice a day for a few weeks. This causes a temporary maturation of the lining membranes and they just come apart. The only problem is that fat babies who have gotten vulvar adhesions once tend to get them again. If too much estrogen is used for too long, sufficient absorption can take place to cause some temporary but impressive breast enlargement and nipple darkening. Be sparing.

Foreskins: Their Virtues, Misadventures, and Maintenance.

Medical people get into heated arguments about all kinds of issues; we debate the significance of cholesterol, the possible virtues of alcohol, even the care of the newborn navel. Some topics really stir up the animals; you should hear the decibel level in discussions concerning the Fate of the Foreskin. As is often the case in medical disagreements, the less real information we have, the louder the debate.

What do we really know about the function of foreskins? They are clearly part of the standard male package, and a fair number of people want to stop the debate right here. They argue that the design is pretty good; if it ain't broke, don't fix it. The trouble with this position is that the design, although serviceable, is not perfect. An analogous example is the appendix, which is also part of the standard human package. A leftover from an earlier and long since discarded method of making colons, its major function now seems to be developing appendicitis. Maybe the foreskin is an equally redundant leftover from the times when the human penis was out there without any significant protection, and a bit of extra skin seemed to the Designer like a neat idea. The people who want to leave foreskins alone also argue that removing the foreskin leaves the head of the penis (the glans) so unprotected that it loses sensitivity, reducing the pleasure of sexual intercourse. This is an argument that is going to be hard to prove. Where do you find enough men to volunteer sometime in midcareer to undergo circumcision, and then report back a few years later about the effect

EVERYDAY PEDIATRICS FOR PARENTS

on their sex life? Or is there any way for circumcised and uncircumcised men to compare notes? "I like it better than you do!" This does not seem to be likely to yield usable data. Then there is the argument that circumcision hurts like the blazes, and it's a barbaric thing to do to a defenseless baby. Some people think circumcised men carry the psychic scars for life. Well, it hurts, all right. Using a tiny injection of a local anesthetic before the circumcision is now increasingly the practice, and that seems to me to be a good thing. As far as the psychic scars, I've never noticed that the ownership of his very own foreskin conferred much specific emotional balance on a man, but then maybe I've failed to look hard enough.

Is there any good reason to get rid of foreskins? Surely the most compelling reason for circumcision is that it is a visible sign of belonging to a group. This may sound like a bizarre notion, but that has been the function of circumcision among many peoples for millenia. It may be the sign of having reached manhood, as in various primitive tribes today, or it may be the sign of having been born into a particular group, as it is with Jews and Muslims. For a few decades in the United States, circumcision became such a standard procedure that uncircumcised young men would sometimes undergo the procedure just to look like everyone else in the locker room. I expect this will no longer occur, since circumcision has become less common in this country. Another less parochial reason for circumcision is that the foreskin can sometimes become too tight to withdraw from its resting place over the glans; this is termed **phimosis.** When this happens it can become infected, a painful business indeed, and even interfere with sexual intercourse. These problems can be avoided if, every day during infancy, the baby's foreskin is gently pulled back as far as it will comfortably go, stretching it a little bit at a time until it can be fully retracted. If the foreskin happens to be unusually tight, this process may actually take many months, but there is no hurry at all. This should never be done with so much force that it causes pain. It is difficult to clean the inside lining tissue of a tight foreskin, and therefore smegma, the normal secretion of the foreskin, tends to accumulate. The irritating effects of the trapped smegma may be the reason why cancer of the penis is more common among men who have not been circumcised. As a reason for routine circumcision, this does not impress me. Make sure that the foreskin can eventually be retracted, and teach the kid to wash himself; that is not asking too much. There is uncertainty over the relationship of male circumcision to cancer of the cervix in women. Some evidence indicates that women whose sexual partners have been circumcised are less likely to develop cervical cancer, but this association may not be cause and effect. The real correlation is probably with exposure to the sexually transmitted, cancer-causing strains of wart virus (human papillomavirus). The significant equation is likely to be: Increased number of sexual partners = increased likelihood of exposure to the virus. Another reason on offer in favor of circumcision is a puzzler: Kidney infections are more common in uncircumcised than in circumcised infant boys. This *does* seem to be true, *but* kidney infections are really quite uncommon in infants, so the argument does not carry a great deal of weight.

Conclusions:

1. If your tribe or religious group believes in circumcision, go ahead.
2. If the foreskin cannot be made to retract easily by midchildhood, circumcision or at least a minor procedure to loosen it may be in order.
3. If Dad and all the other males in the family are circumcised, you may want to circumcise your son just to avoid invidious comparisons. Frankly, I don't see this last point as a major matter. The adult penis is so much different than the penis of the child that the presence or absence of a bit of foreskin probably will be unimportant to all the potential observers.

Menstruation

Menstruation is such a complicated process, and so responsive to all sorts of interference that it is amazing that it functions at all. So much equipment is required: a normal vagina, a properly matured uterus, functioning fallopian tubes, ovaries supplied with all the necessary ova and capable of secreting the right amounts of estrogen and progesterone, a pituitary gland to provide hormonal control, the hypothalamic region of the brain to control the pituitary, and all of this enclosed in a healthy female body, neither too fat nor too thin, with properly adjusted adrenal and thyroid glands, an adequate diet, and the right balance of physical activity. Despite the opportunities for error inherent in the system, most girls manage the entire developmental sequence without a hitch.

Sexual maturation is a long process, beginning in late childhood and extending well into the teens. It begins when some unknown mechanism signals the hypothalamus, an area at the base of the brain, to manufacture and release a hormone (gonadotropin-releasing hormone) which acts on the pituitary gland. The pituitary increases production of two hormones (follicle stimulating hormone and luteinizing hormone) which act on the ovaries. The ovaries increase their output of estrogen and become ready to produce progesterone as well.

EVERYDAY PEDIATRICS FOR PARENTS

These sex hormones are the agents that act directly on the breasts, uterus, and vagina, causing sexual maturation and proper sexual functioning, including menstruation.

The initiation of this cascade of events is influenced by all sorts of forces and circumstances. Good nutrition, living in warmer climates, perhaps increased exposure to artificial light, freedom from serious illness these—are all associated with earlier sexual development and an earlier onset of menstruation. Inadequate diet, lack of sufficient body fat, excessively strenuous physical activity, and various chronic diseases have the opposite effect. For healthy girls, the first sign of sexual development is usually nipple and breast change, late in the first decade or early in the second. Within 2 to 3 years sexual development can be expected to have progressed to the point where the first menstrual periods will arrive; in the United States today this is commonly around age 12½ or 13. Especially during the first years of menstruation, cycles can be wildly erratic; it may be many months after the first period that the second period occurs. This annoying and sometimes anxiety-provoking lack of regularity may persist well into adolescence.

Menstrual Hygiene. I hope that women readers will not take it amiss if I, as a male physician, offer some advice about menstrual hygiene, a subject about which I obviously lack firsthand information. First, **tampons vs. menstrual pads** for young girls. Most girls start with the use of pads until they get used to the business of dealing with their menstrual discharge. After familiarity and some degree of comfort has been achieved, the use of small, soft tampons is worth learning. Along with their practical advantages, tampons have the virtue of requiring that girls develop a more precise understanding of their genital anatomy. Second, regarding **douching.** In case the word had not gotten around yet, ***routine douches are out.*** There is simply no need for any kind of vaginal douche for healthy girls or women. Third, **toxic shock syndrome.** A new disease, occurring mostly in menstruating girls and women, was recognized in the late 1970s. It was marked by fever, a rash, vomiting, and a shocky state of cardiovascular collapse. The cause was found to be an infection most often due to the use of certain types of highly absorbent tampons. If worn for long periods of time, they allowed the growth of dangerous bacteria within the vagina. These tampons have now been taken off the market and the kinds of tampon now available are safe if used with reasonable care. Change tampons when they are soaked with blood, and at least twice daily. Wash external genitals daily during a period.

Disorders of Menstruation. Menstruation is the process of shedding a portion of the inner lining of the uterus. Under the influence of estrogen and progesterone, the uterine lining changes in preparation for receiving and nourishing a fertilized egg. If no fertilized egg appears and implants, the uterine lining begins to break down and bleed, thus producing a menstrual period. Early in puberty, the ovary often does not produce eggs; this results in what are termed **anovulatory cycles.** When no egg is produced, the ovary makes estrogen but no progesterone. The effect on the uterine lining is to produce abnormal thickening, and this may lead to irregular and often excessive menstrual bleeding. This is the most common cause for what is called **dysfunctional uterine bleeding.** Hormone treatment is sometimes needed to control this problem until the normal maturation of reproductive function occurs.

Amenorrhea means the absence of menstrual periods. Sometimes periods do not begin at the expected time in a girl whose sexual development has appeared to be normal; rarely, sexual development in general fails to get underway at the usual age. These two categories of failure to menstruate are termed **primary amenorrhea.** It can be appreciated from the complexity of the entire process of sexual development and function that all kinds of things can occasionally go awry. Unraveling the cause usually requires thoroughgoing gynecological and endocrinological study. The term **secondary amenorrhea** describes the situation of a teenager who has been having normal periods and stops having them. Here the causes are relatively clear cut: pregnancy; excessive weight loss associated with dieting, anorexia nervosa, or bulimia; excessive physical activity, usually from competitive sports; psychological stress. Rare causes include various hormonal problems and chronic diseases.

Dysmenorrhea (Menstrual Cramps). Cramping pain during menses has been a part of the female human condition for a very long time. During the millenia when dysmenorrhea was not understood, a rich growth of lay and medical folklore developed concerning its causes and control. It is no surprise that this has turned out to be mostly nonsense. Unfortunately, scientific understanding takes time to percolate through the culture. The result is that a considerable amount of confusion is still commonplace, and many girls and women have not taken advantage of what is currently known.

Menstrual cramps are due to an excess amount of a substance called **prostaglandin F_2,** produced within the uterus, which causes painful contractions of the uterine muscle. (The prostaglandins are a large family of naturally occurring body chemicals which have scores of different functions; they stimulate or regulate processes such as blood flow, inflammation, pain sensitivity, kidney and stomach function.) Prostaglandin F_2 production is apparently stimulated by the occurrence of ovulation. Many young girls have menstrual cycles without ovulation for the first months or even years of adolescence; these anovulatory cycles are typically free of any cramping pain. Later, when ovulation gets underway, menstrual cramps may appear. Why some women produce too much prostaglandin F_2 is not known. A few have some abnormal process like endometriosis, a condition in which small islands of uterine lining tissue develop away from the uterus, within the pelvis or abdomen. Most girls and women with menstrual cramps are otherwise perfectly healthy.

Until these facts were discovered, theories concerning the causes of dysmenorrhea ranged from the bizarre to the punitive, and the suggested therapies were equally inappropriate. The application of accurate understanding has cleared away all this rubble. For the large majority of girls and women, the control of prostaglandin F_2 by the use of nonsteroidal, anti-inflammatory drugs (NSAIDs) reduces the discomfort of menstruation to a manageable level. The newer and more powerful NSAIDs like ibuprofen (Motrin, Nuprin, Advil) and naproxen (Naprosyn, Aleve) are much more effective than the old standby, aspirin. They work best if the first doses are given *before* the period starts. Try experimenting with different preparations and dosages until you discover what works. Some women get better results with other, prescription-only NSAIDs. The addition of caffeine in the form of strong coffee or tea may also be helpful. For a few women, the inhibition of ovulation by birth control pills is needed.

Attitudes Regarding Menstruation. It was not all that long ago that menstruation was commonly referred to as **The Curse,** and it is worth considering the significance of the word. No doubt about it, menstruation is an inconvenient, messy, and often uncomfortable process. Menstruation is also the signal of women's sexual being, and in a culture that has been suspicious of and worried about sex, it is a danger signal. In many cultures women are perceived by men to be unsafe, unclean, and even unholy during menstruation. And I imagine that menstruation has often meant to women that they are trapped in a subservient, repressive relationship with men, at the mercy of men's bodies and without control of their own. Whether for these reasons or not, generations of young women have somehow learned that menstruation is frightening and unmentionable. Equally, generations of boys have been raised with discomfort and ignorance about menstruation.

My point is to remind parents that even if we still carry some of the old fear, shame, and discomfort, we do not have to pass on these out-of-date and hurtful attitudes to the new generation. In today's culture most of us are less afraid of sex, more willing to talk about it to our kids, more accepting of the necessity of teaching them about sex in our schools. My impression is that more and more girls and their families now welcome the first periods as a rite of passage, the sign of their growing into womanhood. Menstruation need no longer be one of the great unmentionable topics.

Chapter 42

Hearing and Speech Problems

Like so many other aspects of childhood development, hearing and speech are dependent on an amazingly complex web of interconnected and interdependent structures. The opportunities for mistakes and malfunctions are many; the fact that it all works so well for so many is astounding. Just to list the equipment needed is impressive: a normally formed outer ear to allow the access of sound to the middle ear; a middle ear outfitted with a nicely movable ear drum and a set of tiny bones to help direct the sound to the inner ear; a properly constructed and connected inner ear to turn sound waves into nerve impulses; an auditory nerve to whisk the information to the hearing centers of the brain; and a hearing processing center in the brain to decode and make sense out of the nerve impulses. The developing brain then has the further task of making the leap between the understanding of incoming speech and the expression of ideas as outgoing speech, that is to say, learning to talk. The apparatus required for this includes speech centers and muscle control centers dedicated to working the various muscles that control breathing, the vocal cords, eating, and swallowing (so that those functions can be smoothly coordinated with speech), and the face, mouth, and lips. In addition, there are the nerves that carry these commands, and the organs of speech themselves.

The acquisition and assembly of all this paraphernalia starts early. There is some evidence that babies in utero can hear sounds coming from the outside world by the middle of pregnancy, around 26 weeks. They may not hear very much or very clearly, however. The inside of the uterus is a noisy place, what with the roar of the uterine and placental blood flow, and all the bubbling and gurgling emanating from Mom's intestinal tract. By the last month or two of pregnancy, the unborn baby can hear quite a bit. (Some mothers "teach" songs to their babies in the months just before birth. The babies seem to respond to the familiar music when they hear it after being born. I doubt that this is important, but it's fun.)

Newborns hear quite well. They pay most attention to sounds within the usual range of human speech, which is certainly sensible. They are particularly responsive to high-pitched voices, and it is nearly universally the case that adults choose to speak to newborns in a high-pitched "baby talk" style. Within a few days, babies have learned to respond more to their mothers than to anyone else. At a later stage, babies prefer their fathers' voices to those of other men. Clearly, the normal infant rapidly undertakes the process of learning to understand and differentiate the sounds he hears.

He also embarks instantaneously on the tasks of learning to speak. Within a very few days, he will have developed different cries, depending on whether he is reacting to hunger or discomfort. He will also make noncrying noises, and within a very few weeks, a limited but expressive repertoire of goos and gurgles can be expected. Real laughter comes soon thereafter, usually in the second or third month. Much of this talking will be in response to his mother and other caretakers. There can be quite a conversation of reciprocal babbling and baby talk. In the ensuing months babies will practice a variety of sounds. And by the latter part of the first year many infants are speaking their first words. They also clearly understand a number of words, especially their own names, the words "Mama" and "Daddy," words for milk or nursing and food, and "No!" The **receptive** or **passive vocabulary** appears before the **expressive** or **active vocabulary.** The baby who can say nothing more complicated than "Dada" may well *understand* a dozen or more words, let alone all sorts of nonverbal communications including facial expression, body posture, and gesture.

Like everything biological, these processes vary immensely from one child to another. Perfectly normal babies may have their first words as early as 6 months of age or as late as 18 months. The early acquisition of speech is the source of a considerable amount of unearned parental pride; we all tend to think that a child of ours who speaks at an early age is giving evidence of verbal and intellectual brilliance. In fact, the only implication one can legitimately draw is that his intelligence is at least at a normal level; mentally retarded children will generally start to speak at later than normal ages. Whether the early talker will continue to amaze his delighted parents by continued verbal accomplishments can never be assumed. Early speech is fine, but it does not necessarily predict a National Merit Scholar.

Variability of development continues to be a problem in our understanding of language development. Children must master all the **sounds of speech,** consonants and vowels alike; this can take as long as 5 or 6 years, especially for some of the consonants. They must also learn **syntax,** how words go together in phrases and sentences, and **grammar,** the rules of how words are used. And they must develop the **social skills of speech:** how to use speech as a social tool, what rules govern conversation, and the differences in speech depending on whether one is talking to peers, teachers, family, or friends. For each of these separate skills there are normal variations in both speed and eventual degree of mastery. There are also innumerable opportunities for the process to go awry because of abnormalities in structure or function, or because of interference by disease or other environmental factors. This is what makes it tricky to know when to worry about a child's speech development, and when to watch and wait. Observers, both parental and professional, are likely to be quite content with the child whose first words are spoken at 10 to 12 months, who puts two-word phrases together by 18 months, has two-word sentences (noun or pronoun plus verb) at 2 years, puts all the parts together in what sounds and feels like everyday speech by about 4 years, and has all the consonants in place by 5 or 6 years. As the child diverges from this average, normal pattern, we begin to wonder if all is well. The temptation for the doctor is to say "Don't worry; he'll grow out of it." The danger is that serious and permanent deficits may develop if major abnormalities of hearing or speech are allowed to persist. This is particularly true for hearing loss during the first year or so. If the developing brain is not supplied with intelligible sound at the right time, it may never be able to organize itself properly for dealing with speech even if hearing is restored later.

The Assessment of Hearing

Whose hearing should be tested, and how, and when? Like most screening tests available today, testing hearing requires equipment, time, and skilled people to do the tests and interpret the results. Too much testing is a waste of money and has the unintended effect of making normal child development seem to be a hazardous undertaking, requiring professional assistance at every turn. It seems to me that this medicalization of human life is nearly unavoidable. I regret it, but I don't want to miss the chance to help a hearing-impaired baby have a normal life.

The newborns who are most at risk for hearing problems should have the earliest and most precise testing. These include premature babies, sick babies, babies whose close relatives have congenital hearing loss, and babies with abnormalities known to be associated with hearing loss. The best available test at this age is the **brainstem auditory evoked response (BAER),** a method of monitoring an infant's brain waves while presenting him with sounds. This method has the disadvantage of picking up transient abnormalities that prove to be of no lasting importance, but it serves to alert everyone to the infants who will require careful follow-up observation.

During early infancy, the most sensitive observer of hearing problems will usually be the mother who notices that her child does not seem to notice or respond to music, the doorbell, or her own voice. Many babies with hearing loss will start out producing the same vocalizations as babies who hear. However, after a few months without normal auditory stimulation, the cooing and gurgles may subside. This can be a subtle change and easily missed. Formal testing at this age and during the first few years of childhood requires an audiologist with experience in infant hearing evaluation. This is a complex procedure because it requires the measurement of nonverbal responses to a variety of sounds. By age 3 or 4 years, when a child's voluntary cooperation is a possibility, hearing testing can easily be done with the use of earphones and pure-tone audiometry. Pediatricians routinely incorporate this kind of screening into well child care.

An additional tool for hearing evaluation is **tympanometry (imped- ance audiometry).** This clever device measures the physical response of the ear drum to a sound wave. It can detect the most common hearing problem of childhood, fluid within the middle ear, and associated problems like plugged eustachian tubes. Tympanometry is a neat little tool which can produce useful guidance to the doctor, but it can also be vastly misleading. Many an "abnor- mal" tympanogram is the result of a hurried, inexpert measurement or a strug- gling child. A tympanogram is never a substitute for the pediatrician's skillful visual examination of the ear with an ordinary **pneumatic otoscope.**

Doctors must really know how to use this instrument which allows us to see the entire ear drum and watch it move when we puff air down the ear canal. This simple sounding process is not in the least simple. The ear canal is tiny in small children, it is curved, and often partly or completely occluded with ear wax. Ear wax is the Almighty's way of keeping pediatricians humble. We are prevented from having too exalted an opinion about ourselves by spending hours at one end of a wax-removing curette while the ear wax, hidden half an inch away, refuses to budge. This takes a ridiculous amount of time, and it absolutely *has* to be done right. The medical examination also involves careful observation of the rest of the child. We look for hints of illness or abnormality of structure that might interfere with hearing, and we also need to keep a continuing eye on the general processes of growth and development that may impinge on hearing and speech.

Fluid in The Middle Ear (Serous Otitis) and Hearing Loss.

The general topic of ear infections and the problem of fluid remaining in the middle ear is discussed in Chapter 30. The aspect of this problem which concerns us here is the hearing impairment that accompanies any middle ear fluid collection. When a middle ear is infected, the lining membranes ooze secretions into the middle ear space. That is no problem if the eustachian tube is open and the fluid can drain away down the back of the throat, but commonly the eustachian tube is swollen shut and the fluid stagnates. Its presence dampens the movements of the ear drum and the tiny middle ear bones, and prevents sound form being transmitted freely to the inner ear. The effect is muffled hearing, quite like the diminished hearing we are all familiar with when water gets trapped against the outside of our ear drum after a swim or a shower. The difference is that the child with middle ear fluid can't shake his head and free the trapped water. He remains partly deaf; soft and high-pitched consonant sounds are particularly well absorbed by the fluid, so that what he hears is both muted and distorted. Many middle ear infections clear promptly; the child tolerates a week or so of poor hearing, usually without anyone noticing that he isn't hearing as well as usual. But what if the fluid remains? There are three concerns if it does. 1) The middle ear space can't completely heal, and reinfections are likely. 2) The fluid may become thicker, more glue-like, and stiffer, so that it cannot drain out spontaneously when the eustachian tube finally opens. Furthermore, its continued presence may injure the middle ear bones and the delicate little joints connecting them, thereby causing permanent damage to their sound transmitting function. 3) The continued hearing loss may interfere with learning. I've mentioned that prolonged hearing loss in the first year of life is particularly serious because the brain needs auditory input to organize itself; we make sense of the world of sound because our developing brains have had practice dealing with it during the crucial early months of life. This becomes less

EVERYDAY PEDIATRICS FOR PARENTS

of a concern during toddlerhood and early childhood; by then the organizational work within the brain has probably been completed. But the remaining tasks of auditory learning are just beginning. The young child has many words to learn, explanations to understand, commands to heed, songs to sing. It is no small impediment if he is wrapped in a fog of impaired hearing. It is worth considering how the child himself perceives his hearing. This kind of hearing loss may develop slowly as a middle ear infection worsens, or it may occur nearly explosively, as a severely infected middle ear abruptly fills with pus. In the latter case, the child is likely to attend to the pain rather than the diminished hearing. Oddly enough, it appears that most children accept the new state of partial deafness without comment; it is rare for a child to complain about his hearing. Sometimes parents or teachers will notice an increase in irritability as the only sign of deafness. More often, the first symptom is the TV or radio turned up louder than usual.

As is so often true in medical matters, the urgency of this issue is still a matter for argument. Some observers believe that repeated episodes of middle ear fluid in early childhood cause intellectual or at least scholastic damage that cannot be repaired. Others of us have more faith in the power of the small child to heal and to make up for the periods of lost auditory clarity. All of us agree that persistent fluid in the middle ear is a serious matter requiring careful evaluation and sometimes vigorous treatment. How this is to be accomplished is something you and your child's physician must work out.

Other Causes of Impaired Hearing. Hearing impairment has a multiplicity of causes. Some cases are associated with various abnormalities in the structure of the ears and face. Some are familial, with multiple family members having hearing loss on an inherited basis. Deafness due to infection during fetal life with rubella virus is now much less common because of the widespread use of rubella vaccine. We still see congenital cases due to other viral infections, especially cytomegalovirus (CMV). Bacterial meningitis in infancy and childhood continues to cause deafness, but the control of Haemophilus influenzae type b infection by the Hib vaccine has decreased the number of these cases.

Educating the Hearing–Impaired Child. No matter what the cause of the deafness, the education of these children requires complex and coordinated effort. Special education classes and teachers, regular classroom teachers, audiologists, speech therapists, psychologists, social workers, and physicians are all involved. There has been considerable controversy over the best way to educate the child who has little if any usable hearing. The "oral" method uses **lip reading** and stresses the development of usable speech. Oral training of the deaf is difficult for teacher and student alike, and it really does not work very well. Within the deaf community there has been resistance to this approach, and "manual" communication with **sign language** has been preferred. This is much more easily mastered, and excellent communication between people who can sign is typical. But signing is not a skill likely to be learned except by the deaf, despite efforts to teach it to the hearing. "Total communication" attempts to meld both approaches, so that a deaf child can **sign, lip read,** and **speak** to the best of her ability, thus maximizing her ability to relate both inside and outside the deaf community. The "total" approach appears to have become the standard, but the difficulties and limits of any and all of these educational methods must be recognized.

The Assessment of Speech

Speech and hearing are two aspects of one process, verbal communication. Whenever we study progress or problems in either sphere, we must pay attention to the other. During the first years of life, the expected development of verbal skills is relatively simple and straightforward: cries and cooing, laughing, experimenting with sounds, repetitive simple syllables, real words, simple phrases, and, finally, sentences. As the child gets older, we expect increasing precision in pronunciation, mastery of more and more consonants, and better sentence structure. We also expect pronouns to fit, tense and number and gender to be expressed, and a pattern of adult-type language to start emerging. If this sequence fails to unfold in the usual fashion, the first place we look will be at the input side of the equation: Can he hear? If hearing is found to be normal, we must consider the rest of the circuit. The mechanics of speech itself are fairly amenable to study. The structures needed for breathing and the production of sound are either directly or indirectly visible. It is rare that nerve or muscle dysfunction is an impediment to normal speech. The least accessible area is the most important: the parts of the brain that receive and process what is heard, and the parts that produce speech.

The hearing and speech processing centers in the brain remain the puzzle. Prolonged observation and repeated testing is needed to elucidate those speech problems which result from one or another kind of central nervous system dysfunction. Eventually, they can be categorized in several groups.

1. **Normal but slow speech development.** These kids are perfectly okay,

but their timetable is off. I recall stewing about one little boy who seemed absolutely fine in every respect except that he had nothing to say. His mother continued to maintain that he understood and responded appropriately to everything in his world. She successfully resisted my requests for a consultation with a speech and hearing specialist, and eventually Ian burst forth with adequate and indeed, nearly excessive speech in his own good time.

2. **Mentally deficient children.** Children with severe mental deficiency have abnormally slow development in many areas; their social, physical, and verbal skills soon reveal themselves to be far behind the norm. In many cases, there are also abnormalities of appearance that draw attention to the diagnosis. However, children with only minor or moderate mental retardation may show reasonably normal progress in many areas, at least for a year or so. When they eventually fall behind during the second or third year, it is usually clear that their slow speech is part and parcel of a more global deficiency in intelligence. The term "retardation" is somewhat misleading when applied to these children because it may carry the implication of a temporary impediment from which the child may recover, and eventually catch up. I'm afraid that we tend to use words like retardation or "special" or "exceptional" children to avoid speaking truthfully and bluntly to their parents. It is so hard to face the reality that a child is permanently and seriously mentally deficient, and I know that I, and probably other pediatricians as well, avoid saying the harsh and hurtful, but honest words.

3. **Children with autism.** Autism is a rare disorder of brain function characterized by delayed and usually abnormal speech, abnormalities in social behavior, notably withdrawal from others, and peculiar patterns of physical movement. It is exceptionally difficult to know much about the mental processes of autistic children. The intelligence of most of them seems to be markedly deficient, but their speech and behavior is so strange that accurate measurement is impossible. A few autistic people manifest extraordinary ability in a limited area, usually mathematical computation. There is also a high-functioning group (Asberger's syndrome) whose intellectual ability and speech are normal, while their social interactions remain peculiar and problematical.

4. **Children with specific language disabilities.** This is a mixed and confusing group of kids with normal intelligence but one or another prob-

lem with language. These include **central auditory processing dys-functions**—information is received but cannot be handled rapidly and accurately, and developmental **aphasia**—comprehension or expression of speech is imperfect. There may be links between these disorders and **dyslexia**—difficulty in processing written and printed language. As better techniques are devised to study the workings of the brain, light is gradually being thrown on this difficult area.

5. **Cerebral palsy** is the term referring to disorders of muscle function caused by injury or abnormality in the motor control areas of the brain. Children with CP often have speech problems, in addition to many other abnormalities.

Stuttering and Stammering. During the third and fourth years of life, as speech becomes increasingly fluent and complex, children often go through a phase of speech hesitation marked by stuttering. The usual pattern is multiple repetitions of the first syllable of a word, eventually followed by clear speech. The impression one gets is of ideas outrunning the child's ability to express himself; "He seems to be thinking faster than he can talk." This is a fairly common and usually transient stage; after a few months the parents notice that he isn't doing it anymore, and that's that.

Except sometimes it doesn't go away. It is worth noting that the persistent variety of stuttering appears to have a genetic basis in some families. It is also sometimes connected with learning disabilities, including dyslexia, and it is more common in boys. The kids who continue to stammer may become tense and troubled as they notice that their speech pattern brings them all sorts of unwanted attention. Their parents give them unhelpful advice: "Think before you speak. Slow down when you want to say something." Their peers may decide that stuttering is pretty funny. When a child isn't outgrowing stuttering after a few months, when the stuttering is a pervasive aspect of his speech, when it is becoming a focus for family discomfort, or when the child is obviously unhappy about it, consultation with a speech therapist is a good idea.

Lisping, Mispronunciations, and Other Problems with Intelligibility. The common expectation is that small children will have problems with pronunciation. No one is surprised when a 2-year old substitutes or even omits some consonants, and lisping is often perceived as a charming part of babyhood. These failures of fluency are usually of no importance, and they tend to disappear spontaneously by the age of 5 or 6. However, some dysfluencies are important. An occasional toddler develops more and more speech but it becomes less and less understandable. Except in the worst instances, his parents are usually able to make sense of his utterances; sometimes an older sibling is the only person who can translate for him. When speech fluency is this badly impaired the child's social development begins to be put at risk. A peer may decide "If I can't talk to him, I won't play with him." Furthermore, if seriously aberrant patterns of speech remain uninterrupted, eventual remediation may become a difficult undertaking. For these reasons it is important to have a speech therapist evaluate children who do not seem to be progressing toward clear speech. Early intervention in the preschool years can make a major difference.

CHAPTER 43

Diabetes

This is an inherited disorder of the body's ability to utilize carbohydrates (starches and sugars). The metabolism of proteins and fats is also affected, although less importantly, and as the disease progresses abnormalities of the blood vessels often develop. The full name of the illness is **diabetes mellitus,** to distinguish it from **diabetes insipidus,** a rare disorder of the control of urine concentration; the only factor in common between the diseases is the symptom of excessive urination.

For practical purposes, diabetes in kids and teenagers is a different disease from diabetes in adults. Adult-type diabetes is characterized by a gradually increasing resistance to the normal actions of **insulin,** one of the hormones that controls carbohydrate metabolism. This condition can usually be helped by a combination of diet changes plus antidiabetic (hypoglycemic) drugs taken by mouth; most diabetics with the adult-type disease do not need insulin shots. **Adult-type diabetes** (also called **type II** or **noninsulin-dependent diabetes mellitus**) has a strong tendency to run in families; if one identical twin has it, there is an 80 to 90% chance the other twin has it. Rarely, a child or a teenager will develop this adult-type diabetes, but most diabetes that arises before adult life is quite different.

Diabetes appearing in childhood or adolescence typically appears rather abruptly. The underlying problem is the destruction of the insulin-producing cells in the pancreas. When enough of them are injured insulin levels fall, and the body can no longer process carbohydrates. Then the excess sugar builds up in the bloodstream and eventually spills out in the urine. This causes excessive urination and a dangerous loss of body fluids and minerals; the child loses weight and may become dehydrated and acutely ill. Treatment with appropriate fluids and insulin quickly restores a normal metabolic state. Thereafter, insulin is required, given 1 to 4 times a day by injection. (Insulin is a protein: If it were given by mouth, it would be digested and destroyed.) This illness is called **type I,** or **insulin–dependent,** or **juvenile–onset diabetes.** It also has a genetic basis, but other factors seem to contribute in determining who gets diabetes. Unlike adult–onset diabetes, if one identical twin with juvenile–onset diabetes has the illness, there is about a 33% chance that the other twin will have it. If one child in a family has it, a nontwin sibling has a 5% chance of developing it. This type of diabetes is an autoimmune disorder, that is, one in which the body forms antibodies to some of its own constituents. There is an associated increase in other autoimmune illnesses as well, including conditions affecting the thyroid, the adrenals, and the stomach lining. It is not yet known what environmental factors are important although some evidence suggests that certain virus infections can trigger the disease.

Before the discovery of insulin in the 1920s, the treatment of children with diabetes was impossible. All that could be suggested was a diet very low in carbohydrates in a vain attempt to limit the body's losses. The response of the frustrated and frantic physicians sometimes seems to have bordered on religious zealotry. This was exemplified by an illustrated publication from the leading diabetes treatment center called a *Catechism for Diabetic Children.* I recall particularly the picture that showed a child being offered an apple, with the caption "The good child refuses the apple because he knows it is not good for him." This judgmental style permeated diabetic management for decades, and long after the advent of insulin treatment physicians were still talking about "good" and "bad" urines, and describing their patients as "cheating" on their diets. The doctors ordered the parents to assume and maintain utter and complete control over the lives of their chidren. This was especially tough for adolescents with diabetes. At those crucial years when the teenager needed to experience an increase in autonomy, he was faced with anxious parents who wanted to be sure that each insulin shot was accurately and properly given, that every mouthful of food was planned and measured, and that no unauthorized and presumably dangerous binges of milk shakes and pizza were consumed. The result was often that diabetic teenagers acted out adolescent rebellion by fighting about diabetes. They often ended up in the hospital. We termed them "brittle diabetics" and failed to recognize that their metabolic problems were largely due to their struggles for independence. Until quite recently, this peculiar rigidity continued to characterize diabetology. We are now in a happier and more rational era. A great deal has been learned about diabetes in kids, and there is increased agreement concerning management; we no longer need to treat diabetes as a moral issue.

Food for Diabetics. The old, rigid "diabetic diet" with its carefully prescribed amounts of fats, proteins, and starches never worked well. It required an impossible degree of precision in home cooking and eating, and either everyone in the family had to eat a predetermined amount of scientifically chosen food, or the diabetic had to be singled out. The only approach that really makes sense is to help each family develop an eating pattern that will work for *everyone*. The diabetic's food needs are really not much different from anyone else's.

It took the pediatric profession a long time to recover from the carbohydrates-will-kill-you mind set that characterized the preinsulin era. Only recently has the importance of a generous carbohydrate intake been recognized. It is now understood that even concentrated sweets and sugars can quite easily be assimilated by the diabetic—as long as they are taken as part of a meal rather than separately. The diabetic child's catechism no longer needs to exclude that apple.

What the diabetic does require is a reasonably even supply of calories every day, spread out in a fairly predictable fashion so that his insulin can be tailored to his needs. Because so many diabetics end up with vascular diseases associated with fatty deposits in the arteries, a diet avoiding excesses of animal fat and saturated fat is wise. These goals can often be met without forcing major changes in the whole family's patterns of eating. And the diabetic child need no longer go without a piece of cake at his friend's birthday party. Diabetic kids do not need to be made to feel like freaks.

Insulin. As I mentioned above, in juvenile-onset diabetes the pancreas cannot produce enough insulin. A normal pancreas reacts quickly and accurately to changes in the level of sugar in the blood. An increase in sugar triggers an increase in insulin, and the sugar level drops. Excessively high sugar levels may be the cause of the blood vessel complications of diabetes, so it would be desirable to mimic the functioning of the pancreas and thereby attain more regular blood sugar levels. Some implantable devices have been invented which attempt to do this, but they are still in the early stages of development. The best we can do at this time is to use a combination of fast-acting and slow-acting insulins, or multiple injections of insulins to cover the expected ebbs and flows of sugar levels in the blood. This is no simple task because blood sugar is affected by so many factors: Foods, exercise, illness, rate of growth, and emotional state all have profound influences. A further limiting factor is the danger of dropping the blood sugar level so low that brain function is impaired. Hypoglycemic episodes can be frightening and dangerous.

When diabetes begins in infancy or early childhood, the parents must decide the daily insulin dose, and then administer it. At older ages, the child or teenager can learn to give herself the shots; it is a simple procedure which middle-aged kids (over the age of 6 to 8) handle quite well. A little later, the job of deciding on each day's doses will also devolve to the patient herself. This is a tricky business. There is often a high level of parental anxiety bound up with the management of the illness. Especially if the child has had diabetes for years, the pattern of parental control can become powerfully entrenched. Handing over responsibility for a decision like this can be immensely worrisome, but at some point every youngster with diabetes has to fly solo.

Measuring Diabetic Control. Four methods are available to tell the person with diabetes how well his illness is controlled. **Urine testing** used to be the mainstay; simple tests revealed sugar in the urine if the blood sugar had been too high in the preceding hours, and another urine test revealed ketones if inadequate amounts of insulin had forced the body to burn fats instead of sugar. Today these tests are much less important than the direct testing of the blood for sugar. Home **blood sugar testing** is accurate and simple; it allows increased precision in tailoring insulin doses to the body's requirements. Another useful test indicates the average blood levels for the preceding one or two months. This is done by measuring the amount of an altered form of **hemoglobin (hemoglobin A_{1c});** this is blood hemoglobin which has interacted with blood sugar and formed a new compound. The more hemoglobin A_{1c} the higher the average blood sugar has been. This provides a very nice overview of the long term process of control. The fourth method of assessing treatment is clinical rather than chemical. Careful growth measurements will reveal the adequacy of the amount of insulin and food, the two major factors in determining the course of diabetes in kids.

The Family with a Diabetic Child. Diabetes is a challenge to any family. The child's initial illness can be frightening. The diagnosis is usually a shock; hospitalization is often required; the family is faced with a whole series of tasks; there is an immense amount to learn about the illness; a new set of technical medical responsibilities is thrust upon the parents; the other kids are upset. As if this were not enough, many parents feel guilty when they learn about the hereditary aspect of diabetes, and they may worry about the possibility that their other children will develop the same problem.

The long haul is not so easy, either. I've already described the likely necessity for family dietary changes, the daily decisions on insulin doses and interpretion of blood sugar measurements, and the unavoidable infliction of a little pain on your child every time you take a blood sugar measurement or give a dose of insulin. Parents are faced with the conflicting issues of protecting the child's physical health by overseeing the management of the illness, and at the same time, trying to encourage his emotional health by helping him cope with his condition and eventually take day to day responsibility for it. It is a balancing act on a high wire that may stretch over many years. As is true for every chronic condition, the family costs are not inconsiderable and are discussed further in Chapter 48.

Growing Up with Diabetes. The basic problem that the child or adolescent must eventually cope with is: Am I a person who has diabetes? Or am I a Diabetic? That is to say, am I a human being who has a metabolic problem, or does this metabolic problem define my life?

It really helps to talk about this issue, and who better to talk to than other kids with diabetes? Since diabetes in childhood is not a common illness, most kids with newly diagnosed diabetes will be unlikely to know anyone with the same problem. It can be very difficult to discuss with their nondiabetic friends and they may feel puzzled, frightened, and isolated by their illness. Children and teenagers want to feel that they are not different from everyone else, and they want to feel healthy and whole. Having an illness that requires shots, attention to diet, blood tests, and doctor visits hardly supports a comfortable sense of fitting in with the rest of the peer culture.

Many diabetic kids attend diabetic clinics where they can meet others with the same set of problems. Summer camps for children with diabetes provide an even better setting for coming to terms with the illness, and learning to feel more accepting of oneself. The sense of self-reliance combined with the experience of

"I'm not alone; there are lots of others dealing with the same problem" is invaluable. The summer camp experience is also valuable for parents because it reassures them that their children can survive away from home.

The child or teenager with diabetes faces a life with continuing challenges: Damage to blood vessels can impair vision and kidney function; pregnancy poses special difficulties for both mother and baby. We've come a very long way from the preinsulin era, but we still have a distance to go.

Chapter 44

Migraine

Migraine deserves and gets its own chapter, distinct from headaches in general, because it is so much more than just another pain in the head. Migraine is a recurrent form of headache that occurs in distinct episodes lasting hours and even a few days. A migraine may be preceded by an introductory set of symptoms called an **aura;** these may include vague abdominal discomfort, odd visual sensations, including seeing wavy lines or flashing lights, or the sudden appearance of blind spots in the field of vision. Sometimes the aura is nothing more obvious than subtle malaise, or facial pallor. The headache itself typically has a throbbing or pounding character and is usually limited to one side of the head (the word migraine is derived from a Greek word referring to one half of the head.) Nausea and vomiting may precede a migraine or occur after the headache is well under way. The child may complain that loud noises and bright lights are painful. Kids often retreat to a darkened room where they lie quietly or go to sleep.

There are also other ways in which migraine may appear. Small children may have sudden episodes of severe dizziness, sufficient to cause them to fall to the ground. These kids act frightened and confused by their symptoms. Recurrent episodes of acute abdominal pain with or without vomiting sometimes turn out to have been the first hint of migraine developing at a later age. Cyclic vomiting (recurrent episodes of vomiting without any other symptom) may be a manifestation of migraine. Sometimes the earliest symptom of migraine is motion sickness. These instances of migraine without any headache are termed **migraine equivalents.**

Migraine is one of those conditions that truly runs in families. I find that careful questioning usually reveals a parent or grandparent, aunt, or cousin with migraine. Sometimes this travels under the disguise "sick headache," and sometimes I discover that a parent has had migraine for years that has never been accurately studied and diagnosed. It is quite a common disorder. One Scandinavian study found that nearly 1 out of 20 young adults had migraine or had it during childhood; other studies estimate even higher frequencies. It can start at any age, although migraine occurring in early childhood is nearly impossible to diagnose until the child has become old enough to describe his symptoms clearly. Sometimes migraine strikes once or twice and then disappears forever, but it is commonly a years or decades-long affliction.

We are finally learning something about the mechanism of migraine. For a long time it was thought that migraine was caused by a period of abnormal tightness of the tiny muscles surrounding the arteries taking blood to the brain (vasoconstriction) followed by an increased blood flow (vasodilation). More precise methods of measuring brain blood flow have now disproved this theory. The current hypothesis is that nerve impulses cause an irritation of the lining membranes of certain blood vessels in the brain. This seems to lead to a leakage of fluid and subsequent inflammation in the brain tissue, and a temporary depression of the function of the nerve cells of the brain.

It is crucial in understanding and treating migraine to discover the factors that can set off this sequence of events. People with migraine have unusual sensitivity to various chemicals normally present in the blood. Some of these chemical triggers are internal, such as changing levels of normal sex hormones. Some are external, such as birth control pills and constituents of various foods, the most common being chocolate, cheeses, and red wine. Other triggers of migraine include bright or flashing lights, fatigue, excitement, and motion. The role of emotion and of personality style has received some attention but not enough to really increase our understanding. For years, the claim has been made that people with migraine are perfectionists and overachievers, but I don't think too much should be made of this.

How can we tell the difference between a really miserable but otherwise ordinary tension headache and a true migraine? Not easily. Generally speaking, the diagnosis of migraine is based on the entire spectrum of typical symptoms, plus a family history of migraine. It becomes even clearer if the headaches occur in some reasonably predictable fashion; every time after eating a pound of chocolate, for example, or after exposure to flashing lights, or at the same time in every menstrual cycle. Clarifying these causal relationships may require careful observation over a period of months. Furthermore, little kids often have no auras before their migraines, or if they do, fail to tell us about them. And family histories can be hard to obtain. (I recall one child whose mother was sure that her family was free of any migraine history. A telephone call to Grandma revealed that Mom had had quite nasty migraines in her childhood, and that Grandma still had them herself; she had just never mentioned the diagnosis to her daughter.) Basically, if you are not sure that the headache is migraine, it can be treated as such anyway, and the results studied. This form of shooting in the dark is what we physicians dignify with the title "therapeutic test;" it ain't elegant but it is often a good idea.

The treatment of migraine is complex and not completely satisfactory. It has been hard to develop the right medicines in the absence of precise enough knowledge concerning the mechanisms of migraine. And the multiplicity of possible trigger factors complexifies the task of tailoring the proper treatment to each patient. Avoiding known triggers when possible is wise, although it may not always be easy. One teenager in my practice completely controlled his migraines by avoiding chocolate and Coke. When the headaches returned we were all puzzled until Mom found the telltale candy wrappers under his bed. Other behavioral triggers such as excess fatigue, too much schoolwork, and emotional stress may require revamping the child's life style.

Medicines remain the mainstay of migraine treatment. Plain old aspirin or other mild painkillers like acetaminophen and ibuprofen are frequently all that is required. If they fail, the addition of caffeine may help. Stronger painkillers are available for teenagers, but narcotics must be avoided; this is one situation where there is a real risk of habituation. Fortunately, a number of antimigraine medicines are available, and better ones are under development. The newest and most effective is a chemical closely resembling the neurohormone serotonin; it blocks the nerve impulses that set off the migraine.

An alternative method of controlling migraine pain is the use of relaxation techniques, including biofeedback, and my personal favorite, autogenic training. (For more information see *Autogenic Training* by J.H. Schultz and W. Luthe. New York: Grune and Stratton, 1959.) I should warn you that these methods have never been enthusiastically adopted by American doctors. This is in part because the theoretical basis for their use is pretty slim; we have no idea how relaxation protects blood vessels in the head. Furthermore, these techniques take a lot of the doctor's time to teach. It is easier in the short run to reach for the trusty prescription pad. Another problem with these methods is that they do require a certain amount of practice to maintain the skill; this can get pretty boring for impatient teenagers. Autogenic training involves teaching the patient to increase blood flow to the hands, a remarkably simple trick to learn, especially for children and teenagers. One of the advantages of this approach is the wonderful sense of mastery it affords. My first patient who used this was a ten-year old girl with typical migraine. I had told her parents about hand-warming exercises as a alternative to her medication. One night she had a severe migraine at home and the family discovered that they were out of the medicine. They explained how she could control the headache herself by lying quietly and imagining her hands becoming heavy and warm. As she reported later, she pictured hot chicken soup running down her arms; the headache disappeared. The next morning she triumphantly told her parents, "Now I don't need to carry my pills with me anymore; I have something better inside."

The other approach to the control of migraine is preventive medication. There are a number of medications that cut down the frequency of migraines if taken daily. For kids with frequent migraine these are well worth a try. The currently popular list includes ibuprofen (Motrin, Advil, Nuprin, etc.) and propranolol, plus a score of others. As usual, whenever so many medicines are suggested as possible treatments, it means that none of them is uniformly satisfactory; trial and error experimentation is often required to find the right stuff.

This disorder exemplifies an important pattern in medical understanding and therapy. Migraine has been recognized as a distinct entity for centuries, and theories about its causation have been numerous and fanciful. Until quite recently, treatment has been "empiric," the medical term meaning based nearly completely on clinical impressions: Try this, we think it may work. Over the last several decades the application of increasingly precise and probing studies of the neurological, hormonal, and vascular functions of the brain have led to some understanding of what migraine really is. As a result, medicines can be developed that act precisely at the level of the abnormality. This is a wonderful example of true medical progress, and it is by this kind of patient, step-by-step scientific work that many of our ills are gradually coming under control.

Chapter 45

Convulsions and Breath-Holding Spells

Convulsions are surely among the most frightening events that parents must sometimes face. Happily, as bad as they appear, convulsions are rarely life threatening and usually controllable.

A convulsion is the result of a kind of electrical storm in the brain. Our billions of brain cells are linked by electrical impulses, and when these go awry, whole areas of the brain may be affected by a wave of aberrant activity. This can cause a variety of effects including muscle jerking or tightness, loss of consciousness, brief interruptions in attentiveness without complete unconsciousness, and peculiarities in behavior. Convulsions are often referred to as **seizures,** probably because the ancients perceived them to be the result of the person being taken over by evil spirits. The term **epilepsy,** which is still used for recurrent convulsions, means seizure in Greek.

The best known kind of convulsion is one in which the person falls down unconscious, with muscles that are either tightly contracted or rhythmically contracting and relaxing. The technical term for this is **grand mal** or **tonic–clonic** convulsion. Another common kind of convulsion in childhood is called **petit mal** or **absence.** In this condition, the child abruptly seems to lose contact with her surroundings; she becomes silent, stares, may manifest small movements like grimacing or swallowing, and then returns to full awareness, all within a few seconds. There are many other less common types of convulsion, some marked by an abrupt loss of all muscle tone, some by specific patterns of motion, some by uncontrollable rage.

Fever Convulsions. The most common cause of generalized convulsions in early childhood is fever. Very high fever can trigger a convulsion in anyone, but some babies and small children are particularly susceptible. What happens typically is that a previously healthy child will abruptly develop a high fever and have a fairly brief convulsion as the fever is going up. The convulsion usually stops all by itself, and, despite the horrific appearance of the unconscious baby twitching and turning pale or even somewhat blue for a few minutes, no damage is done except to the parents' peace of mind. Heredity plays a role; the majority of these babies have at least one close relative with a similar history. Most babies who have a fever convulsion never have another, but there are a few kids who have several during the first years of life. Among all the children who have fever convulsions about 1 out of 40 go on to develop convulsions without fever, true epilepsy, later in life. The risk of later epilepsy for a normal child who has had only one single, simple fever convulsion is even lower, about 1 out of 100.

Fever convulsions nearly always stop themselves within minutes. While the child is convulsing, lay him down on his side; that position may help ease his breathing. Sometimes a convulsing child may vomit and lying sideways makes it easier to deal with the vomitus. If he feels hot, take his clothes off. Sponging him repeatedly with cool or barely tepid water will help him cool down a bit. (Neither cold water nor alcohol sponging is a good idea; cold water actually does not work as well and alcohol can cause problems from the fumes.) Give him an acetaminophen rectal suppository if one is available. And get on the phone to his doctor! A convulsion that won't stop, or a child who becomes really blue needs emergency care.

Because most fever convulsions are one-time events, prevention is not usually an issue. But if circumstances lead your doctor to suggest preventive medication, effective anticonvulsants are available.

Other Causes of Convulsions. Convulsions can have many different causes. Some are acute reactions to brain irritation, such as the convulsions that can occur during infections in the central nervous system, or those that follow head injuries, or those due to poisons. Then there are the convulsions caused by structural abnormalities in the brain, either built-in defects or tumors. There are also abnormalities in body metabolism that can result in convulsions. Thorough investigation will reveal a specific cause for convulsions less than half the time; the remainder are termed **idiopathic.** The literal meaning of this term is that a disease has its own particular cause; the real meaning is that we don't know what the cause is. We do know that certain types of idiopathic seizure disorders are strongly inherited, but this is not true of all cases.

Treatment of convulsions depends both on the causes and the types of convulsion. The convulsions associated with acute insults to the brain, like infection, injury, and poisoning, require treatment for the underlying cause as well as medication to control the convulsions themselves. Similarly, convulsions due to abnormalities in metabolism or to brain tumors are dealt with by attention to the known causes. For the large group of convulsive disorders where a direct attack on the cause is not possible, anticonvulsant drugs are exceedingly useful. Fitting medicine to patient is a complicated and tricky business. The anticonvulsant drugs are not easy to use; dose adjustment is often a problem, they all have some adverse effects, and it is often hard to know when it is safe to discontinue administration. It takes the best efforts of patient, parents, and physicians to get the most out of them.

Breath–Holding Spells. I have included breath-holding spells in this chapter even though they are not convulsions at all. However, they certainly can look like convulsions, so this is as good a place to discuss them as any.

Breath-holding spells are a transient but dramatic phenomenon of early childhood. In response to a sudden fright or an unacceptable frustration, a child will cry, stop breathing, become pale or somewhat blue, and fall to the ground unconscious. He may briefly be either limp or rigid, his muscles may twitch a few times, and then he will arouse spontaneously or he may relax into a few moments of sleep. Just about the time you have reached 911 on the phone it is obvious that the episode is over.

The most common scenario for breath-holding spells is the response to anger and frustration. These kids generally start with a long scream and a long period of breath-holding. They can get pretty blue before they finally pass out. It is best to consider these spells just a dramatic variation on the common, garden-variety temper tantrum. I see no reason, other than parental terror, to treat them any differently. Once they are underway, you really can't stop a breath-holding spell, so there is no point in intervening. As with any other temper tantrum, allowing the kid to bully you with one of these spells is not useful. These can be learning experiences for everyone concerned. The child learns that his anger is insufficient to blackmail his parents, and that he can live through the frustration of not getting his way. The parents can take the tantrum as a reminder that children sometimes become angry for perfectly sound reasons. Occasionally, there are changes the parents can make to reduce needless frustration in the child's life. (For more comments on tantrums see pages 101–02.)

Breath-holding spells in response to a physical injury or a fright are different. Although they may look a lot like the anger-evoked episodes, these spells are really a peculiar form of fainting. Some of these kids grow up to be easy fainters, and they often have family members who are similarly afflicted. The mechanism that causes loss of consciousness is an abrupt decrease in blood flow to the brain, rather than a lack of oxygen due to breath-holding. In both cases, recovery is automatic and there is no damage to the brain.

In rare instances, breath-holding spells look so much like real convulsions that a full scale investigation is undertaken. Nearly always, this can be avoided if parents are able to observe and subsequently describe a few episodes. Electroencephalograms (EEG) and magnetic resonance imaging (MRI) are expensive and scary; it's nice to avoid them if you can.

Chapter 46

Sudden Infant Death Syndrome (SIDS)

Sudden infant death syndrome, SIDS, crib death, cot death—by any of its names this is a terrible problem. It is not a common event, but for the families of each of these babies, SIDS is a catastrophe.

SIDS is a sudden, unexpected death in a previously healthy infant, unexplained by the child's history or by a thorough post-mortem examination. These babies are usually under 6 months of age, and nearly always under 1 year. This is a diagnosis by exclusion, that is to say, you can't say a child died of SIDS unless you have systematically ruled out all the other causes of unexpected death. These include overwhelming infections, previously unsuspected congenital abnormalities of vital organs, and child abuse. Studies of this sort require time, money, and expert investigators. Since these factors are not uniformly available, public health statistics on the prevalence of SIDS in various parts of the world must be viewed with caution. It appears that the incidence in the United States is in the range of 1 to 2 infants per 1000 per year.

The Causes of SIDS. For over 30 years, SIDS has been the object of intense study all over the world. Literally thousands of research papers have been published in which every conceivable cause of SIDS has been examined. As I write these words in 1996, we do not yet know what causes SIDS. What we do know is that a number of factors are associated with SIDS; families described by these risk factors include a disproportionate number of babies who die of SIDS. Furthermore, we know that some of these risk factors can be changed, and that the risk of SIDS decreases in a community when these changes are instituted.

Risk Factors For SIDS. This list of risk factors should not be interpreted to mean that any of these "cause" SIDS. All we can say is that their presence increases the risk of SIDS. Furthermore, the interrelationships of these factors confuse the issue. For example, in this country, poor people get less prenatal care, so factor 8 and factor 9 are hard to disentangle.

1. Premature birth.
2. Infants of multiple-birth pregnancies.
3. Teenaged mothers.
4. Mothers, fathers, and others in the house who smoke. This is one of the best defined risk factors. **Household tobacco smoke more than triples the risk of SIDS.** It may be linked to SIDS through the greatly increased incidence of respiratory diseases occurring in babies whose adult housemates smoke, or it may be a direct effect of tobacco smoke itself.
5. Mothers who use illicit drugs.
6. Mothers who have had frequent, closely spaced pregnancies.
7. Pregnancies marked by illness.
8. Inadequate prenatal care.
9. Poverty.
10. Formula feeding rather than breast feeding. Some studies show this connection, but some do not.
11. African American and Native American ethnic groups.
12. Winter months.
13. Warmly wrapped babies. The increased incidence during the winter may be related to the increase in respiratory infection during those months, or it may be related to the practice of bundling babies in heavy wrappings.
14. A mild respiratory or intestinal illness in the recent past. Careful investigation has shown that children with SIDS are often recovering from or just over mild viral illnesses. These are the common, trivial, everyday kinds of bugs that usually required no particular medical attention, and certainly would not be expected to be in any way life threatening.
15. Soft and compressible beds. Water beds, old soft crib mattresses, and the use of soft, thick wool or artificial fleeces under the baby all are associated with an increase in SIDS.
16. Having a sibling who died of SIDS. This is associated with a 4 to 5-fold increase in risk.
17. **Sleeping prone (on the belly).** This has been a widely debated risk factor. It is known that in those parts of the world where babies are tra-

ditionally and habitually placed to sleep on their backs fewer cases of SIDS are found. But, it is difficult to compare areas because of differences in the medical standards of diagnosis. However, SIDS rates have fallen by 50% or more in areas where public health campaigns have convinced parents to put babies to sleep on their backs or sides. It is not clear whether this is a simple cause and effect relationship, but it appears to have a substantial impact on the incidence of SIDS. Parents will often discover that many babies sleep less soundly on their backs than on their bellies. For the parents of very fussy infants this may be quite a trial, but this pattern of shallower sleep may also prove to be the reason that fewer back-sleepers die of SIDS.

18. A history of a "near miss SIDS" or "apparent life-threatening event (ALTE)." Sometimes a child will be found limp, or turning blue, or just not breathing. Stimulation or mouth-to-mouth resuscitation is done, and the baby revives. These episodes are often found to have a specific and treatable cause. However, the remaining, unexplained spells seem to be associated with an increased risk of SIDS.

19. Sleeping in a room alone or with other children, rather than sleeping in a room with an adult. A large study done in New Zealand (where SIDS has been unusually common) found that SIDS was much more common in babies who slept in a room without adults. Contrary to what one might expect, this apparent protective effect of an adult presence was *not* found if the adult and the baby shared the same bed! This research finding has not yet been confirmed by other studies, but it is quite consistent with the known low SIDS rates in Southeast Asia where adults and children typically share the same bedroom. Sleeping in a room with another child had no protective effect.

Preventing SIDS. It will be a lot more satisfactory to write these paragraphs in a few more years, when we really understand SIDS. For the present the best we can do is to minimize the risks.

For the mother:
- Get good medical care during pregnancy.
- Don't use illicit drugs.
- Don't smoke, and don't let anyone else in the household smoke.
- Breast feed your baby.

For the baby:
- Put the baby to sleep on his back or side.

- Provide a firm crib mattress.
- Don't use soft, fleecy materials under the baby.
- Keep the baby rather lightly covered rather than heavily bundled when he sleeps.
- Have the baby share a bedroom with an adult at least during the first 7 months when 90% of SIDS occurs.

Infant sleep monitors are devices which attach to the baby and respond to threatening changes in his heart rate or his breathing. The monitors were devised because it is believed that these changes may signal an imminent crib death. It is sometimes suggested that a baby who has been thought to have a "near miss SIDS" should have such a monitor at home so that the parents can be alerted and provide resuscitation if needed. Unfortunately, the monitors don't work very well. They can miss real emergencies and often sound an alarm when none is warranted. The net effect is to drive the family half crazy with anxiety. Enthusiasm for their use has gradually waned.

Chapter 47

Headaches and Other Tension Syndromes

Human beings have put enormous energy into developing vast and nearly inaccessible areas of unconsciousness. Now, it is perfectly sensible that our conscious minds are shielded from the physiologic realities of certain body functions. I am quite content to have my rate of breathing, my blood pressure, my blood sugar, and my kidney functions remain under the control of unconscious processes in my brain or other organs. In the ordinary course of events, I don't need to have access to this information, and I appreciate having it dealt with outside of my knowledge. But the unconscious part of my mind, and everyone else's, has taken over large areas of my emotional life as well. We all go through life incompletely aware of how we feel, at least part of the time. Perhaps this is the result of some kind of evolutionarily useful mechanism, or because that is how we are raised as children, or both, but in any case, that is how it is.

From early infancy, we are taught to ignore, suppress, and lie about our feelings. There is an endless variety of interpersonal scenarios in which these lessons are learned.

A boy falls down, scrapes his knee, and cries.

Father: "You're okay. You're not hurt!"

Child (to himself): "I'm not? I would have sworn I was feeling pain."

A child watches while his mother cuddles the new baby. Waves of jealousy and anger wash through his consciousness.

Mother, to watching child: "Don't you just love your new little sister?"

Child (to himself, while inhibiting the urge to kick his mother in the shin): "I do? This is love?"

Father, at the dinner table: "Finish up your rutabaga. You haven't had enough to eat and I'm sure you're still really hungry."

Child (to himself, while contemplating rutabaga on plate): "Hungry? It seems like I'm full."

I think what happens is that we get so many messages from the powerful adults in our world that contradict our own internal sense of ourselves that we begin to discount our own reality. For one thing, we learn that the adults don't want to hear our views on how we feel. They prefer acquiescence or silence to clear statements that, actually, our knee hurts, we hate our new sister, and we think rutabagas are fairly disgusting, even if we were hungry, which we no longer are.

In terms of getting along with the grownups, ignoring our real feelings actually may be rewarding. The boy who learns to react to pain with stoical silence discovers that his father is pleased with his son's manly demeanor and rewards him with his approval. The child who reaches up and gives the ghastly, interloping new baby a tentative pat gets a warm smile and a kiss from his mother. The little child who eats two more bites of rutabaga is allowed to have dessert. The more repression of feelings, the more rewards. At least some of the time, and for at least some of the feelings, consciously ignoring how we feel seems to turn into an unconscious failure to feel in the first place. We don't hurt, we don't hate, we no longer notice when we are full. We may even learn to appreciate rutabagas.

And so we make our children fit for life in the real world in which there is not all that much room for the unrestrained expression of uncomfortable emotion. Our teachers in school, our bosses at work, our colleagues, even our lovers all have vested interests in our going along with them, on their agendas, for their purposes, filling their needs. So if we neither feel nor express contrary desires, life may seem smoother in the classroom, at work, in social settings, or in bed.

Well, as we all know, it does not work. The dammed feelings have not gone away. They may well have been repressed out of our consciousness, but they have lost none of their force. Denied direct expression in words and behavior, they still have powerful routes through which they can produce effects. Our central and peripheral nervous systems, the sympathetic and parasympathetic nervous systems, and a host of neurohormones are available to carry messages of discomfort and dysfunction to any part of our bodies. Furthermore, an emotional state can change its spots; unacceptable anger can surface as depression, self-hatred can appear in the guise of overeating. Our emotions have lots of tricks.

This is all pretty obvious in adult life; but how about in childhood? Is it possible that bodily symptoms can express emotional states even in infancy? Three examples come to mind: **colic, rumination,** and **hospitalism.** Colic

EVERYDAY PEDIATRICS FOR PARENTS

is really a wastebasket diagnosis; there are surely several different causes for the unhappy, screaming periods in early infancy we term colic. I am convinced that some of these babies are temperamentally tightly wound, hyper-responsive people who seem to funnel their emotional discomfort into gastrointestinal cramping pain. Rumination is a much rarer and therefore, less well-known condition in which an older infant develops the pattern of spontaneous regurgitation of food. These babies sometimes seem unusually apathetic and depressed, and may be reacting to difficulties in mother-child relationships. The third example, hospitalism, is also called **anaclitic depression.** This is a condition seen in orphanages or long-stay hospitals where babies and very young children are separated from their mothers and where the overworked staff have inadequate time to give the children the attention they need. Some of these kids die; they become withdrawn and inactive, refuse to eat, and they waste away. It is difficult to imagine a more dramatic example of the impact of unmet and unexpressed emotional states on the person as a whole.

In older children and in adolescents the most common bodily expressions of blocked emotions are headaches and bellyaches. But this short list does not exhaust the possibilities by a long shot. Skin rashes, pains in the chest, back, arms, or legs, areas of abnormal skin sensation, partial paralyses, the abnormal pattern of breathing known as hyperventilation—all of these physical symptoms and others may spring from emotional causes.

The ways in which our bodies can react to emotions have been the subject of study for many decades, and the neural and hormonal pathways are fairly well worked out. What is often much less clear is *why* a particular child reacts in his or her particular fashion. After all, there are lots of ways to show discomfort. One factor can be the pattern of emotional expression in a given family. If the adults react to stress with headaches, they provide convenient object lessons for their children, and it is no surprise if the kids learn to have headaches just like Dad. Sometimes an injury or illness sets the stage for future symptoms by focusing the attention of child and parent alike on an area of perceived vulnerability. And, of course, sometimes the choice of symptom remains simply mysterious.

Tension Headaches. Headaches of any kind are something of a rarity in early childhood, but by middle childhood, say ages 6 to 8 years, ordinary, grown-up type tension headaches begin to crop up. By adolescence, they are a dime a dozen. These are usually my-whole-head-hurts headaches. They are described as tightness or pressure, in contrast to the pounding or throbbing of migraine. There is often associated tightness of neck and shoulder muscles, and it may be that muscle tension is the underlying mechanism of the pain. These headaches vary in severity and duration, but it is not unusual for them to persist for hours. They may recur nearly every day. Typically, they occur during periods of high emotional stress, and it is usually clear to everyone involved that they are straightforward expressions of otherwise blocked emotion. This simplifies the doctor's approach to management. If he does not have to give serious consideration to causes like brain tumors and sinusitis, he can direct the attention of the child and the family to the real questions: What is going on in this person's life? How can he learn to deal with his life situation without turning it into a pain in the head? (A few suggestions can be found later in this chapter.)

Abdominal Pain Due to Emotional Causes. Bellyaches due to family conflict, school problems, and interpersonal struggles of all kinds have been discussed in Chapter 40, Gastrointestinal Problems. Suffice it to say that this is a very common middle and late childhood and adolescent complaint, and by no means an easy one to sort out. There are so many organic reasons why kids can have belly pain that the physician is duty bound to look for the usual suspects. The hints that emotional tensions are the cause include the location of the pain near the navel, the lack of associated symptoms of illness such as fever and weight loss, the generally healthy appearance of the child, and the absence of any physical findings of disease. There may be other hints as well such as information about new or continuing problems in the family or at school, signs of strain between child and parent during the office consultation, and the demeanor of the child herself. Of course, this kind of information is all potentially misleading. A child who appears to be sad, or tense, or angry may be having belly pain because of her emotional state, but she may also be sad, or tense, or angry because she is fed up with having belly pain from an unequivocally organic illness.

One Approach to Management. I hope that you have noted the tentative flavor of the title of this section; a little humility seems appropriate. These are not simple issues, and I don't think that anyone has yet mapped the road to success in the management of tension syndromes, either in kids or in adults.

The only rule of which I am reasonably sure is **Grossman's Law of Childhood Psychotherapy:** *Don't throw pills at emotional discomfort.* In our medicine-taking society, the first impulse of the physician and the patient is often palliation: Make it feel better. In consequence, the largest selling prescription drugs by an overwhelming margin are tranquilizers and other mood-altering agents. This is a pretty dubious business even when applied to adults. It hardly needs to be said that a feel-good pill does not make the problem go away. These pharmaceutical Band-Aids may keep the real issue hidden for a few hours, but that is about all. When we are dealing with children and adolescents the use of sedatives and tranquilizers seems to me unutterably foolish. Children are malleable and tough. They are capable of rapid learning. **Give them the tools to understand and cope with their environments and their emotional lives; don't blunt their senses with medication and don't teach them that inner peace comes in a screw-cap bottle.**

Does this advice sound preachy, impractical, and cruel? Am I really arguing that you should never give an aspirin to a kid with a headache? Well, no. It is a matter of balance and direction. When our kids are in emotional pain I think our response should be guided by, first and foremost, a willingness to sit down and *listen* to them. There are just an awful lot of miseries that need to be vented, shared, explained, and explored. It can be exceedingly hard to listen to a child telling you how meanly her friends are treating her, how jealous he is of his smart, verbal older sister, or how ashamed she is that her parents are getting a divorce. Parents can sometimes open up these subjects just by telling their children that they wonder if something is bothering them, and what it might be. It is worth trying simple listening, without arguing with the child, without telling her that her feelings are wrong, without defending your own role as a parent. I guarantee you, it isn't easy, but it can truly help. It can substitute words and tears for pain or fatigue, and it can lead to understanding on both sides.

Younger children can be amazingly explicit in identifying and explaining their emotional problems. When they can't get at them directly with words alone, they can sometimes use play instead. This occurs in a kind of low-key, informal, family-style version of the play therapy used by psychotherapists. Children will often express their feelings with a few dolls, or action figures, or stuffed animals, with the parent as a mostly silent but sympathetic onlooker.

Middle-aged and older children can use some interesting verbal games to explore and relieve emotional tensions. A stomachache is addressed by sending a message to it, asking the stomach what the trouble might be, and requesting a reply. These interchanges may be in the form of letters to and from the unhappy organ, or as pictures illustrating the problem. When a child has identified a problem area, you can try playing the game Catastrophic Expectations. This is a "what-if" game that attempts to defuse anxiety provoking situations.

The parent asks what is the worst thing that can happen if the feared event takes place. When the child responds, the parent ups the ante, "And then what is the most awful thing that could happen?" And so forth. When it works, this weird interchange has the effect of leading the child progressively through his fears and letting him experience them in comparative safely. It requires a light touch, and a willingness to encourage some playful exaggeration of the imagined worst. Sometimes a parent can help a child find ways to deal with difficulties. When one of my granddaughters was having trouble with an anxiety provoking situation, her mother asked her to imagine what the powerful although fictional girl Pippi Longstockings would do. Leia quickly invented a series of responses that she could use by herself.

The point of any and all of these techniques is to allow the child to express emotions and relieve symptoms, and, most importantly, to teach the child that there are ways to deal with anger, fear, jealousy, conflict, and all the other scary feelings that will surely come along in the future. Emotional expression is a muscle that needs exercise, and it helps to have a friendly, parental, personal trainer in the family.

Chapter 48

Chronic Illness and Fatal Illness

Somehow, no one expects babies and children to have really bad illnesses. Kids appear to have such a firm hold on health and on life; their vigor and vitality seem nearly to preclude chronic or fatal illnesses. Well, the reality is that children are susceptible to major illnesses, some of them chronic and some of them fatal. In this modern era, our experience with children leads us all to expect that any new illness is likely to be acute and relatively brief, either treatable and curable with medication, or self-limited and not needing much, if any, treatment at all. So all of us, parents and doctors alike, are taken aback when it turns out that an illness is of a quite different sort. That this illness is going to be chronic, that it will be part of the child's life, perhaps for years, perhaps forever, was not part of anyone's expectations when the appointment with the doctor was made. That this illness is going to be fatal is nearly unthinkable.

Equally unthinkable is the possibility that a longed-for new baby may be seriously abnormal. I suppose that all parents have some concerns during pregnancy about the developing baby. We all know that some babies are born with problems, but it seems so unlikely that such a thing could happen to us and ours. No one can possibly be prepared for the devastating reality that our new infant has a major developmental defect or a serious illness. To be thrown from joyous expectation to fearful and bitter mourning in a matter of minutes is nearly too much to bear.

The response of the child's parents to the diagnosis of a chronic illness or a serious birth defect is not unlike the response to a death. Anger, denial, sorrow, and often guilt may dominate for days and weeks. During this time parents are often deluged with necessary and well-meant medical information, but their psychological disorganization may make it nearly impossible for them to take it in. The natural tendency to deny the diagnosis leads some parents to embark on lengthy and usually futile searches for a better opinion or the promise of a cure. Eventually, most parents are able to make some sort of peace with the bad news. Support groups for families with similar problems of illness or disability are absolutely invaluable in this. It is an immense help to meet other parents who have heard the same terrible words and lived with the same terrible reality.

Soon after such a diagnosis is the time when the child's doctor can be crucially useful to the family, as a source of information, as a guide to other medical care when it is needed, and as a helpful and attentive friend. Unfortunately, it is often the case that the child with a newly diagnosed major illness is whisked off to specialist physicians, different hospitals, and a whole new cast of medical characters. Just when the support of a familiar and trusted medical advisor would be most welcome, he is no longer there. Part of this discontinuity is inevitable. Pediatricians and family doctors really do rely on our specialist colleagues to handle some of the uncommon and serious problems. But part of the difficulty is that doctors often fail to make clear among themselves just who is supposed to be in charge of what aspects of the patient's care. All too often the child and the family may find themselves without a medical home base, a place where they know their questions will be answered and their needs addressed. Another problem is that pediatricians and family doctors are used to working with the expectation of *cure*; when we are faced with a child whose need is now for *care* instead, we often feel frustrated and inadequate. I know that we should not let this stand in the way of giving good care, but I am afraid that it does. Our chronically ill patients remind us that we have failed them, and the result is sometimes that we withdraw, medically and psychologically, just when our presence is needed most. I think there may be situations where a parent needs to say to the doctor "Look, I know you can't cure my child, but I don't blame you, I'm not mad at you, and we need you. Please don't abandon us."

Needless to say, the parents of a chronically ill child have other problems to deal with than how the doctors are coping. Both the immediate and the long-term consequences are profound. Illness requires time, money, and loving care, items in limited supply in every family. Family resources that were once available to everyone are now sucked into the care of the sick person. And for many families, this becomes an ongoing disaster. I will never forget the parents of one little girl with cystic fibrosis, a chronic and eventually fatal lung disorder. Her family was consumed by the illness, their savings spent, their energy drained dry. I can hear the exhausted mother saying, "We have no money to buy a rug for the floor, no time for the other children, we worry about her all the time. We don't even make love anymore." The family facing such an illness needs all the help it can get if it is to survive. Friends, relatives, parent support groups, religious congregations—all can play important parts in making life bearable. There are also resources like community health workers, visiting nurses, home health aides, and respite programs to give the parents some time off.

The other kids in the family have particularly poignant needs. Inevitably, they resent the attention that must go to the sibling with the illness. *He* gets to stay home from school, *he* doesn't have to do his share of the chores, *he* is the one friends and relatives make a fuss over. And, inevitably, they will feel guilty about their anger. They may well wish the sick one dead, and then will feel guilty about that, too. Younger children who are still in the stage of magical thinking may believe that their angry thoughts can actually cause injury. Quite often the healthy brothers or sisters develop symptoms themselves. Sometimes, these will vaguely resemble the real illness. This **sick sibling syndrome** can crop up any time during or after any prolonged illness. These kids are not faking; their symptoms are a cry from the heart. Children with the sick sibling syndrome need to be handled gently; they have enough to deal with already.

The issues for the sick child himself are even more complex. He must somehow deal with the illness and its attendant disabilities of limited energy, pain or other unpleasant symptoms and sometimes miserable treatments. If the illness is very serious, he will have to deal with fear. There is a real possibility that a chronic illness will take over the life of the child. This may be due, in part, to the day-to-day necessities imposed by the disease or its treatment. This could be as small a matter as remembering to take his asthma inhaler to school every day, or it may be as all-consuming as staying home to receive another round of intravenous chemotherapy for cancer. In either case, the child may be pushed into a sort of identification with the disease. Rather than feeling that "I am a kid who has asthma," the child can begin to feel that "I am an Asthmatic." The disease can define the person. At the other extreme is the refusal to recognize reality. Serious illness can pose such a threat to the developing sense of oneself that some older children and teenagers resist acknowledging that they are sick. Like their healthy peers, they want to feel powerful and invulnerable. The same impulse that leads teenagers to race motorcycles leads some teenagers with diabetes to skip their life-sustaining doses of insulin. Both the motorcycle racers and the defiant diabetics are likely to find themselves in the hospital. It is a challenge to help these kids steer a course between denial on the one hand and being taken over by the illness on the other.

Understanding Death

Children begin to think about death from a very early age. Lately, I've been watching two of my granddaughters observing snails. At the age of 2, they noted the difference between live, mobile snails and the inert shells of dead snails. It was clear that they were in the process of developing a new mental category—dead things. They are urban children, so they will not have the many opportunities that the children of farmers might have. They will witness neither the births nor deaths of farm animals. They may see a dead bird in the park or a dead cat at the side of the highway, but that is probably all the direct experience with death that they will have in their early childhood. For children like my granddaughters Kate and Emma, death today is likeliest to be simply an experience of disappearance; the snail is no longer in his shell. When their great-grandmother died last year they said, "Grandma Mimi's gone," and pointed to the heavens.

Somehow, very gradually, children have to amplify this idea of death, and eventually they begin to think about death in relation to their parents and themselves. For children, as for most of the rest of us, these are frightening thoughts. Death means loss, abandonment, and loneliness, all feelings that children can understand. Starting at around the age of 3, many children ask about death; they are clearly trying to make sense of the concept.

But what of the feelings of the dying child himself? During and after middle childhood, approximately age 5 and above, it becomes possible to talk directly to children about their illnesses and even about their deaths. To do so requires that you have sufficient faith in the ability of the child to cope with this worst of all possible news. And it helps if the adults in the child's world have chosen to be honest with him throughout the illness. Being honest does not always come easily in these situations. To tell a child that he has a disease which we cannot cure is to give up our aura of adult omnipotence. It means that we are saying to the child, "I can no longer protect you from all the bad things in this world." Doctors have a very hard time giving this message to our child patients. Many years ago an 8-year old patient in my practice was dying of a brain tumor. At the end of one visit he asked me, "Am I going to die?" It was a question for which I was wholly unprepared. He had only recently been referred to me, and I had no idea what he had been told by his neurosurgeon and his parents. How much could he understand about death? He watched me and his parents watched me while I hesitated and then responded, "Yes, you are going to die. There is no medicine that can make you better." That was about twenty-five years ago, and the memory still hurts. I am your doctor, and I cannot help you to live. Perhaps the dilemma for the parents can be softened by religious faith. If one believes that death is followed by an afterlife and that parents and children can look forward to being reunited, then the task of talking about death with the child may be eased.

Home Death and Hospital Death

We may have no choice at all concerning where a death takes place; lives often end abruptly and unexpectedly. But some deaths can be anticipated, and we should give some thought to the setting. The increased power of medicine to diagnose, treat, and even to heal has meant that treatment for a life-threatening illness is usually moved into a hospital, where the newest tools and technology are most readily available. This makes very good sense if there is the possibility of cure—we all want the best odds. But what of the situation where there is no longer any possibility of cure? Part of the problem is that we often do not know what the outcome will be when a patient is admitted to the hospital. Maybe she can be pulled through, maybe she will have a chance for another remission. And then, when it has become clear that this time is the last time, it is exceedingly difficult for anyone to say "Okay, it is time to stop; let her go home to die." So no one says it, and then there is another death in the hospital, often in an Intensive Care Unit (ICU), with all the paraphernalia of life support, when there is no longer any life. Hospitals, in general, are not good places to die. There are too many people, too much noise, the lights are too bright, it is terribly anonymous. It is true that in some circumstances, death can be softened a little. A private room can be found, the medical staff people who helped care for the child can rally around. But, by and large, it is the wrong place.

Of course, there is no right place. The death at home of an old person, surrounded by family and friends, can become a celebration of a long life well lived. The death at home of a child can never have that quality of the completion of life's cycle. But at least there is the possibility that death can be peaceful and comfortable, in surroundings familiar and well loved by the child, without the intrusion of the bustling, noisy, overpopulated, hospital environment. I am aware that the picture I am sketching is an ideal; I have seen innumerable homes unfit for either the living or the dying. But at least some of the time, home is best for the child who is dying and for the family left behind to live.

After A Child Dies

I have already mentioned how important it is for families to get all the support they can in order to cope with the ongoing strains of a chronic or terminal illness. If anything, emotional support is even more important after a child dies. No matter what the age of the child, whether the loss was a tiny, midpregnancy fetus, a toddler, or a teenager, the parents will be grievously hurt. They may be overwhelmed by the depth of their feelings, and they may be distressed to find that their grief lasts and lasts. Somehow, people seem to expect themselves to "get over" a death and get on with life within a matter of weeks; it doesn't happen that way. It takes as long as it takes, and for most parents, it takes a very long time.

The brothers and sisters of a dead child will have an entirely different range of emotions. In even the happiest families, the feelings of siblings toward one another are a tangled web; love is part of it, and so is jealousy and hatred and competition. The result is that siblings may feel both sorrow and relief upon the death of another child in the family. Some families have a strong enough tradition of sharing their feelings that even these shameful and guilty emotions can eventually be expressed, but I suspect that in most situations the surviving siblings simply play the expected game of mourning as best they can.

Parents sometimes react to a child's death by reaching for a replacement child. Overcome by the long and painful process of mourning, they may attempt the shortcut of a new pregnancy or an immediate adoption. There can be problems with this tactic. Fears and expectations properly attached to the child who has died may adhere to the replacement child. Parents may also become understandably but unduly fearful and overprotective with the health of the remaining family. It is never easy for parents to be objective in assessing the seriousness of a child's illness. But after the death of one child, illness in any of the other children may stir so much anxiety that good judgment may become nearly impossible for awhile.

I only wish I could end this necessary but grim chapter with some sort of healing, helping summary. You can see that decades of medical practice have left me indelibly imprinted with the inner expectation that I should always be able to offer a cure. However, the questions that surround the subjects of chronic disability and disease and fatal disease are not truly medical questions at all. They are issues of existence, of what life means to us, of what life is, and how we bear ourselves in the bad times that every life must bring. These issues reside in the province of philosophers, priests, and rabbis, rather than pediatricians. Doctors can help at the edges, we can point those who suffer in the directions where help may be found. But, in the long run, the problems must be met with the help of our families, our dearest friends, and from within our own innermost souls.

Chapter 49

Drugs to Induce Sleep and Control Anxiety

Homo sapiens is a drug-taking animal. That is not a complete definition of our species, but it is an important one. Our forebears discovered millenia ago that fermented beverages induced interesting and pleasurable changes in mental state, that certain plants could be dried and smoked with similarly desirable effects, and that various other plants yielded substances which deadened pain, or lowered fever, or helped heart failure. I heard recently

EVERYDAY PEDIATRICS FOR PARENTS

that some of the great apes also seek out and use medicinal plants; apparently we are not the only species that has figured out that drugs can be useful.

In recent years, our use of drugs has expanded rapidly, especially in the area of mood-altering, anxiety-masking, and sleep-inducing substances. The United States has been a particularly fertile field for this aspect of the pharmaceutical business. Americans have a remarkable record of interest in and consumption of mind-altering substances, and an equally impressive history of ambivalence about them. Travelers to our country in the early nineteenth century commented on the widespread use of alcoholic spirits, and this pattern continues to the present day. Until the early twentieth century morphine, heroin, marijuana, and cocaine were liberally included in hundreds of freely available patent medicines. And a favorite treatment for teething discomfort was a solution of opium.

Our current patterns of drug consumption may look different, but the search for psychological peace through chemical means is still going on. Nowadays, we go the doctor and obtain a prescription for an antidepressant or an antianxiety medication instead of picking up a bottle of a cocaine-laced alcoholic "medicine" at the druggist. I am not wholly convinced that this is progress. Having decided that certain classes of mood-altering drugs are evil, we have made them illegal and therefore immensely lucrative. The only major industry with higher profits than the legal drug industry is the illegal one.

What has all this to do with children? The American drug culture is omnipresent in their lives. From their earliest years American kids see the advertisements that promote the use of drugs. Whether it is to get a good night's sleep, stop a headache, become popular with the opposite sex, or exhibit one's manliness, there is a drug being peddled to do the job. Kids also watch adults, and they see that we drink alcohol, use tobacco, drink coffee and Coke, and pop pills. We form their expectations of adult life, and they cannot fail to notice that grownups "do drugs." Depending on circumstances, it may be Prozac or it may be crack, but any way you slice it, it is still a drug.

This is part of what America teaches its children, and I see no way to avoid these lessons. However, parents may want to teach some alternative lessons as well, and you can do that by the way you use drugs in your home. I have already mentioned that the problem with giving vitamins to kids is the implicit message "Good health comes out of a bottle." The same issue must be faced when we are tempted to administer mood-altering agents to **control anxiety.** Kids get thoroughly upset about all sorts of problems in their lives, and the Dad who uses Halcion to get to sleep may decide that he can smooth things out for his son with a tablet or two. In the short term, drugs work. Give them a dose of Valium and the teenager hysterical about an upcoming test calms down and goes to sleep, and the little girl mourning the death of her pet hamster feels better. But the lesson implicit in the offering of those little yellow tablets is "Peace of mind comes out of a bottle." This lesson not only misleads the child; it also demeans the child by saying, in effect, "You are too weak to handle reality; this pill will shore up your feeble defenses." Of course, there are some extreme situations where using drugs to control anxiety makes sense. Helping children to tolerate frightening and painful medical procedures is an example that comes to mind. In general, though, I think we should be wary of putting these drugs into our children. There is a lot to be said for the experience of coping with reality, no matter how sad or tough or confusing it may be, without the assistance of chemicals.

In addition to the ordinary stresses of daily life imposed on our kids, there are also some chronic, severe psychiatric syndromes of a quite different nature. Children can suffer from the same sort of depressive disease that can afflict adults; they can have panic attacks, and even schizophrenia. I have no doubts at all about the necessity and wisdom of drug therapy in these situations. Coping is an important part of learning how to live, but it is simply insufficient with diseases like these. Children with major psychological problems need all the support they can get, whether it is psychological, chemical, or from friends and family.

Back in Chapter 27 I discussed **relieving pain,** and I argued that there was no virtue at all in letting kids suffer unnecessarily. Here, on the other hand, I am arguing that most kinds of acute psychologic discomfort should be left unmedicated. It appears that I am saying that ***physical pain deserves to be controlled, but acute psychic pain should often be experienced and borne.*** That is, in fact, just what I mean. We learn and grow by coping with the psychological difficulties of life. They provide important opportunities for interacting with others, and encourage personal maturation. The test anxiety experienced, lived through, and survived may help the teenager confronted with his next test; "I made it okay last time, and I guess I can make it again." The death of the hamster, deeply felt, and thoroughly mourned, is a lesson in the cycle of life that includes us all. It will not be the only death that child must deal with. In both of these examples the parents can be supportive and possibly provide insight *without* handing out medicine. Enduring physical pain, on the other hand, seems to me to bring only meager rewards, and for young children no rewards at all. Some parents may wish to inculcate into their children a degree of stoicism in the face of physical pain. That is a reasonable choice when you are dealing with older kids or teenagers who can be expected to understand what enduring pain means and why it may be acceptable. But allowing small children to be in needless physical pain makes no sense at all.

The other popular use of brain-altering drugs is for **sedation.** There are times when we may desperately want our children to sleep. Generally, this is for the convenience (or the survival) of the adults in the family; less often sedation is used with the direct benefit of the child in mind. One common reason to sedate a child is a long airplane trip. This seems to me to make perfect sense, and I only wish that better sedatives were available for this sort of use. The old-fashioned barbiturate sedatives (phenobarbital, Seconal, etc.) worked erratically; sometimes the child slept peacefully and sometimes not. One mother reported to me that the phenobarbital I had prescribed for her daughter had hopped her up so badly that "I had to walk her all the way to South Africa." Mildly sedating antihistamines like diphenhydramine (Benadryl) and promethazine (Phenergan) are often used, but their effects are inconsistent and often inadequate. Tranquilizer drugs like hydroxyzine (Atarax, Vistaril) are rather weak but can usually provide at least a few hours of peace. The benzodiazepines (Librium, Valium, etc.) are available only in tablets which makes them hard to administer. We could use a palatable liquid sedative with a predictable length of action, but we don't really have one yet.

A word about other means to relieve pain and control anxiety: Drugs are not our only tools. In Chapter 47 I discussed various ways you can help your children deal with psychological distress. Some of these techniques can also be used to help relieve physical pain. In addition, **hypnosis** and **self-hypnosis** methods are remarkably useful, especially in dealing with repeated, painful, and frightening medical procedures. The common thread here is the attempt to help the child achieve a sense of mastery and control. American doctors have been slow to adopt the use of psychological pain control. We are trained to *do* things *to* people, rather than to help people do things for themselves. Furthermore, it is unquestionably faster to write a prescription for a medication than it is to embark on a training program with a child on self-hypnosis or the use of guided imagery. If your doctor knows how to use nondrug methods, you may want to give them a try; if he doesn't, he may be able to refer you to a practitioner with the appropriate skills.

Chapter 50

Schools, Learning, and Learning Problems

Every generation of parents seems to have its favorite subjects to worry about. One of the most popular parental obsessions today is about formal education. I am impressed with this every time I see the tense, furrowed brow of a mother or father agonizing over the importance of admission to the right nursery school. Obviously the education of our children is important, but I think that parental overconcern is partly based upon an underestimation of the contributions of the family and the child to the educational process. From the family the child learns whether learning is desirable, whether questions can be posed and answered, whether books are valued, and whether one must sometimes work quite hard to reach a distant goal. The child contributes her own styles of thought, patterns of activity, ability to focus, interests in the world, peculiarities of temperament, and her own intelligence. With these raw materials the schools and teachers must struggle.

If you spend a little while browsing in the education section of your local bookstore you will see a startling array of books describing brilliantly successful approaches to teaching our young. The range of theories and the diversity of methods is extraordinary. These books are probably all written by honest and highly competent teachers, all of whom are describing what has worked for them. Unfortunately, they are stressing the effect of the message and forgetting the importance of the messenger. Given a happy, energetic, dedicated teacher working in a reasonably decent school environment, one can confidently expect better than average success with the children. I know that the teacher may believe that her results are directly related to the theory which she is applying, but the only way to explain the approximately equivalent successes gained with contradictory methods is by giving credit to the teachers themselves.

This also may explain why new approaches to teaching work so well in the laboratory setting, and are such dismal failures when transferred to the real world. Same theory, different teachers (and also different schools, principals, children, parents, and environment). Professional educators need to do controlled experiments, matching teachers, classes, and schools, and then testing the effects of various educational methods. Until they do, neither they nor the rest of us will have any idea what kinds of schooling are best.

Starting School

The question "When should children start formal education?" receives different answers depending on when and where the question is being asked. In this country, school used to start at about age 6, the time of entry into first grade. Then kindergarten was invented, designed to be a gentle bridge between home and the academic life, and 5-year olds marched off to school. A few decades ago the nursery school movement developed, claiming that social skills could and should be inculcated into preschoolers, and thus 3 and 4-year olds became students. Then, as mothers increasingly became workers out of the home, it became necessary to do something with all those toddlers, and preschool began to incorporate younger and younger children. Eventually, the differences between infant day care and preschool became blurred, and today the children dropped off every morning at "child development centers," family day care homes, and the like range down to the newborn period. Even for the children fortunate enough to stay at home, formal instruction begins earlier and earlier. Toy manufacturers promote devices to accelerate infant learning; books are published which urge parents to teach their babies to read. Even prenatal learning is advised. At this point, only the sperm and the egg are exempted from pedagogy. At the risk of appearing cynical, I must say that the interest in "learning toys" and the like is based more on the needs of the toy manufacturers and the book writers than on those of the child.

One problem with collecting very young children in institutions termed "schools" is that some of their caretakers may be tempted to expose them to a formal, academic curriculum at much too early an age. It is an understandable impulse. The kids are right there; why not teach them? Furthermore, teaching may feel like a more valuable undertaking than ordinary child care. And, of course, the academic prowess of the toddlers reflects favorably on the institution and its workers. The disadvantage of this premature pedagogy is the inevitable, predictable failure of some of its intended participants. Children vary enormously in the ages at which they develop the ability to sit still and absorb concepts like letters and numbers. The earlier a group of kids is exposed to these tasks, the more of them will fail. If the effort to instill these skills is sufficiently persistent, the continued failure of some children will be noted by everyone, especially the failures themselves. This is not a terrific way to start an academic career. In some Scandinavian countries this fact is appreciated and children are not exposed to formal reading instruction until age 7. They have many fewer children with reading disabilities than we do.

The conclusion I draw from all this is that the day care of babies and toddlers should be primarily a play-based social learning experience with academic instruction postponed until at least kindergarten or first grade. I don't mean that these little people can't learn; on the contrary, they are learning all the time. Introducing the crucial subjects of reading and writing is a matter of timing; there is just no hurry.

In many schools, kindergarten has become the place where the academic big push begins. One effect of this is that many parents keep their kids in preschool an extra year so that they will be more fully ready to cope with the demands of teachers who want every child to graduate from their classes already literate. Generally, the kids held back are boys because their parents are aware that academic readiness develops a year or so later in boys than girls. When one of these boys finally starts regular school he has the undoubted advantages of being more socially skilled, better prepared to do the academic work, and more physically developed. In the short run, all this may make school life easier. However, in the long run, it means that he may always be somewhat out of step with his classmates. In modern American classrooms, where everybody is supposed to be just about the same age, being older often means that his interests will be different than those of the other kids. Some of these older-than-the-average children become the odd men out. For the parents who do not want their 5-year olds pushed into reading, the better option is to find kindergarten teachers who agree with them. It is also possible to let the school principals and teachers know that not every parent is in a hurry to put her children prematurely on the academic treadmill. Consumer demand is a powerful tool.

The Unhappy Student. Even in the best of all possible schools, there are bound to be times when a given child is not happy or thriving in a given classroom. The signs are varied: Some children become morose and withdrawn, both at school and at home; some act out their discontent on the playground or in class. It may take awhile before it becomes clear that there is some sort of mismatch between the child's needs and the academic environment. When parents come to that conclusion, your protective, and understandable, impulse may be to move the child to a different class. If the problem is an incompetent teacher or an uncontrolled and chaotic classroom, a rapid transfer may be the best solution. But if the problem is intrinsically that of the child herself, a change

EVERYDAY PEDIATRICS FOR PARENTS

of scene will not be the answer. You need to ask what the child brings to the classroom. It may be her own anxiety, her lack of social aptitude, her unhappiness about a situation at home, or the first signs of a learning disability. The first step for the parent toward sorting all this out should be a conference with the teacher. No matter what reports the child has brought home, the teacher's observations are bound to be useful. It is often possible for a parent to spend some time in the classroom, acting as a teacher's aide. By all means, take this opportunity to get an impression of the total situation. Investing a few hours will provide insight into the society of the classroom and the way your child functions within it. The school psychologist and possibly a teacher specializing in learning problems may be needed. It may also prove helpful to involve your pediatrician in this. He can bring a knowledgeable and neutral perspective to what may sometimes be a sticky problem, and school people are usually pleased to have help from the child's doctor.

Learning Disabilities of Attention and Behavior. There are all sorts of reasons why a child may have trouble learning. These include a lack of teachers and books, dreadful schools, and disordered families or communities. Other causes are specific to the child himself, such as anxiety, nearsightedness, impaired hearing, or true mental retardation. In addition, there is a group of children whose learning is impaired in specific and sometimes subtle ways that appear to reflect limited but important problems in brain function. These are children with normal intelligence in general who have difficulty with any of a large variety of mental tasks such as the mental processing of symbols, or transferring information between visual and auditory modes. Such specific learning disabilities, especially **dyslexia**—difficulty in reading, writing, and spelling— have been the subject of study since the early decades of this century, but progress in understanding and in treatment has been slow. Another group of children have learning problems because they are too hyperactive, impulsive, or unfocused to attend to academic work. These kids were initially said to have "minimal brain damage." The term was then changed to the slightly less horrific "minimal brain dysfunction," which was later dropped in favor of "attention deficit disorder" (ADD), which has most recently been changed to **attention deficit hyperactivity disorder (ADHD).** To confuse matters further, there is a substantial overlap between these groups of children; quite a few dyslexic kids have ADHD as well.

About these problems of attention and behavior, we have a rather small store of what appears to be real information. Incidence figures are unreliable;

we do not even know how many kids we are talking about. Depending on how the problem is defined, between 1 and 15% of children are said to have specific learning disabilities. The incidence of ADHD is similarly unclear; estimates vary form 3 to 15% of American children. I find it disturbing that these diagnoses are much more popular in the United States than in the rest of the world. Does this mean that we are so much smarter at recognizing problems of learning and behavior, or that we are doing something wrong with our children, or that we have less tolerance for normal variations in classroom conduct and achievement, or what? It used to be thought that boys were much more likely than girls to have specific learning difficulties, but recent studies now suggest that the incidence is about equal in the two sexes. Because girls with problems of attention and of learning tend to be quieter and cause less trouble than similarly afflicted boys, the girls are often overlooked and underdiagnosed. Family studies have shown that some forms of learning disability and ADHD are inherited. Anatomic and physiologic research indicates that, in some cases at least, these kids' brains are wired differently; this should give pause to anyone proposing a quick-fix panacea.

Dyslexia and Other Learning Disabilities. Teachers are likely to suspect specific learning disabilities when academic tasks begin in earnest in the early grades. Very early diagnosis is difficult; testing is a lot easier when the child is older and more mature. However, the diagnosis should be made as soon as possible: The child who fails and fails inevitably suffers in self-esteem. One 7-year old girl in my practice was seen by her mother saying to her reflection in a mirror, "You're stupid." The sooner this kind of repetitive failure can be stopped, the better. (It is a pleasure to report that this child is currently a wonderful high school girl who plays basketball, raises guide dogs, and still has time to work extra hard for her straight A's. Sarah has had skillful and intensive special educational help because her parents would not let her school provide anything less.) Figuring out whether a child has a specific learning disability is a real challenge. Ordinary medical and neurological examinations are either entirely useless or, at most, reveal a modest excess of what are termed "soft" neurologic signs, which are often just a measure of immaturity. Observation of the child in his normal habitat by teachers, parents, psychologists, or physicians may reveal short attention span, impulsivity, distractibility, irritability, physical awkwardness—or nothing at all. Psychoeducational tests are the best tools to define the learning problem. This requires a skillful psychologist or a pediatrician trained in developmental problems who will not be misled or distracted by variations in behavior and functioning due to socioeconomic or ethnic differences.

In short, when a child in the early years of school is doing poorly, we need to find out whether the cause is a ghastly classroom situation, subcultural differences in expectations, a devastated home life, a major or minor disorder of psychological health, simple mental deficiency, poor vision or impaired hearing, a specific disorder of reading, speech or motor activity, attention deficit disorder, or any combination of these. No one involved in making this determination should rush to judgment; too much depends on getting the right answers.

Treatment remains difficult. I don't want to sound unduly pessimistic but the history of failed therapies is impressive. Years ago, a theory of the importance of mixed laterality or mixed dominance had a vogue. Mixed laterality means simply that the dominant hand is not the same side as the dominant eye or foot. Treatments were invented that claimed to retrain the brain into more normal patterns by teaching the children to crawl "properly," or to walk on a balance beam with greater grace. Unfortunately, the researchers who promulgated this notion had failed to notice that mixed dominance is equally common in kids with no learning problems at all. Then there were (and still are) practitioners who prescribe special eyeglasses, or esoteric eye exercises, or "vision training." And, as always when standard treatments are unsatisfactory, there are the purveyors of high-dose vitamins and mineral supplements with their exciting claims.

The children who have a specific learning disability benefit from the best special education programs. It is as if they learn alternative ways to do the mental work required. In later life, they often continue to have the same basic difficulties; their reading or spelling or whatever may never amount to much, but this is not always a disaster. One lawyer father whose son had dyslexia told me that he had the same problem: "All through Harvard Law School my reading was so slow that I had to hire other students to read the cases aloud to me." For many children, special education should include psychotherapy. The child who has felt stupid for years may need some help to get over the blows he has suffered to his self-esteem.

Attention Deficit Hyperactivity Disorder (ADHD). The child who eventually earns the diagnosis of attention deficit hyperactivity disorder may exhibit some suggestive patterns of behavior at an early age, but these are not easy to differentiate form the normal toddler vigor. Unfocused, distractible, impulsive, often hyperactive conduct may lead parents or teachers to wonder if something is wrong. School work in particular demands consistent, focused, organized, and sustained attention. Furthermore, life in the classroom requires taking turns, being quiet much of the time, and staying in confined spaces doing prescribed tasks—all difficult for the ADHD child. In addition to the pediatric, neurologic, and psychoeducational evaluation, such children should be the subjects of careful observation inside and outside the classroom. Helpful tools include behavior rating scales which have been devised for use by parents, teachers, and psychologists.

As with dyslexia, there have been various unsatisfactory attempts to explain and cure problems of attention and behavior. A popular dietary therapy popular for awhile was the Finegold diet, based on the idea that salicylates in foods caused an allergic reaction leading to hyperactivity. When careful studies were eventually undertaken, the results were a grave disappointment. Very few if any children improved. In short, both in theories and therapies, there have been many efforts but few successes.

The children with problems of attention and behavior typically benefit from **drug treatment.** Caffeine, usually taken in the form of coffee, dextroamphetamine (Dexedrine) and its chemical cousin methylphenidate (Ritalin) all have the paradoxical effect of keeping them calm and focused.

There are several other drugs which can be used if those fail. But these drugs are no cures; when the medicines are stopped, the kids continue to struggle with the same impulsivity and distractibility that made their teachers and parents want to strangle them years before. It is difficult to know when they should be discontinued, if ever. Public discussion of drug therapy for ADHD has been increasingly noisy, although not necessarily helpful. The specter of a generation of perfectly healthy and normal kids being drugged by impatient parents, overwhelmed teachers, and foolish physicians continues to appear in articles and books. These concerns are real, and I have no doubt that some children are given these agents on inappropriate indications. But if you give Ritalin or Dexedrine to kids who *don't* have ADHD, they get completely wired. Any parent or teacher who makes that mistake will stop in one hell of a hurry. The second aspect of treatment is **special education** to remedy the academic losses already incurred, to structure the learning situation in a way that more closely meets the special needs of the child, and to help the child overcome the specific learning problems that often exist coincidentally with ADHD. The third approach is **psychological management** at home and at school. This is most often in the form of behavior modification by rewards and punishments.

Both teachers and parents may need instruction and support in this endeavor. The field of learning disabilities and attention-behavioral problems remain in an unsatisfactory state. There is an awful lot we do not yet understand.

Chapter 51

Television and Other Electronic Distractions

Several hundred pages ago I solemnly stated that I was not going to tell you how to raise your children. I said that this is a book meant to show the breadth of possibilities of childrearing, and that you, the parent, really had to be the expert regarding your own kids. Well, I suppose I've already breached that contract here and there. Concerning some issues, my favorite prejudices (otherwise known as soundly based, scientifically validated conclusions!) are so strong that they have a tendency to creep in. Here they come again.

Television and computer games are disasterous for all of us, and for children they are even worse. Even if you already believe this, read on, if only to strengthen your resolve to do something about it. If you don't believe it, consider the following.

First, the message. **1) Grownups are fools:** Attractive, coherent-sounding human beings have so little sense that they get excited about the effectiveness of a floor polish and act as though a hair rinse were changing their lives. If possible, the men are even bigger fools than the women. Fathers are generally portrayed as bumbling and obtuse; moms are caring but ditzy; and the kids are wise-beyond-their-years smart-alecks. **2) Consumption is what really counts:** Happiness comes from owning a new car, going on an expensive cruise, or owning the right pair of basketball shoes. **3) Sexual intercourse is usually devoid of consequences:** So one must be ready for sex at any time; it is deliriously passionate; and nobody ever seems to get herpes. **4) Violence is the key to survival:** Expect life to be filled with knives, fists, guns, and a variety of explosives; when you kill someone, they just fall down; death doesn't often seem to matter much to anyone.

As if the mayhem on television wasn't enough, violence is now attractively packaged for our children in home video games such as Nintendo. In case you have been hibernating for the last decade and missed this, the basic scenario is deadly and violent confrontation with enemies. It is the player's task to destroy, (kill), the bad guys. The object of the game is to become a competent killer with good eye-hand coordination. One of my partners told me about a new game to which a friend had introduced her children. The storyline was simplicity itself; three teenaged gangs (yellow, white, and brown) fight each other on a high school playground. They use switchblades and other weapons to kill each other. The winner is rewarded with the girlfriend of the murdered leader of the defeated gang. When my horrified partner returned the video game to the store, the clerk said dismissively, "It's certainly getting harder to be politically correct here in Berkeley."

Does any of this matter? There can hardly be any doubt about the immediate and powerful effect of television on children. A number of studies have demonstrated that exposure to TV violence is followed by an abrupt increase in violent behavior among the children. In addition, studies in the United States, Canada, and South Africa show that murder rates more than doubled about 10 to 15 years after TV became popular in each country—after just one generation of watching TV violence. It is true that Americans have always had a violent society, celebrating frontier-style aggression and making heroes out of our outlaws. And for most of the last century the world has been an incredibly violent place, never free from wars, coups, riots, or revolutions. Television has brought war right into our homes with the evening news. Our politics and our entertainment are in complete agreement; both systematically teach our young to expect and therefore to accept killing as the norm. And they learn fast. Homicide is now the second leading cause of death of young American males between the ages of 15 and 35, and most of the killers are themselves young.

The old saying "You are what you eat" applies to the diet of the mind as well as the body. A diet of television has been shown to increase aggressive tendencies, to increase callous indifference to the sufferings of others, and to increase a generally fearful, mistrusting, and hopeless view of life. In short, our children are watching a lot more than Sesame Street and Mister Rogers.

So much for the message; the second issue is the medium itself. Quite apart from their content, the electronic media teach a silent but powerful lesson: "Expect excitement and entertainment, and even learning, without any effort at all." Our children bathe every day in this culture of passivity. Experienced school teachers report that the television-reared child is easily bored by the monochromatic, quiet effort needed to master academic skills. Quite apart from its effect on willingness and ability to learn, what is the result of this indoctrination on one's whole approach to life?

The third issue concerns what is lost; what would your children be doing if the TV or the Nintendo were not there? As our children get fatter and softer, decade by decade, it is obvious that a substantial amount of physical playtime is lost. This should come as no great surprise; children are awake about 12 to 16 hours a day, and school kids are away from home about half of that time. The few hours of daylight that remain after school are easily invaded by the tube and the video game. Reading and homework are also obvious candidates for eclipse. One or two favorite programs after dinner, and it's nearly time to go to sleep. When does the homework get done? When does the family spend time together without the distraction of TV? How much time is left to read to your kids? If they spend more time with the adults on television than they spend with you, the TV adults will become their role models. Are those the people you want to teach your children how to be grownups?

By now you are probably saying, "What an unbalanced and one-sided presentation of the situation!" Well, I plead guilty. There are indeed some charming and informative aspects to television. A very few children's shows, some nature and science programs, an occasional presentation of serious music, dance, or drama, coverage of the few truly important news stories—it is a short list. I don't think it amounts to anything against the immense damage done by television, hour after hour, day after day, to hundreds of millions of watchers of all ages.

"But, TV is such a great babysitter! How could I ever get anything done at home if I couldn't sit the kids down in front of the cartoons?" This is a really tough question, the unsatisfactory answer to which is that parents managed before television. One mother I know became alarmed about the invasion of Monday night football, cops and robbers, situation comedies, and cartoons. She took the unusual step of disabling the family TV, and announced to everyone that the repairman had the necessary part on backorder. The results were instant: Books were read, craft projects undertaken, noisy and active outside play resumed, father and children did things together. After two months, the TV was "repaired" but stringent rules for viewing kept the beast at bay. It was one of the most useful lies I've ever seen.

I think it is worth while deciding how many hours a week you are willing to have your children watch TV or play video games. A mother in my practice and I actually had the following conversation not long ago.

Grossman: "How many hours is Betsy awake during an average day?"

Mother: "Well, she sleeps from 9 to 7:30 and she takes a 1 hour nap, so that leaves 12½ hours awake."

Grossman: "So, meals and baths and the like take about an hour and a half a day, and she's at school from 8:30 until 3:30, that's another 7 hours; she has about 4 hours a day left for everything else in her life?"

Mother: "That sounds about right."

Grossman: "And you say she watches TV at least 2 hours every day? That means that half of her available time is in front of the tube."

Mother: "Sometimes she plays her video games for a while, too."

Grossman: "Does that leave enough time for playing and reading and being with the family and everything else you'd like your child to be doing? Does spending 50% of her free time watching TV seem appropriate?"

Mother: "You're making me feel awfully guilty!"

Well, there's nothing wrong with a small dose of accurately placed guilt—but guilt is not enough. Parents also need to *enforce* whatever limits they decide are appropriate, although this is not easily accomplished. When they were forbidden TV at home, my kids watched the tube when they were at the homes of their friends, and there was nothing I could do about it. I assume that other parents who wish to limit TV will have the same problem. (Before I became aware of the extent to which my children were continuing to indulge in this subterfuge, I used to worry lest their supposed lack of information about popular television programs might make them feel somehow estranged from the culture of their peers. They eventually relieved me of that illusion.) Nor can one expect the rules to be followed when the adults are out of the house. In short, we may as well be realistic about the extent of our ability to shape the environment in which our children grow. But we do have some say in the matter, and if we value the contents of our children's hearts and minds, now is the time to say it.

Chapter 52

Summing Up

Be not afraid of greatness: some are born great, some achieve greatness, and some have greatness thrust upon them.

—William Shakespeare. *Twelfth Night. Act II, Scene 5.*

Shakespeare might well have been talking about parenthood. For some mothers and fathers it is as natural as falling off a log; for others it is something of a struggle; and for quite a few it comes as a surprise. For all parents, I trust it will be a complex, infinitely rewarding, sometimes painful, always challenging, and ultimately fulfilling framework around which your lives are constructed. It has been, and continues to be, for me.

Our individual family journeys start in so many different ways. We get pregnant by mistake, or just when we planned to, or only after years of trying. Some of us become parents through adoption or through marriage with a ready-made family of stepchildren. There are so many kinds of households, filled with the limitless alchemy of parents, siblings, relatives, and friends. The extremes of wealth or poverty, the influences of class and culture and community—what an incredible and nearly unimaginably diverse world of possibilities for new human infants. Our babies arrive into circumstances as varied as human experience. And, needless to say, the babies themselves are an equally heterogeneous lot.

So, here we are, at the start of the life of a new human being, with our own personal ideas and ideals of what it is to be mothers and fathers and families. What had we better keep in mind? I have no more Grossman's Laws to offer, but I will restate a few of my favorite ideas. First, **observe and respect your child.** Try to gain a realistic appreciation of your child's strengths and weaknesses, and discover what sort of temperament she came with. Second, **aim to know yourself;** no easy matter but a great endeavor. Having a clear idea of who you are and what you want will protect you from the winds of parental fashion and the pressures to conform to someone else's ideas of raising kids. It is also a good idea to become acquainted with your own particular obsessions and peculiarities and guard against them getting in the way of the larger goals of family life. Third, **remember that square pegs don't fit in round holes.** At one time or another, most families come up against a peg/hole mismatch. There is no single solution to the dilemmas that arise when the wishes or standards or needs of parent and child are at cross purposes. Sometimes there is no solution at all. Fourth, **being a parent does not mean being a doormat.** You are older, more experienced, and, with any luck at all, at least temporarily wiser. Don't let the little people bully you. Fifth, **remember that your goal is to graduate mature, responsible, independent people after a couple of decades of tender, loving care at home.** That means giving them lots of practice at being mature, responsible, and independent. Start as early as you can manage, and enjoy their growth. Sixth, in the words of a wise psychiatrist friend, **we all have a choice of meeting life with either excitement or anxiety.** Without doubt, there are times when anxiety is impossible to avoid. But for most of that part of life we call parenthood, meeting life with excitement means meeting it with hope and joy.

On the front cover of this book are my five grandchildren. From them I am learning a keener appreciation of the privilege of living. Watching them grow has deepened my sense of the way an individual's life is wholly immersed in the life of family, friends, community, country, and world. John Donne told us that no man is an island. Nor are our families; in the long run, we survive or suffer or thrive with the rest of humankind. Our children and our grandchildren show us our place in the great chain of existence, and they remind us to cast our nets wide and play our roles in the wider world.

End of sermon, end of book.

Index

EVERYDAY PEDIATRICS FOR PARENTS

EVERYDAY PEDIATRICS FOR PARENTS